P9-DDI-884

LIBRARY-LRC
TEXAS HEART INSTITUTE

Plasma Lipoproteins
and Coronary Artery Disease

CURRENT ISSUES IN ENDOCRINOLOGY AND METABOLISM

Series Editor

JEROME M. HERSHMAN MD
Chief, Endocrinology Section,
Wadsworth Veterans Administration Medical Center,
Los Angeles, California;
Professor of Medicine,
University of California, Los Angeles,
California

Previous volumes in the series

Graves' Ophthalmopathy
JACK R. WALL AND JACQUES HOW

Molecular and Clinical Advances in Pituitary Disorders
SHLOMO MELMED AND RICHARD J. ROBBINS

Thyroid Hormone Metabolism: Regulation and Clinical Implications
SING-YUNG WU

Polycystic Ovary Syndrome
ANDREA DUNAIF, JAMES R. GIVENS, FLORENCE P. HASELTINE AND
GEORGE R. MERRIAM

Plasma Lipoproteins and Coronary Artery Disease

Edited by

ROBERT A. KREISBERG MD
Professor of Medicine,
University of Alabama at Birmingham,
Birmingham, Alabama

and

JERE P. SEGREST MD, PhD
Director, Atherosclerosis Unit;
Professor of Medicine,
University of Alabama at Birmingham,
Birmingham, Alabama

BOSTON

BLACKWELL SCIENTIFIC PUBLICATIONS

OXFORD LONDON EDINBURGH

MELBOURNE PARIS BERLIN VIENNA

We would like to dedicate this book to all of our authors and the other talented and creative scientists and investigators who have made this such a dynamic and exciting field. Their observations allow us to continuously adjust our understanding of the roles of lipoproteins in human disease and, most importantly, the process of atherosclerosis. It is a privilege and a pleasure to be a part of this whole process.

© 1992 by
Blackwell Scientific Publications, Inc.
Editorial offices:
238 Main Street, Cambridge
  Massachusetts 02142, USA
Osney Mead, Oxford OX2 0EL, England
25 John Street, London WC1N 2BL
  England
23 Ainslie Place, Edinburgh EH3 6AJ
  Scotland
54 University Street, Carlton
  Victoria 3053, Australia

Other editorial offices:
Librairie Arnette SA
2, rue Casimir-Delavigne
75006 Paris
France

Blackwell Wissenschafts-Verlag
Meinekestrasse 4
D-1000 Berlin 15
Germany

Blackwell MZV
Feldgasse 13
A-1238 Wien
Austria

All rights reserved. No part of this book may be
reproduced in any form or by any electronic or
mechanical means, including information storage
and retrieval systems, without permission in
writing from the publisher, except by a reviewer
who may quote brief passages in a review.

First published 1992

Set by Excel Typesetters, Hong Kong
Printed in the United States of America by
Book Crafters, Chelsea, Michigan

93 94 95 96 5 4 3 2 1

DISTRIBUTORS

USA
  Blackwell Scientific Publications, Inc.
  238 Main Street
  Cambridge, Massachusetts 02142
  (*Orders*: Tel: 800 759-6102
             617 876-7000)

Canada
  Times Mirror Professional Publishing, Ltd
  5240 Finch Avenue East
  Scarborough, Ontario M1S 5A2
  (*Orders*: Tel: 416 298-1588
             800 268-4178)

Australia
  Blackwell Scientific Publications
  (Australia) Pty Ltd
  54 University Street
  Carlton, Victoria 3053
  (*Orders*: Tel: 03 347-0300)

Outside North America and Australia
  Marston Book Services Ltd
  PO Box 87
  Oxford OX2 0DT
  (*Orders*: Tel: 0865 791155
             Fax: 0865 791927
             Telex: 837515)

Library of Congress
Cataloguing-in-Publication Data

Plasma lipoproteins and coronary artery disease/
  edited by Robert A. Kreisberg, Jere P. Segrest.
      p.   cm. — (Current issues in
  endocrinology and metabolism)
  Includes bibliographical references and index.
  ISBN 0−86542−206−0
    1. Coronary heart disease—Pathophysiology.
    2. Blood lipoproteins—Pathophysiology.
  I. Kreisberg, Robert A.
  II. Segrest, Jere P.   III. Series.
    [DNLM: 1. Atherosclerosis—etiology.
    2. Coronary Disease—etiology.
    3. Lipoproteins—blood.   WG 300 P715]
  RC685.C6P58 1992
  616.1'232071—dc20

Contents

List of Contributors

JOHN J. ALBERS PhD, *Research Professor of Medicine, Department of Medicine, Northwest Lipid Research Laboratories, University of Washington, Seattle, Washington*

PHILIP J. BARTER MD, PhD, *Professor of Cardiology, Department of Medicine, University of Adelaide, Adelaide, Australia*

WILLIAM A. BRADLEY PhD, *Professor, Department of Medicine; Associate Director, Atherosclerosis Research Unit, University of Alabama at Birmingham, Birmingham, Alabama*

JOHN C. CHAMBERLAIN MA, BM, BCh, *Clinical Research Assistant and Honorary Lecturer, Medical College of St Bartholomew's Hospital, West Smithfield, London, England*

GUY M. CHISOLM PhD, *Staff member, Department of Vascular Cell Biology, Cleveland Clinic Foundation, Cleveland, Ohio*

BYUNG H. CHUNG PhD, *Associate Professor, Department of Medicine, Atherosclerosis Unit, University of Alabama at Birmingham, Birmingham, Alabama*

DAVID J. GALTON MD, DSc, *Professor and Head, Department of Human Metabolism and Genetics, St Bartholomew's Hospital, West Smithfield, London, England*

DAVID W. GARBER PhD, *Assistant Professor, Department of Medicine, Atherosclerosis Research Unit, University of Alabama at Birmingham, Birmingham, Alabama*

SANDRA H. GIANTURCO PhD, *Professor, Department of Medicine; Chief, Lipoprotein Metabolism, Atherosclerosis Unit, University of Alabama at Birmingham, Birmingham, Alabama*

HENRY N. GINSBERG MD, *Associate Professor of Medicine, Department of Medicine, Columbia University College of Physicians and Surgeons, New York, New York*

SCOTT M. GRUNDY MD, PhD, *Director, Center for Human Nutrition; Chairman, Department of Clinical Nutrition; Professor, Departments of Internal Medicine and Biochemistry, University of Texas Southwestern Medical Center at Dallas, Dallas, Texas*

YAAKOV HENKIN MD, *Fellow and Associate, University of Alabama at Birmingham, Birmingham, Alabama; Ben-Gurion University, Beer-sheva, Israel*

D. ROGER ILLINGWORTH MD, PhD, *Professor of Medicine, Division of Endocrinology, Diabetes and Clinical Nutrition, Department of Medicine, Oregon Health Sciences University, Portland, Oregon*

JOHN P. KANE MD, PhD, *Department of Medicine and Biochemistry, University of California at San Francisco, San Francisco, California*

ROBERT A. KREISBERG MD, *Professor of Medicine, University of Alabama at Birmingham, Birmingham, Alabama*

CORA E. LEWIS MD, MSPH, *Assistant Professor of Medicine, Division of General and Preventive Medicine, Department of Medicine, University of Alabama at Birmingham, Birmingham, Alabama*

SANTICA M. MARCOVINA PhD, DSc, *Research Professor of Medicine, Department of Medicine, Northwest Lipid Research Laboratories, University of Washington, Seattle, Washington*

ALBERT OBERMAN MD, MPH, *Professor and Director, Division of General and Preventive Medicine, Department of Medicine, University of Alabama at Birmingham, Birmingham, Alabama*

JOHN F. ORAM PhD, *Research Associate Professor, Department of Medicine, University of Washington, Seattle, Washington*

KERRY-ANNE RYE PhD, *Research Associate, Department of Medicine, University of Adelaide, Adelaide, Australia*

ANGELO M. SCANU MD, *Professor, Departments of Medicine, Biochemistry and Molecular Biology, University of Chicago, Chicago, Illinois*

DONALD M. SMALL MD, *Chief, Biophysics Institute, Boston University School of Medicine, Boston, Massachusetts*

GEORGE A. TALLIS MD, *Visiting Assistant Professor, Department of Medicine, Atherosclerosis Unit, University of Alabama at Birmingham, Birmingham, Alabama*

Preface

Although we are far from understanding atherosclerosis we have come "light" years in a relatively short time. The field is an exciting and dynamic one in which lipids and lipoproteins remain as important factors both from the standpoint of pathogenesis and therapy. There are, however, other emerging areas that are, or will prove to be, equally important. We refer to a better understanding of the fundamental biology of the vessel wall and the roles of growth factors, cytokines, and concomitant abnormalities in fibrinolysis. In the future it may be possible to treat or prevent atherosclerosis by intervening at multiple sites in the process. For example, drugs may be used to: (i) reduce the levels of detrimental lipoproteins; (ii) increase the levels of protective lipids and lipoproteins; (iii) reduce atherogenicity of lipids and lipo-proteins by use of antioxidants; (iv) reduce levels of lipoproteins (Lp(a)) that may inhibit fibrinolysis; (v) reduce levels of lipids and lipoproteins that increase the levels of inhibitors of fibrinolysis (PAI-I); and (vi) prevent the release, or block the action, of cytokines or growth factors that result in smooth-muscle proliferation and/or the migration of monocytes or macrophages into the vessel wall.

This book is divided into four functional sections. Section one sets the stage for section two and deals with the clinically important issues of the epidemiology of coronary heart disease and the effects of lipid-lowering therapy on primary and secondary prevention. Section two emphasizes the biochemistry and physiology of lipoproteins and their potential roles in atherogenesis. The chapters in this section discuss the basic structure and function of lipoproteins: low-density lipoproteins, high-density lipoproteins, triglyceride-rich lipoproteins, postprandial lipoproteins, Lp(a), and oxidized lipoproteins. The final chapter of this section discusses the importance of lipoprotein receptors in lipoprotein transport as well as in atherogenesis. Section three provides an in-depth review of lipoprotein classes and subclasses further emphasizing the heterogeneous nature of lipoproteins, the important and divergent properties of apolipoproteins, and finally the use of molecular tech-niques for better understanding lipoprotein disorders. The final section brings us back to the important clinical issues of the treatment of patients with hypercholesterolemia, hypertriglyceridemia, and low high-density lipoprotein levels.

Overall, this book presents an up to date review of the very important but continuously changing field of lipoproteins and coronary heart disease. The authors have attempted to provide succinct and focused reviews of their assigned topics in an easy to read style that we hope is helpful. The authors were selected for their knowledge and expertise in their specific areas. We believe that they have done an admirable job and we thank them for their effort.

Section I
Introduction

Chapter 1

Epidemiology of Lipid Disorders in Special Populations

CORA E. LEWIS & ALBERT OBERMAN

Major clinical trials clearly indicate that a 1% reduction in an individual's total serum cholesterol level leads to a 2% reduction in coronary heart disease (CHD) risk [1]. While generalized to both sexes and all age and race groups, this compeling evidence of treatment efficacy has been derived mainly from middle-aged white males with hypercholesterolemia. An important issue is whether these effects differ across age, race, and sex groups and whether different treatment criteria should be employed for primary vs. secondary prevention.

Using data from the second National Health and Nutrition Examination survey (1970–1980) Sempos *et al.* [2] estimated that 41% of adults in the USA should have lipoprotein analysis after initial measurement of total cholesterol based on the recommendations of the Expert Panel on Detection, Evaluation and Treatment of High Blood Cholesterol in Adults [1] (Table 1.1). There was little difference between blacks and whites but it appeared that more men (45%) than women (36%) were candidates for lipoprotein analysis, attributed mainly to the higher prevalence of CHD or two or more risk factors among men. Based on these criteria, 36% of all adults aged 20–74 years need medical advice and intervention for high levels of blood cholesterol alone. This translates into about 60 million Americans aged 20 years and older who potentially require therapy for hypercholesterolemia based on screening for total cholesterol and risk factors. However, current estimates of the number of individuals requiring lipoprotein analysis by these guidelines may be too conservative. A recent analysis suggests that 41% of those at high risk due to high levels of low-density lipoprotein cholesterol (LDL-C) or low levels of high-density lipoprotein cholesterol (HDL-C) would be undiagnosed using screening based on total cholesterol levels alone [3]. This suggests that lipoprotein analysis be used among all those with total cholesterol levels of 200 mg/dl (5.16 mmol/l) or more, further increasing the number of candidates for lipid-lowering therapy.

Cholesterol studies including the major clinical trials have focused on middle-aged men for a variety of reasons. Men develop CHD about

10–15 years earlier than women and much more information is available on related CHD risk factors in men. There is also the complexity of hormonal variation in women and its influence on both lipids and CHD. Dealing with elderly participants makes these trials more complex in view of comorbidity, nutritional issues, and the ability to retard or regress advanced lesions over time, while younger people have few CHD events. Additionally, differences in lipid profiles and other CHD risk factors have been noted among blacks which might cause one to manage these patients differently. However, the recommendations and "cutpoints" in the Expert Panel report were intended to apply to all adults over the age of 20, although it was recognized that modifications based on physician judgment might be necessary when dealing with individual patients, particularly young adults, the elderly, and women. In this chapter we report differences in patterns of lipid disorders and related CHD risk among the elderly, women, minority groups, and those with manifest CHD, with particular emphasis on implications for screening and treatment.

Differences among population groups

Age

Mortality rates in the USA have markedly declined among older persons since 1968 [4]. There is a mistaken notion that a 75-year life expectancy at birth dictates that individuals at that age have no further life expectancy; actually the life expectancy of a 50-year-old female exceeds 30 years [5] and even an 85-year-old now has a life expectancy of over 6 years [6]. Consequently, the 65 and over population is itself aging; it is projected that by the year 2000, 49% of this group will be 75 years of age or older [4]. This has led to an increase in both the proportion of the population over the age of 65 and the absolute numbers of these individuals. Thus, an increasing number of cardiovascular events will be postponed to the later years of life. Given the increased lifespan of the elderly, prevention of cardiovascular disease among them will be important in determining the quality of these additional years for a growing segment of the USA population.

CHANGES IN LIPID METABOLISM

Mean total cholesterol values increase among men and women through middle age. The average annual increase has been calculated as approximately 2 mg/dl (0.05 mmol/l) among men aged 20–30 years and

Table 1.1 Percentage of USA adult population by ATP classification based on total serum cholesterol value. (Adapted from [2])

Population group	Desirable (<200 mg/dl)	Borderline high (200–239 mg/dl with two risk factors)	High (≥240 mg/dl)	Total needing lipoprotein analysis*	Candidates for intervention†
All persons	43	30	27	41	36
Race					
Black	48	28	24	39	34
White	42	31	27	41	36
Sex					
Male	44	31	25	45	41
Female	42	29	28	36	31
Age (years)					
20–39	61	26	13	22	20
40–59	28	35	37	54	46
60–74	22	33	44	64	58

ATP, Adult Treatment Panel.
* Sum of those with borderline high level and two risk factors and those with high level total cholesterol.
† Based on percentage of those needing lipoprotein analysis whose LDL-C level required intervention by ATP guidelines.

1 mg/dl (0.025 mmol/l) for those aged 30–60 years, while the increase among women is 1.5 mg/dl (0.04 mmol/l) from 20 to 40 years and 2 mg/dl (0.05 mmol/l) from 40 to 60 years of age [7]. Age-related increases in the lipoproteins also occur. LDL-C levels increase as a consequence of lower rates of LDL catabolism and fewer hepatic LDL receptors. After peaking in the late 50s among men and a few years later among women (Fig. 1.1), serum total cholesterol and LDL-C levels gradually decrease among the elderly of both sexes [8]. This decline may reflect differential survival (a survival advantage from lower cholesterol levels), changes in dietary habits with age [9], or the presence of chronic disease among the frail elderly [10,11]. HDL-C levels increase approximately 5 mg/dl in men after age 50 years and in women between 40 and 50 years due to decreases in hepatic triglyceride lipase activity and possibly decreases in hepatic HDL-C catabolism [12]. In men, this may also reflect a survival artifact.

LIPOPROTEIN RISK FACTORS AMONG THE ELDERLY

The issue of greatest interest is whether LDL-C is a determinant of CHD risk in the elderly and, consequently, should the same therapeutic

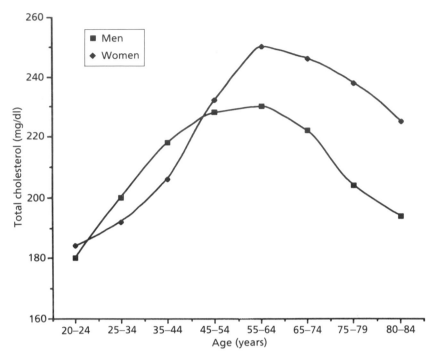

Fig. 1.1 The change in mean total cholesterol with age in men and women. After age-related increases peak in the 50s, mean levels decrease with age in both sexes. (Adapted from [8].)

"cutpoints" used for the middle-aged be applied. Results from earlier studies have indicated that the strength of the relationship between cholesterol and CHD is present in the elderly but is weaker [13,14], especially in women. More recently data from several sources [15–18] indicate that the association is just as strong in older men as in the middle-aged. HDL-C also remains an independent predictor for CHD in the elderly, more so among women [9]. There are several possibilities for the inconsistent findings in terms of relative risk at older ages: failure to measure lipoprotein fractions, misclassification of individuals based on single cross-sectional measurements, comorbidity, and selective survival [16].

A related concern is whether prediction at older ages is best based on repeated temporal measurements over a broad age span, or a single measurement at an earlier age or at current age. In the Honolulu Heart Study the prediction of disease was not age dependent but equally useful in proximity to or remote from the event. However, Hawaiian men of Japanese ancestry develop CHD later in life than do non-Orientals and thus these results may be misleading in a white population. In the Whitehall Study [19] cholesterol measurements obtained at an earlier age were much more predictive of CHD in old age than those measured at an older age. Appropriate data on lipid trends and prognosis are unavailable from women, but hormonal changes in lipid levels and the generally low risk at younger ages complicate the prediction of subsequent CHD.

Even if the relative risk of CHD with increasing cholesterol levels is lower with increasing age, the more clinically relevant attributable risk is greater. The attributable risk reflects the number of CHD events that could be theoretically prevented by lowering cholesterol levels. The risk of CHD attributable to elevated cholesterol is considerably higher in older individuals because of the much higher probability of CHD in a shorter period of time. Excess risk, the absolute difference in disease rates at different risk factor levels, is a measure of the risk due to elevated cholesterol values. In pooling data from 23 study populations to compare excess risk associated with cholesterol $\geqslant$240 mg/dl ($\geqslant$6.20 mmol/l), Manolio et al. [8] found that the contribution of excess CHD in men under 65 years of age averaged 710 cases/10 000 while in men 65 and older the excess risk averaged 995 cases/10 000. Using Framingham data, Gordon and Rifkind [16] calculated the effect of lowering cholesterol from 285 mg/dl (7.37 mmol/l) to 200 mg/dl (5.18 mmol/l) among 1000 men and women. Among 35–44-year-olds, risk was reduced by 77% and 1.8 deaths per year per 1000 men were prevented (0.7 deaths for women). Among the elderly, 75–84 years of age, risk was reduced only 23%, but 12.7 deaths per year per 1000 men (6.5 for women) were prevented. In a study of a cohort of over 2500 white males aged 60–79, Rubin et al. [20] calculated the relative and excess risk of CHD death among those whose cholesterol levels were in the highest quartile relative to those whose cholesterol levels were in the lower three quartiles. Although the relative risk associated with cholesterol did not change greatly with age, total mortality and the excess risk of death due to CHD increased markedly across the age groups (Fig. 1.2).

Although risk reduction is highest among the young, many more CHD events are preventable among the elderly in absolute terms. Hypercholesterolemia cannot be ignored as a risk factor among the elderly, and some are recommending that the National Cholesterol Education Program (NCEP) guidelines be extended to individuals up to 75 years of age [21]. Well designed clinical trials to examine the effect of drug treatment for hypercholesterolemia among the elderly are now underway.

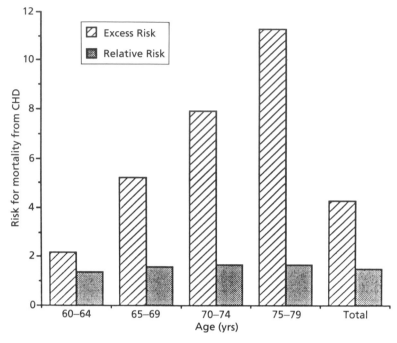

Fig. 1.2 Relative vs. excess risk for CHD mortality by age, comparing men in the highest quartile of serum cholesterol to men in the three lower quartiles. Although relative risk demonstrated little change, excess risk of mortality due to high cholesterol increased with age. (Adapted from [20].)

Gender

Women have a low incidence of CHD before menopause, after which the occurrence of CHD quickly accelerates to approximate the rates for men. The incidence among adult men, on the other hand, is much less age dependent. Consequently, morbidity and mortality rates, as well as the overall prevalence of CHD, are nearly equal in elderly men and women. The sex difference at younger ages does not apply to all women. The presence of diabetes in younger women eliminates the sex differential for CHD [22]. Also, younger women who use oral contraceptives and smoke have an increased risk of CHD. Further, women have a survival disadvantage once CHD is manifest with higher mortality following myocardial infarction and technical difficulties with performing angioplasty or coronary artery bypass grafting [23].

Although CHD is the predominant cause of death in women as in men, few data examining CHD and lipids relate to women [24]. Evidence exists from epidemiologic studies that extrapolation of the available data across gender is not always appropriate.

LIPOPROTEIN RISK FACTORS AMONG WOMEN

The effects of the lipoprotein risk factors on CHD incidence differ between men and women. At high levels of LDL-C the relationship to CHD appears to be similar for both sexes [24], but at lower elevations the relationship is weaker in women than in men [25]. Epidemiologic studies have also documented that women tend to develop CHD at higher levels of total cholesterol than men [25], possibly due to the higher proportion of HDL in the total cholesterol of women. Another explanation for this discrepancy may be differences in LDL particles between males and females, as women appear to have more particles that are larger and less dense than the more atherogenic small and dense particles found in men [26,27].

Adult women have HDL-C levels about 10 mg/dl (0.25 mmol/l) greater than men, a possible explanation for their relative protection from CHD until menopause. After menopause, lipoprotein profiles become more atherogenic [28] and CHD rates increase. The effect of HDL-C levels among women appears to be very powerful; the inverse correlation of HDL-C and CHD is stronger in women than men. In the Framingham study a decrease of 10 mg/dl in HDL-C was associated with a 50% increase in coronary risk among women and in the Lipid Research Clinic follow-up a comparable 42% increase in risk was noted [29]. High levels of HDL-C also appear to offset in part the risk of high total cholesterol levels while low levels of HDL-C (considered as <45 mg/dl among females) increase risk even in women with a desirable total cholesterol value of less than 200 mg/dl (5.18 mmol/l) [25].

Although most studies were conducted in men, those in women have found triglyceride to be at least a univariate risk factor [30]. Scandinavian studies consistently demonstrate a strong relationship among women between triglyceride and myocardial infarction but not angina pectoris, while in other studies the relationship appears less significant after adjusting for other lipoproteins, especially HDL-C. While these epidemiologic studies have shown that HDL-C and triglyceride levels are inversely correlated [30], experimental studies reveal that triglyceride metabolism directly affects both HDL [31] and LDL [32] particles, suggesting a primary role of triglyceride in atherogenesis. Given the evidence that postprandial and not fasting triglyceride levels are more predictive of CHD [33], the relationship between CHD and triglyceride may become stronger when studies employ standardized protocols for measuring nonfasting values.

In addition to the qualitative differences in lipoprotein risk factors between the sexes noted previously, quantitative differences also exist.

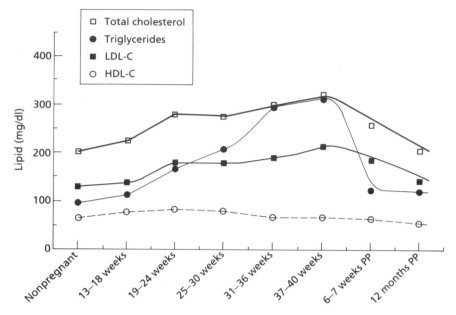

Fig. 1.3 Lipid changes during pregnancy (by weeks gestation) and in the postpartum period. Lipid levels, except for HDL-C, increase through pregnancy and peak in the third trimester. After delivery the return to baseline is rapid for triglyceride but prolonged for LDL and total cholesterol levels. (Adapted from [34].)

Lipid and lipoprotein values in adult women differ from those in men, and fluctuate through various phases of their lives. This variability is due in a large part to alterations in hormone levels such as with pregnancy, menopause, and use of hormonal therapy.

MENSTRUATION AND PREGNANCY

Despite the marked changes in hormone levels during the menstrual cycle, changes in lipoprotein levels are modest. Some evidence suggests that the associated estrogen level changes may affect the triglyceride content of very low-density lipoprotein (VLDL) particles. No effects on HDL-C or LDL-C have been described. The cyclic fluctuations in progesterone associated with menses do not appear to alter lipoprotein levels [26].

In contrast to the relative stability of lipoproteins associated with menses, normal pregnancy is associated with dramatic alterations in lipids. Potter and Nestel [34] described these changes throughout the pregnancies of 43 women (Fig. 1.3). Total cholesterol increased 50%, mainly during the second trimester, while triglyceride increased threefold and peaked during the third trimester. Total cholesterol levels were still significantly elevated at 6–7 weeks postpartum, requiring several months to return to baseline while triglyceride levels were only minimally elevated at 6 weeks postpartum. In VLDL lipoproteins, both cholesterol and triglyceride rose in proportion to the ratio in nonpregnant women while the ratio of triglyceride : cholesterol increased in LDL and HDL particles. LDL-C levels increase throughout pregnancy by nearly 50%, accounting for much of the increase in total cholesterol levels [35], and remain elevated at 8 weeks postpartum with or without lactation. HDL-C levels rise to a maximum of 45% at midgestation and then drop to 15% above prepregnancy levels [26]. Compositional changes in HDL occur after midterm, leading to increases in the protein fraction of the particles. Some data suggest that postpartum HDL-C levels may remain lower than prepregnancy levels [36]. The pregnancy-associated changes in lipoprotein metabolism are amplified in certain pathologic states. Greater increases in VLDL lipids occur with hypertension or preeclampsia, while greater increases in total and LDL cholesterol levels characterize women with antecedent hypercholesterolemia [34]. Excessive alterations in lipids associated with pregnancy (above the 95th percentile) may suggest either an underlying genetic hyperlipidemia or predict dyslipidemia in later life [35,37].

ORAL CONTRACEPTIVES

The formulations of oral contraceptives available in the USA are either progestin only or combinations of an estrogen (ethinyl estradiol or mestranol) and a progestin (norethindrone, norethindrone acetate, ethynodiol diacetate, norethynodrel, norgestrel, or levonorgestrel). Ethynodiol diacetate, norethynodrel, and norethindrone acetate are metabolized by the liver to norethindrone, the active estrane progestin. The gonane progestins, norgestrel and its active isomer levonorgestrel, have greater progestational potency and have greater androgenic effects than the estranes [38]. Norgestrel is 5–10 times, and levonorgestrel 10–20 times, as potent as the estranes [39]. As all of these progestins also have estrogenic, antiestrogenic, and antiandrogenic activities, the net metabolic effects of a combination agent depend upon the dosages and types of estrogen and progestin contained in it. Data are insufficient to determine if the newer triphasic formulations are superior in terms of their metabolic effects to older formulations.

The effects of oral contraceptives on lipids and lipoproteins are thus complex and somewhat dependent upon the specific compound used [40]. Generally, LDL-C is elevated with all preparations, as is apopro-

Table 1.2 Mean changes in lipids and lipoproteins with menopause and age. (Adapted from [28])

	Menopausal women	Premenopausal controls
Cholesterol (mmol/l)		
Total	0.25 (9.7)	0.17 (6.6)*
HDL	−0.09 (−3.5)	0.00 (0.0)[†]
HDL$_2$	−0.04 (−1.5)	0.01 (0.4)
HDL$_3$	−0.06 (−2.3)	−0.01 (−0.4)
LDL	0.31 (12.0)	0.14 (5.4)*[†]
Triglycerides (mmol/l)	0.08 (7.0)	0.05 (4.4)*
Apoproteins (g/l)		
A-I	0.04	0.06*
A-II	−0.02	−0.03*
B	0.06	0.05*

Values in parentheses are mg/dl.
* Baseline vs. follow-up for both groups, $p \leq 0.05$.
[†] Cases vs. controls, group × examination interaction term, $p < 0.05$.

tein B where it has been measured. The relative elevations are dependent on the dose and potency of the progestin. Norgestrel appears to lower HDL-C or HDL$_2$ even in the lowest dose triphasic combinations. Norethindrone may also lower HDL$_2$. Apoprotein A-I levels are increased by oral contraceptives, with norgestrel having less effect than the estranes [26]. Although available data from epidemiologic and animal studies have not documented an acceleration of atherosclerosis with oral contraceptive use to date [39], the possible impact of these lipid changes on CHD risk is unresolved [40]. However, studies of experimental atherosclerosis in primates indicate that oral contraceptives protect against disease despite adverse lipid changes, suggesting that estrogen exerts a protective effect independent of lipoproteins.

MENOPAUSE AND POSTMENOPAUSAL HORMONE REPLACEMENT

The menopause is a time of marked change in the lipid profiles of women. In a prospective study with 2.5 years of follow-up, Matthews *et al.* [28] found significant decreases in HDL-C and increases in LDL-C among women who became menopausal in comparison to their premenopausal controls (Table 1.2). These changes, in excess of the changes due to age observed in both groups, remained significant after adjustment for age, body-mass index, and smoking. The changes in both groups over time, given their similar ages, are consistent with the gradual decrease in endogenous estrogen that occurs during the perimenopausal period [26]. Cross-sectional studies also document strikingly increased LDL-C levels among postmenopausal women [23]. The presence of obesity and the distribution of body fat (waist:hip ratio reflecting central obesity) may independently add to the adverse effects of menopause on lipids [41,42]; however, further data will be needed to clarify this issue. Whether the type of menopause experienced is natural or surgical makes little difference in the lipid profile changes [43]. Finally, qualitative lipid changes also occur with menopause. Postmenopausal women appear to have higher numbers of small, dense and consequently more atherogenic LDL particles than premenopausal women [26,44]. These findings, coupled with the high rate of CHD in postmenopausal women, indicate that the postmenopausal state is an independent risk factor for CHD.

Postmenopausal hormonal therapy can modify the lipoprotein profile. Oral estrogen use increases triglycerides in a dose-dependent fashion, decreases LDL-C $10-20$ mg/dl, increases HDL-C $5-10$ mg/dl, and increases apoproteins (particularly A-I) [23]. Estrogen replacement therapy (ERT) also attenuates the age-related increase in LDL-C and decrease in HDL-C levels [28]. These effects appear to be mediated through an increase in hepatic lipoprotein secretion of VLDL and an increase in LDL receptor activity. The mechanism for the HDL change is unclear, but probably involves hepatic lipase activity and a reduced catabolic rate. The route of administration also affects lipid responses. Because transdermally applied estrogen is not subject to the "first-pass" through the liver, there may not be an effect on lipoprotein levels with this formulation [45]. Finally, the beneficial effects of ERT on lipids apparently persist for over 20 years [46].

BEHAVIORAL FACTORS AFFECTING LIPOPROTEINS IN WOMEN

Obesity, smoking, alcohol intake, and exercise all determine HDL-C levels to some extent. The dose-related decrease noted with smoking may be greater among men [25], while the alcohol-related changes appear to be greater in women [47]. The studies on the effect of exercise on HDL-C have mainly been done in men. However, a cross-sectional study of middle-aged women found that physical activity was not independently associated with any lipid or lipoprotein measured [48], suggesting that the relationship between HDL-C and exercise may be weaker or absent among women. The adverse effect of obesity is most prominent on HDL_2 among women [48].

There is increasing interest in the distribution of body fat and its impact on health. The difference in susceptibility to CHD between women and men has been attributed in part to differences in the distribution of body fat rather than gender [49]. The "male (or central) pattern" of obesity with large amounts of abdominal fat has been related to an insulin-resistance syndrome that includes hypertension, low HDL-C, high triglycerides, and abnormal glucose tolerance with a marked susceptibility to CHD [50–53]. Proposed mechanisms for the influence of central adiposity on CHD include effects on cholesterol levels, plasma insulin, glucose, and hormone levels [49], possibly mediated through differences in metabolic behavior of adipocytes in different body regions [54]. In contrast to men, women tend to maintain body fat along the thighs and buttocks rather than intra-abdominally. This distribution of body weight can be indirectly characterized by the waist:hip ratio, with a low value (<0.72) reflecting lower body fat predominance [55]. Women with male pattern or central obesity (ratio >0.80) do have less desirable lipoprotein profiles and are at greater risk of CHD [56–60]. In a study by Ostlund and colleagues [61], gender did not influence HDL_2 levels significantly when waist:hip ratio, plasma insulin level, and glucose intolerance were entered in a multivariate regression model.

Race

BLACK VS. WHITE

Data from NHANES II participants revealed no differences in the proportions of whites and blacks meeting NCEP treatment guidelines [2], suggesting that the overall total cholesterol and risk factor distributions may be similar between the races. However, the distributions of other lipid risk factors differ between blacks and whites. These differences are not always due to biologic factors.

The Bogalusa Heart Study found higher HDL-C levels in adolescent and young adult black males [62], and higher levels of HDL_2 among black boys and girls aged 11–17 years when compared to their white counterparts [63]. Among adults aged 18–30 years participating in the Coronary Artery Risk Development in Young Adults Study (CARDIA), black males had higher HDL-C and apolipoprotein A-I levels than white males, and lower triglyceride and apolipoprotein B levels (Table 1.3). In comparison to white females, black women had higher LDL-C and apolipoprotein A-I and B levels, and lower triglycerides. Gender differences were more pronounced among the white participants [64].

Table 1.3 Mean (and standard deviation) lipid and lipoprotein values (mg/dl) among CARDIA participants by age group (18–24 years and 25–30 years). (Adapted from [64])

	White men		White women	
	18–24	25–30	18–24	25–30
Total cholesterol	168.1 (31.6)	161.0 (33.9)	173.5 (29.7)	177.8 (31.1)
LDL-C	104.8 (29.0)	115.4 (31.0)	104.6 (28.0)	107.0 (28.9)
HDL-C	46.1 (10.4)	47.4 (11.6)	54.2 (12.5)	54.3 (13.3)
Triglycerides	85.9 (55.6)	92.9 (77.2)	73.1 (35.7)	68.2 (44.0)
Apolipoprotein A-I	130.4 (18.8)	133.1 (19.6)	138.1 (22.1)	140.3 (20.3)
Apolipoprotein B	88.9 (23.0)	96.6 (25.2)	87.8 (21.9)	88.7 (23.0)
	Black men		Black women	
	18–24	25–30	18–24	25–30
Total cholesterol	167.8 (31.5)	183.7 (36.1)	176.3 (34.3)	181.1 (33.1)
LDL-C	102.4 (29.9)	114.4 (33.9)	109.4 (32.2)	112.1 (31.6)
HDL-C	52.7 (12.5)	54.1 (14.8)	54.7 (12.4)	56.9 (13.2)
Triglycerides	63.7 (38.9)	76.2 (44.5)	61.3 (28.0)	65.4 (36.1)
Apolipoprotein A-I	139.5 (22.1)	142.1 (23.0)	140.4 (21.7)	142.8 (21.9)
Apolipoprotein B	85.1 (22.8)	94.2 (24.9)	89.2 (25.8)	91.9 (23.2)

Small groups of black males and females were compared with their white counterparts aged 5–44 years in the Lipid Research Clinics Program Prevalence Study [65]. HDL-C was higher in blacks in each 5-year age group among males, and seven of eight age groups among females. The mean black–white difference was greater for males at each age. Adjustment for triglyceride levels, which were lower in blacks, reduced but did not eliminate the HDL differences. Similar lipid levels found in cord blood samples from black and white infants [66] suggest that other factors may account for at least some of the ethnic difference in HDL-C levels, such as behavioral characteristics [67]. Gender and racial differences in HDL-C levels were found among NHANES II participants [68], with gender, race, alcohol consumption, smoking, and body-mass index strongly related to HDL-C. Years of education were less strongly related to HDL-C while the effect of income varied with race. Higher income whites had higher HDL-C levels, while lower HDL-C levels characterized higher-earning blacks. White female CARDIA participants had more favorable lipoproteins with higher educational attainment [64]. Other data have shown that racial differences in HDL-C levels do not exist among men at higher educational levels [67].

Blacks reportedly have a higher prevalence of elevated lipoprotein-(a) (Lp(a)) levels than whites [69,70]. The distribution of Lp(a) appears to vary across racial groups, being highly skewed in white populations with a predominance of very low values but more normally distributed in American and African blacks [71].

The study by Saad *et al.* [72] found differences in the relationship between blood pressure and insulin resistance by race. Fasting plasma insulin and glucose disposal rate were not correlated with blood pressure in Pima Indians and blacks, suggesting that racial differences may also be present in the relationship of insulin resistance and lipoproteins.

HISPANIC VS. WHITE

Hispanic populations are culturally diverse, making it difficult to draw valid conclusions across all of these groups. Much of the data are derived from Mexican Americans. The San Antonio Heart Study [73], which involved 25–64-year-old Anglo and Mexican Americans, suggested that total and LDL cholesterol levels are similar between these groups. Differences were noted for triglyceride levels among males and females (higher among Mexican Americans) and HDL-C levels among females (lower among Mexican Americans). About half of this difference was explained by obesity. The difference in triglyceride levels disappeared among females after adjusting for centrality of adiposity. Data from Starr County, Texas indicated similar distributions of lipoproteins except higher triglycerides in males and females, and lower HDL-C levels in female Mexican Americans as compared to the general population, again consistent with the frequency of obesity in Hispanic groups [74]. Thus, some differences in lipoprotein levels may exist between Anglo and Mexican Americans, explainable at least in part by behavioral factors.

Lipid screening of 217 Hispanic mothers of young children in New York City found lower age-specific total cholesterol and HDL-C levels than those found in the Lipid Research Clinics (LRC) Prevalence Study. Mean LDL-C levels were 20% lower than in LRC, while triglyceride levels were higher. These results were not adjusted for body mass nor was this sample population-based. Further, the women represented different Hispanic groups: 73% were born in the Dominican Republic, 20% in the USA, 7% in Puerto Rico, and 1% in other Latin American countries [75]. Screening of 458 healthy blood donors in Puerto Rico revealed that 20% had moderate and 12% had high risk LDL-C levels, while 24% and 11% had borderline high and high total cholesterol levels. HDL-C levels below 35 mg/dl (0.9 mmol/l) were present in 30% of the men [76]. These total cholesterol prevalences are lower than those reported using the NHANES II data (14% borderline high and 27% high) [2]; however, almost 40% of the blood donors were aged 30 or less. Further studies are needed among Mexican American and other Hispanic groups to adequately characterize the prevalence of lipid and lipoprotein disorders among these groups.

OTHER EFFECTS OF RACE

Race is often considered a surrogate measure for socioeconomic status, and thus connotes more than just genetic and cultural factors. Additionally, race and socioeconomic status can affect disease patterns indirectly through barriers to medical care and low utilization of preventive services. Although narrowed in recent years, the discrepancy in health status between the poor and the more advantaged remains large [77–80]. A study of school children aged 5–18 years found higher cholesterol levels among schools with a predominantly lower socioeconomic status student body [81]. Blacks had the highest levels of all groups, while Hispanics (Puerto Ricans and Dominicans) also had significantly higher cholesterol levels than whites. Cholesterol screening and awareness was strongly associated with age, race, and educational attainment in the 1989 Behavioral Risk Factor Surveillance System Survey [82]. Other studies have documented that whites are more likely to be aware of and treated for hyperlipidemia than Mexican Americans [83], while blacks [84] and the poorly educated [85] remain less knowledgeable of CHD and its risk factors.

Lipid disorders in those with CHD

As a group, individuals with manifest CHD are at high risk for reinfarction and death. Superimposed on the high absolute risk of recurrent events is an increase in risk attributable to elevated cholesterol [86]. Evidence for the association of cholesterol level with recurrent coronary events or disease progression comes from epidemiologic and secondary prevention studies. Among white males aged 40–69, Pekkanen *et al.* [87] found a markedly different 10-year risk of cardiovascular mortality among patients with cardiovascular disease, varying from 3.8% for those with low risk total cholesterol levels to 19.6% among those with a high risk cholesterol level and disease. The corresponding risks among those without disease at baseline were 1.7% and 4.9%, respectively. High levels of LDL-C (>160 mg/dl or 4.1 mmol/l) as well as low HDL-C (<35 mg/dl or 0.9 mmol/l) also predicted greater mortality among those with CHD. Among survivors of myocardial infarction aged 30–64 years, partial ileal bypass reduced total cholesterol (23.3%) and LDL-C (37.7%) but increased HDL-C (4.3%) in comparison with controls at 5 years [88]. The surgery group had significantly fewer CHD deaths and nonfatal myocardial infarctions (combined endpoints), less disease progression on arteriograms, and underwent fewer coronary artery bypass grafting surgeries than controls. Similar results were found among the female participants in this trial. Diet alterations resulting in lower fat intake stabilized disease progression in the placebo group of the Cholesterol-Lowering Atherosclerosis Study (CLAS) [89]. Among patients with heterozygous familial hypercholesterolemia and coronary lesions followed for 2 years, combined diet and drug therapy decreased LDL-C levels 38.1% in the treatment group and 10.6% in the controls, and increased HDL-C levels 28% in the treatment group [90]. Coronary angiograms documented mean progression of stenosis among controls and regression in the treatment group, both in male and female patients. LDL-C level was the best predictor of outcome, being more powerful than group assignment. While 92% of these patients had no CHD symptoms, other studies of men after coronary artery bypass grafting [91,92] or with a significant proportion of men with CHD symptoms [93] have also documented improvement in lipoprotein risk factors, angiographic assessment of lesions, and clinical outcome with aggressive lipid-lowering drug treatment.

These trials provide strong evidence for the effect of cholesterol level, and particularly LDL-C, on the course of CHD. The failure of treatment studies to date to significantly lower total mortality among intervention groups may be due to lack of statistical power from inadequate sample size and study duration. These same trials have shown increased divergence in mortality rates with time, suggesting that longer follow-up periods may be necessary. It has further been estimated that an 8% change in total cholesterol level is the minimum needed to demonstrate an effect. Overall, however, the data demonstrate that a 10% reduction in cholesterol can reduce the rate of nonfatal reinfarction by 19% and of fatal reinfarction by 12% [86]. Given the potential efficacy of treatment and the continuous nature of the association between cholesterol and outcome in this high risk group, aggressive therapy to lower LDL-C is indicated for most patients with CHD, perhaps to levels of 100 mg/dl (2.59 mmol/l) as indicated by experimental studies. Further trials will be needed to assess the impact of intervention among those with other lipoprotein risk factors, such as low HDL-C levels, as well as among groups other than middle-aged males.

Implications for screening and treatment

Screening

Programs for detecting risk factors involve population-wide screening, case-finding approaches, or a combination of these two strategies. The screening program adopted must consider, among other factors, the underlying prevalence of the risk factor or disease in the population and the efficacy of treatment once a risk factor is found. NCEP guidelines [1] presently recommend population-based screening of total cholesterol for all adults over the age of 20 years. As most disease events occur in persons at a slightly increased risk from several factors rather than those at extremely high risk levels of a single factor, such a screening program could be more useful than programs that only screen individuals for isolated risk factors [24].

In order to examine the potential effects of targeted vs. population-based approaches, investigators have performed computer simulations based on presently available risk and incidence data. Goldman and coworkers [94] constructed their model using relative risk coefficients based on Framingham data. Targeted approaches appreciably lowered CHD incidence among males aged 35–54 years, but had little impact among older men. Similar results were found with a population-based approach of lowering total cholesterol 10 mg/dl in all men. Among women, the targeted approach achieved greater reductions in CHD incidence at all age ranges than among men, but the population-based approach required lowering total cholesterol 23 mg/dl to achieve the same effect. Further analysis with this model revealed greater efficacy of intervention among individuals at risk than among the general population [95]. A combined approach with differing strategies across gender and risk groups is more appropriate with this model. A similar analysis among the population of England and Wales found that targeted treatment reduced CHD mortality by 22%, twice the reduction achieved through population-wide screening and treatment [96]. This model supports the use of targeted intervention. Finally, new data on the relative insensitivity of screening based solely on total cholesterol have been reported [3], suggesting that more widespread use of lipoprotein analysis in screening is required. Screening and treatment strategies thus need to be tailored to the population group, with greater use of lipoprotein analysis among those at high risk by virtue of elevated lipids or nonlipid risk factors.

Excluding the elderly from screening and treatment based solely on such data is not appropriate given their high absolute rates of CHD. A more individualized approach is required in this group, in which quality of life due to CHD and other diseases as well as cost–benefit issues of treatment (e.g., cost of prescriptions, side-effects, presence of CHD, other risk factors, etc.) are considered [97]. The NCEP recommendations for screening, lipoprotein analysis, and treatment should thus be extended to healthy elderly individuals and not limited to the young and middle-aged.

Population-wide efforts to decrease cholesterol levels by dietary change may benefit women less than men. A potential lesser effect of diet in women [27] plus the potential adverse effect on HDL-C levels of adopting the recommended diet [24] argues for a more targeted approach in females, particularly premenopausal. Efforts among women should incorporate more frequent use of lipoprotein analysis to characterize risk status based on LDL-C and HDL-C levels, particularly among women with "borderline high" total cholesterol. One group that may be more likely to benefit from screening and follow-up are women who exhibit excessive, or "supraphysiologic," lipid changes during pregnancy. Women with this trait may require careful surveillance after pregnancy to detect and treat hyperlipidemias. Another high yield group for screening and treatment is the large number of individuals with CHD or at especially high risk of CHD—smokers, diabetics, hypertensives, and those with a strong family history of CHD.

Issues of screening and treatment among minority groups include low levels of awareness and perhaps underlying differences in lipoprotein distributions. The patterns of HDL-C differences between the races, and especially among black women, imply that lipoprotein analysis should be used for risk categorization in blacks. The effect of the suggested racial differences in Lp(a) and apolipoproteins on CHD, and thus screening practices, is as yet unresolved. The high CHD mortality rates of blacks relative to whites [98–100] and of the economically and educationally disadvantaged [101] highlight the importance of risk factor distribution, behavioral risk factors, and access to care among these groups. Given that a considerable number of patients with CHD will have total cholesterol levels below 200 mg/dl (5.17 mmol/l) but LDL-C levels above 130 mg/dl (3.36 mmol/l), and that aggressive treatment of lipid disorders in patients with CHD improves outcome, fasting lipoprotein analysis rather than total cholesterol screening should be performed among all patients with manifest CHD.

Treatment

Although current data are insufficient to clearly demonstrate treatment efficacy among the elderly, lipid lowering probably can benefit men up to the age of 69 as demonstrated in the LRC Coronary Primary Prevention Trial [102] and in the Los Angeles Domiciliary Trial [103]. The prevalence of comorbid conditions and the likelihood of greatly reduced quality of life after a myocardial infarction or stroke points out the need for prevention in this age group, where functionally competent and independent individuals may be disabled by a relatively small insult to the cardiovascular system. Further, some data from secondary prevention studies indicating cessation or slowing of disease progression [88,90] imply potential benefit to the vast majority of older individuals who already have lesions of coronary artery disease. Therefore, although definitive data on the issue of lipid-lowering treatment among the elderly are lacking, the decision to treat or not to treat should be individualized and "physiologic" age should be the predominant consideration. As treatment benefit is not immediately apparent in clinical trials, and since the likelihood of improving functional status by delaying the development of CHD is low in elderly individuals whose activity is already limited by other severe chronic disease, it is essential to carefully select potential candidates for lipid-modifying therapy.

Elderly persons respond to diet and cholesterol-lowering drugs as well as younger individuals [104]. Although some may have difficulties in changing dietary and lifestyle habits that have been acquired in earlier years, many of the elderly are willing to make such changes in order to lower their risk for cardiovascular disease. It is of utmost importance to ensure that any new diet is nutritionally balanced, and does not aggravate preexisting nutritional deficiencies. Finally, many elderly individuals have other coexisting diseases and require multiple medications, thus predisposing them to excessive adverse effects from some lipid-lowering drugs; this may be particularly true of nicotinic acid and the resins.

Although premenopausal nondiabetic women are at much less risk of CHD than men, women who experience coronary events are at a survival disadvantage in comparison to men and the risk of CHD among the postmenopausal approximates that of men. These factors justify special efforts to improve early recognition and treatment of CHD and its prevention among women. To this end, the major cardiac risk factors should reflect the importance of menopause, smoking, low HDL-C levels, and diabetes mellitus among women.

The treatment of dyslipidemias among women may well differ from that among men. As LDL-C levels are possibly less important among women, and as dietary responses among women are potentially less than among men [25], dietary treatment for women may well be less efficacious. The importance of HDL-C levels among women requires attention to obesity, cigarette smoking, and exercise, as well as pharmacologic regimens that raise HDL levels if needed. Dietary or drug treatment of women during pregnancy is generally not attempted. For those individuals experiencing severe hypertriglyceridemia, an appropriate diet appears indicated to prevent pancreatitis. However, hypolipidemic agents are not recommended generally during pregnancy and experience with their use is limited. Oral contraceptives affect lipids, depending on the formulation, but these agents are not known to be associated with increased CHD risk.

Recent reports indicate that ERT in menopausal women may greatly reduce the risk of cardiovascular disease and all-cause mortality. The reduction in CHD is estimated at 50% or more due, in part, to hormonally induced changes in lipoproteins; however, other mechanisms are likely to be involved [105,106]. Although progestins may adversely affect lipids, the combination therapy of estrogen with less androgenic progestin analogs (medroxyprogesterone acetate in the USA) does not appreciably affect lipids [26]. The use of combination therapy has not been shown to favorably affect CHD, as estrogen therapy alone has. Finally, although estrogen use has been associated with breast and uterine cancer in previous studies [107], recent data indicate that ERT can decrease breast and gastrointestinal cancer and result in lower overall cancer mortality [108].

Aggressive therapy of dyslipidemia can improve the outcome of persons with manifest CHD. In these individuals, treatment at lower lipid levels is warranted given the high absolute risk for recurrent events and the success of clinical trials in reducing the risk. The goal should be to achieve stabilization at a minimum, or promote regression of coronary artery lesions. LDL-C levels should be reduced to 100 mg/dl (2.58 mmol/l) or less with pharmacologic and/or diet therapy if indicated by the patient's age, cardiac, and overall health status, and other risk factors [109].

Summary

The relationship between CHD and cholesterol and the effect of cholesterol-lowering therapy on the primary and secondary prevention of CHD has been examined mainly in middle-aged white males. Differences exist between this more commonly studied group and the elderly, minorities, and women in terms of CHD risk, lipid and lipoprotein distributions, and response to treatment.

Although the association between CHD and cholesterol may not be as strong among the elderly as among the younger age groups in relative terms, the high absolute risk of CHD and the age-related increases in lipids merit consideration of screening and lipid-lowering treatment in these individuals, based on the presence of other risk factors and comorbid conditions. Clinical trials directly assessing the efficacy of such treatment are underway.

CHD incidence rates are low among young women relative to similarly aged men, but increase markedly among postmenopausal women while women's lipid and lipoprotein levels fluctuate in response to hormone levels and hormonal therapies. Further, qualitative and quantitative lipoprotein differences exist between the sexes, particularly with regard to the importance of HDL-C. Given the differences in lipoprotein risk factors and distributions, targeted screening and treatment with greater reliance on lipoprotein analysis is required, particularly among younger women. Hormone replacement therapy in postmenopausal women has other benefits (e.g., prevention of osteoporosis) and risks (e.g., uterine cancer). Clinical trials will be required to demonstrate the most efficacious regimens in terms of agents and doses that maximize benefits and minimize risks.

The distributions of some lipids and lipoproteins such as HDL-C and Lp(a) may vary between the races although implications of these differences for CHD risk are not as yet clear. The presence of these differences suggests a greater need for lipoprotein analysis among blacks than required by the present recommendations for the general population. More data are needed on lipids and lipoproteins in other groups, such as Hispanics, as well as on the effects of Lp(a), triglycerides, and other lipoproteins on CHD risk. Minorities and low socioeconomic status persons also require targeted efforts to increase awareness of the importance of cholesterol as a CHD risk factor if progress in treatment is to be made.

The presence of manifest CHD places an individual at high risk for acute coronary events and death. This risk is associated with LDL and HDL cholesterol, as suggested by the secondary prevention trials using angiography that have demonstrated at least a slowing of disease progression among treated groups. Available evidence suggests that all individuals with CHD or at high risk should be considered for lipoprotein analysis and aggressive treatment of LDL-C levels. The epidemiology of lipid and lipoprotein risk factors for CHD varies greatly among different populations. These differences require modification of the original Adult Treatment Panel screening and treatment guidelines in order to maximally benefit all segments of the population.

References

1 National Cholesterol Education Program Expert Panel. Report of the National Cholesterol Education Program expert panel on detection, evaluation, and treatment of high blood cholesterol in adults. *Arch Intern Med* 1988;148:36–69.
2 Sempos C, Fulwood R, Haines C *et al*. The prevalence of high blood cholesterol levels among adults in the United States. *JAMA* 1989;262:45–52.
3 Bush TL, Riedel D. Screening for total cholesterol. Do the National Cholesterol Education Program's recommendations detect individuals at high risk of coronary heart disease? *Circulation* 1991;83:1287–93.

4 Brody JA, Brock DB, Williams TF. Trends in the health of the elderly population. *Annu Rev Public Health* 1987;8:211–34.
5 Olshansky SJ, Carnes BA, Cassel C. In search of Methuselah: Estimating the upper limits to human longevity. *Science* 1990;250:634–40.
6 Brody JA. Prospects for an ageing population. *Nature* 1985;315:463–6.
7 Center for Disease Control. Predicting future cholesterol levels for coronary heart disease risk assessment. *MMWR* 1989;38:364–7.
8 Manolio TA, Pearson TA, Wenger NK *et al*. Cholesterol and heart disease in older persons and women: Overview of an NHLBI workshop. *Ann Epidemiol* 1992;2: 161–76.
9 Zimetbaum P, Frishman W, Aronson M. Lipids, vascular disease, and dementia with advancing age. *Arch Intern Med* 1991;151:240–4.
10 National Center for Health Statistics, Cohen BB, Barbano HE, Cox CS *et al*. Plan and operation of the NHANES I Epidemiologic Follow-up Study, 1982–84. Vital and Health Statistics. Series 1, No. 22. DHHS Pub. No. (PHS)87-1324. Public Health Service. Washington: US Government Printing Office, 1987.
11 Coroni-Huntley J, Brock DB, Ostfeld AM, Taylor JO, Wallace RB. Established populations for epidemiologic studies of the elderly: Resource Data Book. DHHS. NIH Publication No. 86-2443:1–10.
12 Kasim S. Cholesterol changes with aging: Their nature and significance. *Geriatrics* 1987;42:73–82.
13 Anderson KM, Castelli WP, Levy D. Cholesterol and mortality: 30 years of follow-up from the Framingham Study. *JAMA* 1987;257:2176–80.
14 Mariotti S, Capocaccia R, Farchi G *et al*. Age, period, cohort and geographical area effects on the relationship between risk factors and coronary heart disease mortality: 15-year follow-up of the European cohorts of the Seven Countries Study. *J Chron Dis* 1986;39:229–42.
15 Benfante R, Reed D. Is elevated serum cholesterol level a risk factor for coronary heart disease in the elderly? *JAMA* 1990;263:393–6.
16 Gordon DJ, Rifkind BM. Treating high blood cholesterol in the older patient. *Am J Cardiol* 1989;63:48H–52H.
17 Zimetbaum P Frishman W, Ooi WL *et al*. Relationship between the plasma lipids and the incidence of cardiovascular events in the old: The Bronx Longitudinal Aging Study. *Circulation* 1990;82:III-619.
18 Castelli WP, Wilson PWF, Levy D, Anderson K. Cardiovascular risk factors in the elderly. *Am J Cardiol* 1989;63:12H–19H.
19 Rose G, Shipley M. Plasma cholesterol concentration and death from coronary heart disease: 10 year results of the White Hall Study. *Br Med J* 1986;293:306–7.
20 Rubin SM, Sidney S, Black DM *et al*. High blood cholesterol in elderly men and the excess risk for coronary heart disease. *Ann Intern Med* 1990;113:916–20.
21 Kafonek SD, Kwiterovich PO Jr. Treatment of hypercholesterolemia in the elderly. *Ann Intern Med* 1990;112:723–5.
22 Barrett-Connor E, Cohn BA, Wingard DL, Edelstein SL. Why is diabetes mellitus a stronger risk factor for fatal ischemic heart disease in women than in men? The Rancho Bernardo Study. *JAMA* 1991;265:627–31.
23 Knopp RH. Effects of estrogen on serum lipoproteins and significance for arteriosclerotic disease. *Cholesterol and Coronary Disease . . . Reducing the Risk* 1990;2:8–10.
24 Crouse JR III. Gender, lipoproteins, diet, and cardiovascular risk: Sauce for the goose may not be sauce for the gander. *Lancet* 1989;ii:318–20.
25 Bush TL. Influences on cholesterol and lipoprotein levels in women. *Cholesterol and Coronary Disease . . . Reducing the Risk* 1990;2:1–6.
26 Miller VT. Dyslipoproteinemia in women. Special considerations. *Endocrinol Metab Clin North Am* 1990;19:381–99.

27 McNamara JR, Campos H, Ordovas JM *et al.* Effect of gender, age, and lipid status on low density lipoprotein subfraction distribution; Results from the Framingham Offspring Study. *Arteriosclerosis* 1987;7:483–90.
28 Matthews KA, Meilahn E, Kuller LH *et al.* Menopause and risk factors for coronary heart disease. *N Engl J Med* 1989;321:641–6.
29 Bush TL, Fried LP, Barrett-Connor E. Cholesterol, lipoproteins, and coronary heart disease in women. *Clin Chem* 1988;34:B60–B70.
30 Austin MA. Plasma triglyceride and coronary heart disease. *Arterioscler Thromb* 1991; 11:2–14.
31 Patsch JR, Prasad S, Gotto AM Jr, Bengtsson-Olivecrona G. Postprandial lipemia. A key for the conversion of high density lipoprotein$_2$ into high density lipoprotein$_3$ by hepatic lipase. *J Clin Invest* 1984;74:2017–23.
32 Deckelbaum RJ, Granot E, Oschry Y, Rose L, Eisenberg S. Plasma triglyceride determines structure–composition in low and high density lipoproteins. *Arteriosclerosis* 1984;4:225–31.
33 Patsch JR, Hopferwieser T, Muhlberger V *et al.* Postprandial lipemia in patients with coronary artery disease. *Arteriosclerosis* 1990;10:766a.
34 Potter JA, Nestel PJ. The hyperlipidemia of pregnancy in normal and complicated pregnancies. *Am J Obstet Gynecol* 1979;133:165–70.
35 Knopp RH, Bergelin RO, Wahl PW *et al.* Population-based lipoprotein lipid reference values for pregnant women compared to nonpregnant women classified by sex hormone usage. *Am J Obstet Gynecol* 1982;143:626–37.
36 van Stiphout WAHJ, Hofman A, de Bruijn AM. Serum lipids in young women before, during, and after pregnancy. *Am J Epidemiol* 1987;126:922–8.
37 Montes A, Walden CE, Knopp RH *et al.* Physiologic and supraphysiologic increases in lipoprotein lipids and apoproteins in late pregnancy and postpartum: Possible markers for the diagnosis of "Prelipemia." *Arteriosclerosis* 1984;4:407–17.
38 Crook D, Godsland IF, Wynn V. Oral contraceptives and coronary heart disease: Modulation of glucose tolerance and plasma lipid risk factors by progestins. *Am J Obstet Gynecol* 1988;158:1612–20.
39 Mishell DR. Contraception. *New Engl J Med* 1989;320:777–87.
40 Henkin Y, Como JA, Oberman A. Secondary dyslipidemia. Inadvertent effects of drugs in clinical practice. *JAMA* 1992;267:961–8.
41 Wing RR, Matthews KA, Kuller LH, Meilahn EN, Plantinga PL. Weight gain at the time of menopause. *Arch Intern Med* 1991;151:97–102.
42 Scheidt-Nave C, Barrett-Connor E. Adverse effect of early natural menopause on lipid profile among postmenopausal women. *Circulation* 1990;82:III–467.
43 White AD, Ephross SA, Hutchinson RG, Patsch W. Surgical and natural menopause and risk factors. *Circulation* 1990;82:III–468.
44 Campos H, McNamara JR, Wilson PWF, Ordovas JM, Schaefer EJ. Differences in low density lipoprotein subfractions and apolipoproteins in premenopausal and postmenopausal women. *J Clin Endocrinol Metab* 1988;67:30–5.
45 Walsh BW, Schiff I, Rosner B, Greenberg L, Ravnikar V, Sacks FM. Effects of postmenopausal estrogen replacement on the concentrations and metabolism of plasma lipoproteins. *N Eng J Med* 1991;325:1196–204.
46 Barrett-Connor E, Wingard DL, Criqui MH. Postmenopausal estrogen use and heart disease risk factors in the 1980s: Rancho Bernardo, Calif, revisited. *JAMA* 1989;261:2095–100.
47 Weidner G, Connor SL, Chesney MA *et al.* Sex differences in high density lipoprotein cholesterol among low-level alcohol consumers. *Circulation* 1991;83:176–80.
48 Meilahn EN, Kuller LH, Stein EA, Caggiula AW, Matthews KA. Characteristics associated with apoprotein and lipoprotein lipid levels in middle-aged women. *Arteriosclerosis* 1988;8:515–20.
49 Reaven GM. Role of insulin resistance in human disease. *Diabetes* 1988;37:1595–607.

50 Zavaroni I, Bonora E, Pagliara M *et al.* Risk factors for coronary artery disease in healthy persons with hyperinsulinemia and normal glucose tolerance. *N Engl J Med* 1989;320:702–6.

51 Krotkiewski M, Bjorntorp P, Sjostrom L, Smith U. Impact of obesity on metabolism in men and women. Importance of regional adipose tissue distribution. *J Clin Invest* 1983;72:1150–62.

52 DeFronzo RA, Ferrannini E. Insulin resistance. A multifaceted syndrome responsible for NIDDM, obesity, hypertension, dyslipidemia, and atherosclerotic cardiovascular disease. *Diabetes Care* 1991;14:173–94.

53 Wingard DL. Sex difference and coronary heart disease: A case of comparing apples and pears? *Circulation* 1990;81:1710–12.

54 Kissebah AH, Vydelingum N, Murray R *et al.* Relation of body fat distribution to metabolic complications of obesity. *J Clin Endocrinol Metab* 1982;54:254–60.

55 Hartz AJ, Rupley DC, Kalkhoff RD, Rimm AA. Relationship of obesity to diabetes: Influence of obesity level and body fat distribution. *Prev Med* 1983;12:351–7.

56 Peiris AN, Sothmann MS, Hoffmann RG *et al.* Adiposity, fat distribution, and cardiovascular risk. *Ann Intern Med* 1989;110:867–72.

57 Lapidus L, Bengtsson C, Larsson B *et al.* Distribution of adipose tissue and risk of cardiovascular disease and death: A 12 year follow up of participants in the population study of women in Gothenburg, Sweden. *Br Med J* 1984;289:1257–61.

58 Thompson CJ, Ryu JE, Craven TE, Kahl FR, Crouse JR III. Central adipose distribution is related to coronary atherosclerosis. *Arterioscler Thromb* 1991;11:327–33.

59 Freedman DS, Jacobsen SJ, Barboriak JJ *et al.* Body fat distribution and male/female differences in lipids and lipoproteins. *Circulation* 1990;81:1498–506.

60 Bjorntorp P. Obesity and the risk of cardiovascular disease. *Ann Clin Res* 1985;17:3–9.

61 Ostlund RE, Staten M, Kohrt WM, Schultz J, Malley M. The ratio of waist-to-hip circumference, plasma insulin level, and glucose intolerance as independent predictors of the HDL_2 cholesterol level in older adults. *N Engl J Med* 1990;322:229–34.

62 Srinivasan SR, Rerichs RR, Webber LS, Berenson GS. Serum lipoprotein profile in children from a biracial community: The Bogalusa Heart Study. *Circulation* 1976;54:309.

63 Srinivasan SR, Freedman DS, Webber LS, Berenson GS. Black–white differences in cholesterol levels of serum high-density lipoprotein subclasses among children: The Bogalusa Heart Study. *Circulation* 1987;76:272–9.

64 Donahue RP, Jacobs DR Jr, Sidney S *et al.* Distribution of lipoproteins and apolipoproteins in young adults: The CARDIA study. *Arteriosclerosis* 1989;9:656–64.

65 Tyroler HA, Glueck CJ, Christensen B, Kwiterovich PO Jr. Plasma high-density lipoprotein cholesterol comparisons in black and white populations: The Lipid Research Clinics Program Prevalence Study. *Circulation* 1980;62(Suppl IV):99–107.

66 Frank FA, Brown RF, Franklin CC. Screening diagnosis and management of dyslipoproteinemia in children: Strategies for reduction of adult cardiovascular disease starting in childhood. Lipid disorders. *Endocrinol Metab Clin North Am* 1990;19:1.

67 Freedman DS, Strogatz DS, Eaker E, Heosoef R, DeStefano R. Differences between black and white men in correlates of high-density lipoprotein cholesterol. *Circulation* 1990;81:715.

68 Linn S, Fulwood R, Rifkind B *et al.* High density lipoprotein cholesterol levels among US adults by selected demographic and socioeconomic variables: The Second National Health and Nutrition Examination Survey 1976–1980. *Am J Epidemiol* 1989;129:281–94.

69 Pearson T, Davidson L, Jenkins P *et al.* Lipoprotein (a) levels in blacks versus whites: Marked differences in levels and correlations with other lipids. *Circulation* 1990;82:III–120.

70 Srinivasan SR, Dahlen GH, Jarpa RA, Webber LS, Berenson GS. Black–white differences in serum Lp(a) levels and its relation to parental myocardial infarction among children. Bogalusa Heart Study. *Circulation* 1990;82:III–20.

71 Uterman G. The mysteries of lipoprotein (a). *Science* 1989;246:904–10.

72 Saad MF, Lillioja S, Nyomba BL *et al*. Racial differences in the relation between blood pressure and insulin resistance. *N Engl J Med* 1991;324:733–9.

73 Haffner SM, Stern MP, Hazuda HP, Rosenthal M, Knapp JA. The role of behavioral variables and fat patterning in explaining ethnic differences in serum lipids and lipoproteins. *Am J Epidemiol* 1986;123:830–9.

74 Hanis CL, Hewett-Emmett D, Douglas TC, Schull WJ. Lipoprotein and apolipoprotein levels among Mexican-Americans in Starr County, Texas. *Arterioscler Thromb* 1991;11: 123–9.

75 Shea S, Basch CE, Zybert P *et al*. Screening using national cholesterol education program guidelines in a population of urban Hispanic mothers. *Prev Med* 1989;18:824–32.

76 Marcial MA, Carbia AF. Serum cholesterol levels in Puerto Rican volunteer blood donors. *Bol Asoc Med P R* 1989;81:297–9.

77 Department of Health and Human Services. *Report of the Secretary's Task Force on Black and Minority Health*. Washington, DC: US Government Printing Office (GPO #017-090-00078-0), 1985.

78 Blendon RJ, Aiden LH, Freeman HE, Corey CR. Access to medical care for black and white Americans: A matter of continuing concern. *JAMA* 1989;261:278.

79 Feldman JJ. Health of the disadvantaged: an epidemiological overview. In: Parron DC, Solomon F, Jenkins CD (eds) *Behavior, Health Risks, and Social Disadvantage*. Washington, DC: National Academy Press, 1982: 13.

80 Davis K, Gold M, Makus D. Access to health care for the poor: does the gap remain? *Annu Rev Public Health* 1981;2:159.

81 Resnicow K, Morley-Kotchen J, Wynder E. Plasma cholesterol levels of 6585 children in the United States. Results of the Know Your Body Screening in Five States. *Pediatrics* 1989;84:969–76.

82 Centers for Disease Control. Factors related to cholesterol screening, cholesterol level awareness—United States, 1989. *JAMA* 1990;264:2985–6.

83 Stern MP, Patterson JK, Haffner SM, Hazuda HP, Mitchell BD. Lack of awareness and treatment of hyperlipidemia in type II diabetes in a community survey. *JAMA* 1989;262:360–4.

84 Gillum RF, Grant CT. Coronary heart disease in black populations. II. Risk factors. *Am Heart J* 1982;104:852–64.

85 Pierce DK, Conner SL, Sexton G *et al*. Knowledge of and attitudes toward coronary heart disease and nutrition in Oregon families. *Prev Med* 1984;13:390–5.

86 Rossouw JE, Lewis B, Rifkind BM. The value of lowering cholesterol after myocardial infarction. *N Engl J Med* 1990;323:1112–19.

87 Pekkanen J, Linn S, Helss G *et al*. Ten-year mortality from cardiovascular disease in relation to cholesterol level among men with and without preexisting cardiovascular disease. *N Engl J Med* 1990:322:1700–7.

88 Buchwald H, Vargo RL, Matts JP *et al*. Effect of partial ileal bypass surgery on mortality and morbidity from coronary heart disease in patients with hypercholesterolemia. Report of the Program on the Surgical Control of the Hyperlipidemias (POSCH). *N Engl J Med* 1990;323:946–55.

89 Blankenhorn DH, Johnson RL, Mack WJ, Zein HA, Vailas LI. The influence of diet on the appearance of new lesions in human coronary arteries. *JAMA* 1990;263:1646–52.

90 Kane JP, Malloy MJ, Ports TA *et al*. Regression of coronary atherosclerosis during treatment of familial hypercholesterolemia with combined drug regimens. *JAMA* 1990;264:3007–12.

91 Blankenhorn DH, Nessim SA, Johnson RL *et al*. Beneficial effects of combined colestipol–niacin therapy on coronary atherosclerosis and coronary venous bypass

grafts. *JAMA* 1987;257:3233—40.

92 Cashin-Hemphill L, Sanmarco ME, Blankenhorn DH. Augmented beneficial effects of colestipol—Niacin therapy at four years in the CLAS Trial. *Circulation* 1989;80:II—381.

93 Brown G, Albers JJ, Fisher LD *et al*. Regression of coronary artery disease as a result of intensive lipid-lowering therapy in men with high levels of apolipoprotein. B. *N Engl J Med* 1990;323:1289—98.

94 Goldman L, Weinstein MC, Williams LW. Relative impact of targeted versus populationwide cholesterol interventions on the incidence of coronary heart disease: Projections of the Coronary Heart Disease Policy Model. *Circulation* 1989;80:254—60.

95 Tsevat J, Weinstein MC, Williams LW, Tosteson A, Goldman L. Expected gains in life expectancy from various coronary heart disease risk factor modifications. *Circulation* 1991;83:1194—201.

96 Khaw K-T, Rose G. Cholesterol screening programmes: How much potential benefit? *Br Med J* 1989;299:606—7.

97 Denke MA, Grundy SM. Hypercholesterolemia in elderly persons: Resolving the treatment dilemma. *Ann Intern Med* 1990;112:781—92.

98 Haywood LJ. Coronary heart disease mortality, morbidity and risk in blacks. II. Access to medical care. *Am Heart J* 1984;108:794—6.

99 Gillum RF. Coronary heart disease in black populations. I. Mortality and morbidity. *Am Heart J* 1982;104:839—51.

100 Adams L, Africano E, Doswell W *et al*. Summary of workshop. I: working group on epidemiology. *Am Heart J* 1984;108:699.

101 Harlan WR, Stross JK. An educational view to lower plasma lipid levels. *JAMA* 1985;253:2087—90.

102 Gluek CJ, Gordon DJ, Nelson JJ, Davis CE, Tyrolen HA. Dietary and other correlates of changes in total and low density lipoprotein cholesterol in hypercholesterolemic men: the lipid research clinic coronary primary prevention trial. *Am J Clin Nutr* 1986;44:489—500.

103 Dayton S, Pearce ML, Hoshimoto S, Dixon WJ, Tomiyasu V. A controlled trial of a diet high in unsaturated fat in preventing complications of atherosclerosis. *Circulation* 1969;60(Suppl 2):1—63.

104 Shear CL, Franklin FA, Stinnett S *et al*. Expanded clinical evaluation of Lovastatin (EXCEL) study results. Effect of patient characteristics on Lovastatin-induced changes in plasma concentrations of lipids and lipoproteins. *Circulation* 1992;85:1293—303.

105 Knopp RH. Cardiovascular effects of endogenous and exogenous sex hormones over a woman's lifetime. *Am J Obstet Gynecol* 1988;158:1630—43.

106 Ross RK, Paganini-Hill A, Mack TM, Henderson BE. Cardiovascular benefits of estrogen replacement therapy. *Am J Obstet Gynecol* 1989;160:1301—6.

107 Steinberg KK, Thacker SB, Smith J *et al*. A meta-analysis of the effect of estrogen replacement therapy on the risk of breast cancer. *JAMA* 1985—1990;265:191.

108 Henderson BE, Paganini-Hill A, Ross RK. Decreased mortality in users of estrogen replacement therapy. *Arch Intern Med* 1991;151:75—8.

109 Oberman A, Kreisberg RA, Henkin Y. A practical approach to patient management. In: Oberman A, Kreisberg RA, Henkin Y (eds). *Principles and Management of Lipid Disorders*. Baltimore: Williams & Wilkins, 1992:249—50.

Chapter 2
Progression, Stabilization, and Regression of Coronary Heart Disease: Effects of Lipoprotein Modification

YAAKOV HENKIN & ROBERT A. KREISBERG

Laboratory, animal, clinical, and epidemiologic studies support the hypothesis that elevated blood cholesterol is an important etiologic factor in the development of atherosclerotic cardiovascular disease [1]. However, until recently most physicians did not regard the detection and treatment of lipoprotein disorders as high priority. This is because the ultimate proof of benefit from treatment requires evidence that modification of dyslipidemia prevents or improves cardiovascular disease in humans. During the past decade this evidence has finally accrued. Large scale clinical studies from several countries provide convincing evidence that lipoprotein modifications by dietary and/or drug interventions have the potential to prevent the development of coronary heart disease (CHD) in asymptomatic dyslipidemic individuals (primary prevention), as well as retard the progression of CHD in patients with preexisting disease (secondary prevention). This evidence has brought about a new enthusiasm for the detection and management of lipoprotein disorders.

The evidence in these studies can be classified into two broad categories: anatomic and clinical. Anatomic studies use histopathologic (animal) and angiographic (human) techniques to provide evidence that the degree of luminal stenosis in coronary and femoral arterial vessels is reduced by the modification of abnormal lipoprotein states. Such studies have the advantage of demonstrating statistically significant results in shorter time intervals with fewer subjects than primary prevention trials. Ethical considerations prevent the use of these techniques in primary prevention human studies, where coronary angiography before and after treatment cannot be justified. In addition, angiographic evidence of reduced plaque formation and luminal stenosis does not necessarily indicate prevention of CHD or clinical benefit. Clinical studies evaluate the actual clinical outcome of lipid modifications, but since the incidence of such endpoints is generally low, large study populations and longer follow-up periods are required to illustrate a treatment effect.

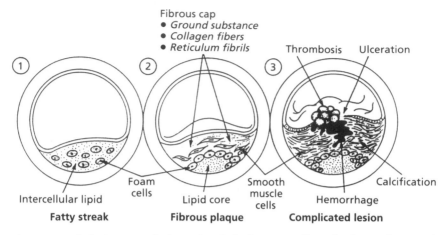

Fig. 2.1 Morphologic stages of atherosclerosis. Lesions generally evolve from a fatty streak which consists of foam cells, to a fibrous plaque, and finally to lesions involving calcification, ulceration, hemorrhage, and thrombosis. (Reproduced from [52].)

Effects on the vascular anatomy

The atherosclerotic plaque

Atherosclerotic lesions are commonly classified as fatty streaks, fibrous plaques, or complicated lesions (Fig. 2.1). Fatty streaks are probably the earliest form of arterial lesions, and are characterized by focal intimal accumulations of lipid-laden smooth-muscle cells and macrophages (foam cells) and fibrous tissue [2]. They appear in early childhood and are believed to be reversible, although there is some evidence to indicate a relationship between fatty streaks and more mature forms of atheroma in later life. Fibrous plaques are palpably elevated areas of intimal thickening and represent the most characteristic lesion of evolving atherosclerosis. Typically they are firm, elevated, and dome-shaped. They consist of a central core of extracellular lipid and necrotic cell debris, covered by a fibromuscular cap containing large numbers of smooth-muscle cells, macrophages, and collagen. The complicated lesion is a calcified fibrous plaque containing various degrees of necrosis, thrombosis, and ulceration. These are the lesions most frequently associated with clinical symptoms.

Animal studies

Both hypercholesterolemia and atherosclerosis can be induced in animals by increasing the cholesterol content of their diet. Although the lesions are often less extensive and complicated than those seen in human atherosclerosis, the degree of complication can be augmented by prolonging the period of cholesterol feeding and combining it with endothelial cell injury [3]. With the exception of cholesterol mono-hydrate crystals and some free cholesterol trapped in altered connective tissue, the bulk of cholesterol in the lesion exchanges with cholesterol in the plasma [4]. Thus, reduction of the plasma cholesterol should lead to a reduction in plaque cholesterol.

Experimental studies using a variety of animals models, including nonhuman primates, have clearly demonstrated that retardation of atherosclerosis, and even regression of existing plaques, can occur when normal cholesterol levels are restored for prolonged periods [2,5]. These studies involved dietary, surgical, and pharmacologic interventions for lipoprotein modification, and have analyzed plaque anatomy and histology in animals sacrificed at various stages of the study. The best results were achieved when intervention was started early, as regression is more easily achieved in early lesions.

The first sign of regression involves a return to normal cellular proliferative pattern and loss of foam cells [2,6]. This is associated with a marked decrease in the lesional content of esterified cholesterol, and somewhat less of a decrease in free cholesterol. The loss of cholesterol is multiphasic, with a rapid loss occurring within the first 6 months that correlates with disappearance of foam cells, and a much slower late phase of removal of extracellular lipid. In fact, extracellular accumulations of cholesterol can persist for many years, or even transiently increase, despite favorable conditions for regression. This suggests the presence of multiple cholesterol pools, some more readily mobilized than others. Mobilization of necrotic material also occurs slowly, the rate being related to the initial severity of the lesion. Regression is associated with a decrease in the elastin content and an increase in the collagen and calcium content of the lesion [7]. These changes are accompanied by considerable plaque remodelling and repair of the endothelial surface.

However, the pathologic lesions in experimental animal athero-sclerosis are different from those in humans, which typically develop over several decades and at lower serum cholesterol concentrations. Human lesions tend to be less fatty and more fibrous, and have more frequent complications such as ulceration and thrombosis. Thus, extrap-olation of results from animal studies to human atherosclerosis should be done with caution.

Human studies

Anatomic studies in humans are obviously more difficult to perform, and require the use of angiographic techniques to demonstrate changes in the luminal diameter and contours. This is an indirect approach to the arterial wall, and the results may be influenced by a variety of physiologic and pathologic processes such as changes in vascular tone and thrombosis, as well as technical artifacts [8,9]. Visual interpretation of coronary arteriograms is also associated with a high degree of inter- and intraobserver variability, thus requiring meticulous methodology to achieve a blinded, unbiased opinion relating to changes. This is especially true when the change in diameter of the stenosis is less than 20% [8]. Evaluations of this technique by the investigators of the National Heart, Lung and Blood Institute (NHLBI) Type II Coronary Intervention Study have shown that the use of a panel of three experienced readers decreases the variability and increases the reliability of the evaluation [10]. However, such assessment is still only semiquantitative and limited to terms such as "definite" or "probable" progression and regression.

The development of computerized coronary arteriography has eliminated many of the problems associated with visual arteriography [11]. These systems digitize the selected cine-frame and correct for distortion. The image is calibrated using the known dimension of the cardiac catheter; automatic programs determine arterial contours and calculate the vessel diameter and degree of stenosis with excellent reproducibility.

The assessment of plaque regression is also liable to other inaccuracies. This is mainly due to lysis and remodeling of thrombi, which may not always be distinguishable from regression of an atherosclerotic plaque [8,9]. Since plaque regression can probably occur spontaneously, adequate controls should always be used in the assessment of intervention effect.

UNCONTROLLED TRIALS

During the 1970s and early 1980s, several uncontrolled trials and case reports described the effects of lipid lowering on atherosclerosis progression (Table 2.1) [12–24]. Various intervention modalities were employed, including surgical (portacaval shunt, ileal bypass), plasma exchange procedures, lifestyle modifications (diet, exercise), and drugs. The results of these studies are difficult to interpret due to the small numbers of participants and the relative nonaggressiveness of their lipid-lowering effects.

Table 2.1 Uncontrolled angiographic studies. (Modified from [12])

Reference	Intervention	No. of patients	Duration (years)	Angiographic changes		
				Regress	=	Progress
[13]	Ileal bypass	30	2–4	3	22	5
[14]	Ileal bypass	31	2	5	21	5
[15]	Ileal bypass	1	10	1		
[16]	Portacaval shunt	1	1.5	1		
[17]	Plasma exchange	2	2	1		
[18]	Diet	39	2		17	22
[19]	NA	31	3.5	3	11	17
[20]	Cholestyramine, clofibrate	1	3.5	1		
[21]	Diet, clofibrate, neomycin, tibric acid	25	1.1	9	3	13
[22]	Clofibrate or NA	30	1.3–1.8		15	15
[23]	Diet, col	25	7		21	4
[24]	Diet, clofibrate, NA	24	7		12	12

Regress, number of patients with regression of lesions; Progress, number of patients with progression of lesions; =, number of patients with no change in lesions; col, colestipol; NA, nicotinic acid.

Two such studies from Europe provided insight to the relationship between lipoprotein levels and progression of atherosclerosis. The Leiden Intervention Trial [18] analyzed the effect of a vegetarian diet on the progression of coronary lesions in 39 patients with stable angina pectoris, but did not include a control group. Changes in luminal stenosis were assessed by both visual and computer-assisted image angiographic analysis. The Helsinki Study [24] employed visual coronary angiographic assessment to study the effects of diet, in addition to clofibrate and/or niacin, in 28 patients with total cholesterol levels above 7.2 mmol/l (280 mg/dl) or serum triglyceride above 2.0 mmol/l (180 mg/dl) and with two- or three-vessel disease. A group of men taking part in a simultaneous study, in which they received medical treatment for their coronary disease but no lipid-lowering therapy, served as a nonrandomized control group. The absence of adequate control groups in both studies prevented assessment of the treatment effects on lesion progression; however, both studies found positive correlations between lesion growth and the total cholesterol:high-density lipoprotein (HDL) ratio. In the Leiden study, disease progression was significant in patients who had a ratio higher than the median in that study (total cholesterol:HDL 6.9), but was absent in all those who had a ratio lower than this median throughout the trial, as well as in those who had initial ratios higher than 6.9 but had significant lowering during the dietary intervention period.

CONTROLLED TRIALS

Although early uncontrolled trials provided encouraging support for the efficacy of lipid lowering in prevention of atherosclerosis progression, the ultimate test of a treatment effect is the blinded, randomized, placebo-controlled clinical trial. Several such angiographic trials have been published since 1984 (Table 2.2), and provide additional evidence for such an effect.

The NHLBI Type II Coronary Intervention Study [25] involved individuals with CHD and Type II hyperlipidemia (low-density lipoprotein cholesterol (LDL-C) in the upper 10th percentile after 1 month of

Table 2.2 Controlled angiographic studies

Name (reference)	Intervention	No. of patients	Sex	Condition	Duration (years)	Angiographic changes vs. control Regress	Progress
NHLBI [25]	Cholestyramine vs. placebo	59 57	M + F	↑ LDL, CHD	5		↓
CLAS [26,27]	Col ± NA vs. placebo	80 82	M	TC 180−350 mg/dl coronary bypass	2−4	↑	↓
Kane [28]	Col ± NA ± lov vs. placebo	40 32	M + F	Heterozygous FH	2.2	↑	↓
FATS [29]	Col + NA, col + lov, placebo ± col	36 38 46	M	↑ Apoprotein B, CHD, family history of CVD	2.5	↑	↓
POSCH [30]	Ileal bypass vs. usual care	137 52	M + F	↑ TC and/or ↑ LDL, previous MI	9.7		↓

Col, colestipol; NA, nicotinic acid; lov, lovastatin; M, male; F, female; FH, familial hypercholesterolemia; CVD, cardiovascular disease; TC, total cholesterol; Regress, regression of lesions; Progress, progression of lesions; MI, myocardial infarction.

dietary therapy) who were randomly allocated to treatment with the bile-acid sequestrant cholestyramine or placebo for a period of 5 years. Sample size calculations during the planning phase of the study indicated a desired study population of 250 participants in order to achieve statistically significant results; however, the entry criteria were rigorous and only 143 patients could be recruited during the 54-month recruitment period, of which 116 completed the study. The treatment resulted in a lowering of LDL-C by 26% and an increase in HDL-C by 8%, compared to a 5% decrease in LDL-C and a 2% increase in HDL-C in the placebo group. Visual, semiquantitative angiographic assessment was performed by three individual blinded panels, each consisting of three experts who evaluated the baseline and 5-year follow-up angiograms in random order. CHD progressed in 49% (with 35% defined as definite progression) in the control group compared to 32% (with 25% defined as definite progression) in the treatment group, the difference not achieving statistical significance. However, when adjustments were made for baseline inequalities in risk factors (alcohol consumption, ventricular regional contractile function, systolic blood pressure, and postdiet triglyceride levels), the effect of treatment was more pronounced and statistically significant. This was most prominent in lesions that caused 50% or greater stenosis at baseline (progression occurring in 33% of placebo and 12% of cholestyramine-treated patients).

The Cholesterol-Lowering Atherosclerosis Study (CLAS) [26] was a randomized, placebo-controlled trial testing combined colestipol and niacin therapy in 162 nonsmoking men aged 40–59 years with previous coronary bypass surgery and baseline cholesterol levels of 185–350 mg/dl (4.78–9.05 mmol/l). This study was unique in conducting a prerandomization trial of the study drugs and selecting responders only, as well as in employing a flexible but aggressive drug-dose regimen in order to achieve maximal responses. Thus, although the patients and the angiographic assessment panel were blinded to the treatment, the clinic staff were not blinded. Angiographic assessment was performed visually by a panel of two angiographers and a moderator. During the first 2 years of treatment there was a 26% reduction in total cholesterol, 43% reduction in LDL-C and 37% increase in HDL-C levels. This was accompanied by a significant reduction in the average number of lesions that progressed per subject, as well as in the percentage of subjects with new atheroma formation, in both the native coronary arteries and the bypass grafts (Fig. 2.2). Atherosclerosis regression, as indicated by perceptible improvement in overall coronary status, occurred in 16.2% of the colestipol/niacin group and 2.4% in the placebo group. Interestingly, beneficial effects were noted in subjects with initial cholesterol

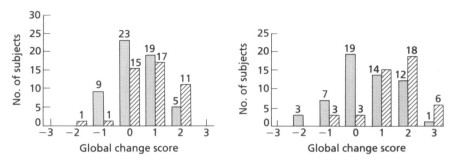

Fig. 2.2 Distribution of global coronary change score by treatment groups at 2 years of follow-up (left figure) and at 4 years of follow-up (right figure) in the Cholesterol-Lowering Atherosclerosis Study (CLAS) [26]. Zero indicates no change from baseline; 1, definitely discernible change; 2, intermediate change; and 3, extreme change. Positive numbers indicate progression; negative numbers, regression; stipple bars, drug-treated group; hatched bars, placebo-treated group. (Reproduced from [12].)

levels in the 180–240 mg/dl (4.65–6.21 mmol/l) range as well as in those in the 240–350 mg/dl (6.21–9.05 mmol/l) range, suggesting that cholesterol lowering has benefit in "normocholesterolemic" individuals with coronary artery disease (CAD). A follow-up of 103 subjects who elected to continue the study for 2 additional years revealed further divergence in disease progression and regression between the two groups [27].

A drug regimen similar to that used in the CLAS was also used in a study by Kane *et al.* in patients with heterozygous familial hyper-cholesterolemia [28]. Seventy such patients between the ages of 19 and 72 years, without evidence of significant CHD, received treatment with a low-fat, low-cholesterol diet. They were then randomized into a control group of 32 patients (treated with diet alone or diet plus low-dose colestipol) and a treatment group of 40 patients treated with niacin and colestipol. When lovastatin became available for clinical use it was added to the drug regimen of 16 of the patients in the drug-treatment group. After a mean follow-up of 26 months, the lipoprotein changes in the drug-treatment group were −38% for LDL-C, −19% for triglyceride, and +28% for HDL-C; the corresponding changes in the control group were −11% for LDL-C and insignificant for triglyceride and HDL-C. The mean change in percent area stenosis, as evaluated by quantitative angiography, was +0.80 for the control group (indicating progression of disease) and −1.53 for the drug-treatment group (indicating regression) (Fig. 2.3). A treatment benefit was seen in both women and men, although it reached statistical significance only in women. This is an

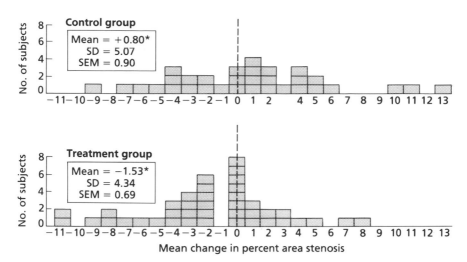

Fig. 2.3 Distribution of within-patient mean change in coronary lesions as percent area stenosis in the control (top, $n = 32$) and treatment (bottom, $n = 40$) groups in patients with heterozygous familial hypercholesterolemia. Asterisk indicates $p = 0.039$ for the difference between groups. (Reproduced from [28].)

important observation since it addresses the issue of whether women benefit from such therapy.

Another study that employed the drugs colestipol, niacin, and lovastatin was the Familial Atherosclerosis Treatment Study (FATS) [29], a randomized, double-blind quantitative angiographic comparison of three lipid-altering strategies. One hundred and twenty men with documented CHD, a family history of premature cardiovascular disease, and elevated apolipoprotein B (apo B) levels ($\geq 125\,\text{mg/dl}$) were placed on a diet and then randomly assigned to one of three treatment regimens for 2.5 years: niacin plus colestipol, lovastatin plus colestipol, or placebo with or without colestipol. Changes in LDL-C and HDL-C were -46% and $+15\%$, respectively in the lovastatin/colestipol group and -32% and $+43\%$, respectively in the niacin/colestipol group. The proportion of patients showing progression only (without regression) was less in the lovastatin/colestipol (21%) and the niacin/colestipol (25%) groups than in the control group (46%), while the proportion of patients showing only regression was greater in the lovastatin/colestipol (32%) and the niacin/colestipol (39%) groups than in the control group (11%) (Fig. 2.4). Clinical events were also less frequent in the two treatment groups (by approximately 85%) than in the control group. Multivariate analysis indicated that a reduction in the level of apo B (or LDL-C) and

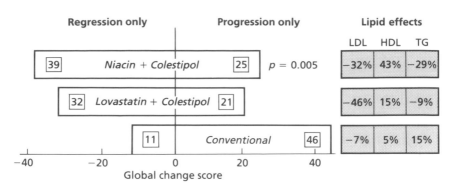

Fig. 2.4 Definite lesion changes in the FATS [29] according to the three treatment groups. The numbers in the horizontal bars on the graph represent percentage of patients. The numbers in the squares on the right represent the lipid and lipoprotein changes in each of the corresponding treatment groups. (Reproduced from [53].)

in systolic blood pressure, and an increase in HDL-C correlated independently with regression of coronary lesions.

Finally, the fact that the method of lipid lowering itself is not the major determinant of benefit was demonstrated by the Program on the Surgical Control of the Hyperlipidemias (POSCH) [30], where partial ileal bypass of the distal 200 cm (or distal one-third, whichever was greater) of the small intestine was used as the means for lipid lowering. The study population consisted of 838 subjects (approximately 15% of the group were women), between the ages of 30 and 64 years, who had survived a first myocardial infarction (MI) and had a total cholesterol of at least 5.69 mmol/l (220 mg/dl) or an LDL-C of at least 3.62 mmol/l (140 mg/dl). The subjects were instructed on a low-fat, low-cholesterol diet and then randomized to either a surgical or control group. After a mean follow-up period of 5 years, the surgery group had a total cholesterol level 23% lower, LDL-C 38% lower, and HDL-C 4% higher than the control groups Arteriographic evaluation, using a protocol similar to that in CLAS, revealed less disease progression in the surgery group at 3, 5, 7, and 10 years. Mortality due to CHD and confirmed nonfatal MI were collectively reduced by 35%, and the number of patients who required coronary-artery bypass grafting or coronary angioplasty was reduced by 62% and 55%, respectively. The number of patients that developed peripheral vascular disease was also reduced by 27%. Although overall mortality in the entire surgical group was reduced by 21%, the difference in overall mortality reached statistical significance only in the subgroup of patients with an ejection fraction ≥50%, where it was reduced by 36%.

Overall, the above studies consistently show that aggressive lipoprotein modification can result in detectable retardation of atherosclerosis, as well as regression of existing atherosclerotic plaques, in both the coronary and peripheral arterial circulations. A common finding in many of these studies was that both elevation of the HDL-C and reduction of the LDL-C correlated independently with such anatomic changes. This fact will be further elaborated later (see p. 50).

Effects on clinical endpoints

While the radiologic studies were exploring the effects of lipid-lowering strategies on the vascular anatomy, large scale clinical studies were being conducted to evaluate the outcome of comparable treatments on clinical endpoints. The complex nature of such studies and the large number of participants required to achieve statistically significant results demand meticulous planning and appreciable resources. This is especially true in primary prevention trials, where the expected incidence of new cardiovascular events is relatively low. The major issue examined was the effect of cholesterol lowering on cardiovascular morbidity (angina, nonfatal MI) and mortality (fatal MI, sudden death). However, there are additional issues that require clarification. What effects do such treatments have on the overall mortality? Is the method of lipid lowering important in determining the outcome? What is the optimum treatment duration? Does the modification of specific lipoproteins (rather than the total cholesterol) confer additional benefit? These and other questions have so far been only partially resolved. The following section will review some of the studies conducted to answer these questions; only controlled studies that employed lipid lowering as their major intervention, with sufficiently large sample size and follow-up periods, will be described.

Primary prevention studies (Table 2.3)

NUTRITIONAL STUDIES

Studies involving dietary interventions as the principal mode of lipid modification are hampered by the unblinded nature of most such studies (which has the potential of applying a different quality of care to the treatment group) and by their relatively modest impact on the magnitude of lipid lowering compared to that achievable with potent

Table 2.3 Primary prevention studies of CHD

Study (reference)	Intervention	No. of patients	Sex	Condition	Duration (years)	Reduction (%) TC	Reduction (%) CHD
VA Study [31]	Diet	846	M	Domiciliary care		13	31
Finnish Mental Hospital [32]	Diet	676	M + F	Mental hospital residents	2–3.5*	15	50
Minnesota Survey [33]	Diet	9057	M + F	Mental hospital residents	1–4.5*	14	NS
WHO [34]	Clofibrate, placebo	10 627	M	↑ TC	5.3	9	20
LRC-CPPT [35]	Cholestyramine, placebo	3806	M	↑ LDL-C	7.4	9	19
Helsinki [36]	Gemfibrozil, placebo	4082	M	↑ Non-HDL-C	5	9	33

TC, total cholesterol; M, male; F, female; NS, not significant.
* The time spent by each participant in the study was variable, depending on the length of their hospitalization.

drugs. Since the incidence of new onset CHD in primary prevention studies is potentially low, many nutritional studies did not achieve sufficient statistical power to detect a treatment effect. Only three of these studies will be mentioned here.

The Los Angeles Veterans Administration Study [31] was a randomized trial in individuals without earlier overt atherosclerotic disease. The diet used was rich in polyunsaturated fatty acids. The mean serum cholesterol was reduced by 13% in the intervention group compared to the control group. At the end of the study, the difference in CHD mortality between the two groups did not reach statistical significance, but the total cardiovascular incidence was significantly decreased by 31% in the intervention group. There was a small increase in non-atherosclerotic deaths (trauma and carcinoma); thus, total mortality was not significantly affected.

The Finnish Mental Hospital Study [32] was conducted on middle-aged men in two mental hospitals. A cholesterol-lowering diet was employed in one hospital while the other hospital served as control; after 6 years the diets were "crossed over" and continued for another 6 years. The average serum cholesterol was significantly reduced in the treatment group (hospital) in each phase, as were the incidences of major electrocardiogram (ECG) changes and CHD mortality. Although this study was not randomized, the results were impressive.

The Minnesota Coronary Survey [33] was a 4.5-year double-blind, randomized clinical trial that was conducted in six Minnesota state mental hospitals and one nursing home. It compared the effects of a 39% fat control diet (18% saturated fat, 5% polyunsaturated fat, and 446 mg dietary cholesterol per day) with a 38% fat treatment diet (9% saturated fat, 15% polyunsaturated fat, and 166 mg dietary cholesterol per day), and involved 4393 men and 4664 women who were institutionalized and received either diet for a cumulative duration of at least 1 year during the study period. All subjects in the institutions who agreed to participate, irrespective of their entry lipid levels, were enrolled. The average fall in total cholesterol during the low-fat diet period (mean duration 384 days) was 14%. For the entire study population, no differences in cardiovascular death or total mortality were observed. A favorable trend for all endpoints occurred in the younger age groups who were on the low-fat diet for over 2 years, but the numbers were small and the difference did not reach statistical significance.

DRUG STUDIES

The World Health Organization (WHO) Trial [34], conducted in three European centers, was one of the earliest drug studies in this area and had an unfavorable impact on future lipid-lowering strategies. The study evaluated the effect of clofibrate on prevention of CHD in asymptomatic, hypercholesterolemic middle-aged men. A total of 10 627 men were randomly assigned to clofibrate or placebo and followed for an average of 5 years. A mean reduction in total cholesterol of approximately 9% was achieved in the treatment group, and was accompanied by a 25% decrease in the incidence of nonfatal MI (Fig. 2.5). However, the incidence of fatal MI and angina was similar in the two groups, while the incidence of all-cause mortality was actually greater in the clofibrate group. This was principally due to a greater number of deaths related to the liver, intestinal, and biliary systems. A follow-up of the study participants after completion of the study revealed that these adverse effects had been confined to the treatment period only.

In contrast to the results of the WHO study, two other primary prevention studies provided encouraging results. The first of these was the Lipid Research Clinics Coronary Primary Prevention Trial (LRC-CPPT) [35], a multicenter, randomized, double-blind study on 3806 asymptomatic, middle-aged men with Type II hyperlipoproteinemia and

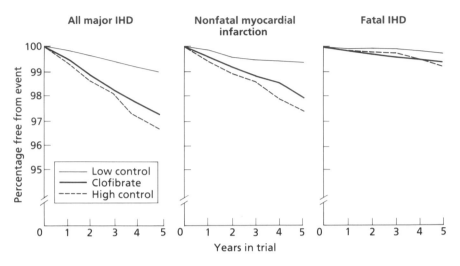

Fig. 2.5 Major ischemic heart disease in the first 5 years of the WHO Clofibrate Study. (Reproduced from [34].)

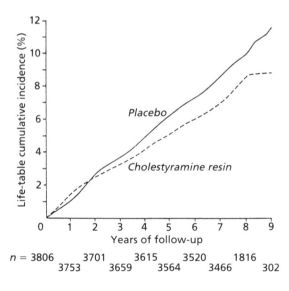

Fig. 2.6 Life-table cumulative incidence of primary endpoint (definite CHD death and/or definite nonfatal MI) in treatment groups, computed by Kaplan–Meier method. *n* equals total number of Lipid Research Clinics Coronary Primary Prevention Trial participants at risk for their first primary endpoint, followed at each timepoint. (Reproduced from [5].)

cholesterol concentrations above the 90th percentile. The treatment group received cholestyramine while the control group received a placebo for an average of 7.4 years. The cholestyramine group experienced on average an 8.5% reduction in total cholesterol, a 12.6% reduction in LDL-C, and a 10% increase in HDL-C compared to the placebo group; this was accompanied by a 19% reduction in incidence

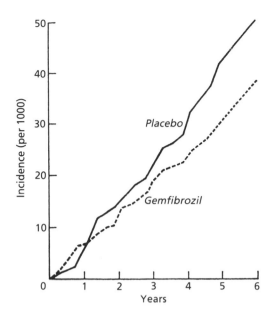

Fig. 2.7 Kaplan–Meier cumulative incidence (per 1000) and annual number of cardiac endpoints, according to treatment group and time in the Helsinki Heart Study. (Reproduced from [36].)

of definite CHD death and/or definite nonfatal MI (Fig. 2.6). This benefit became apparent after 2 years and was proportionate to the decrease in total and LDL cholesterol levels, as well as to the compliance to treatment. The incidence rates for new positive exercise tests, angina, and coronary bypass surgery were also significantly reduced. However, the reduction in overall mortality was not significant due to a greater number of violent and accidental deaths in the cholestyramine group.

The Helsinki Heart Study [36] was also a randomized, double-blind, placebo-controlled trial in 4081 asymptomatic middle-aged men with Types IIa, IIb, or IV hyperlipoproteinemia (non-HDL cholesterol >200 mg/dl). Treatment with gemfibrozil for 5 years resulted in an 11% decrease in LDL-C, a 35% decrease in serum triglyceride, and an 11% increase in HDL-C compared to the control group. This was accompanied by a 26% reduction in definite coronary deaths and a 34% reduction in the cumulative rate of cardiac endpoints (fatal and nonfatal MI and sudden cardiac death) at 5 years in the treatment group compared to the control group (Figs 2.7, 2.8). The changes in LDL-C and HDL-C levels, but not triglyceride levels, were independently associated with CHD reduction. As in the LRC-CPPT study, the benefit became evident after approximately 2 years of treatment. Overall mortality was not reduced due to an increase in the incidence of violence, accidents, and intracranial hemorrhage.

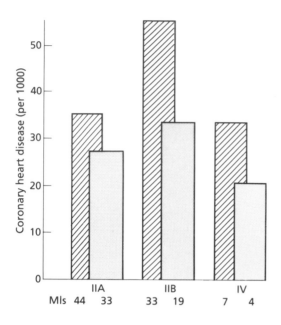

Coronary heart disease (per 1000)

Mls   44   33   33   19   7   4

IIA   IIB   IV

Fig. 2.8 Standardized incidence and number of cardiac endpoints by treatment in different Fredrickson types in the Helsinki Heart Study. Hatched bars, placebo; stipple bars, gemfibrozil. (Reproduced from [36].)

Secondary prevention studies (Table 2.4)

The absolute risk for reinfarction in association with elevated cholesterol levels is substantially higher in patients with coronary disease than in asymptomatic individuals [37]. Since long-standing, complicated atherosclerotic lesions appear to be less susceptible to regression than earlier lesions, the question arises whether patients with existing CHD will also benefit from lipoprotein modifications.

A number of nutritional studies evaluated the effects of lipid-lowering diets in prevention of recurrence of symptomatic disease in men who had sustained a first MI. These were generally of short duration (2–3 years) and limited sample size, and achieved only modest degrees of cholesterol lowering. No significant benefit of treatment on CHD recurrence was demonstrated in these studies.

The Coronary Drug Project [38] was a multicenter, randomized, double-blind, placebo-controlled study of 8341 men with electrocardiographic documentation of previous MI. The participants were randomly allocated to one of the following lipid-modifying drugs: niacin, clofibrate, dextrothyroxine, or one of two estrogen regimens. Treatment with dextrothyroxine and the estrogens was discontinued prematurely because of adverse effects. After an average follow-up period of 6 years, despite a mean decrease in the serum cholesterol (6% for clofibrate and 10% for niacin) and triglycerides (22% for clofibrate and 26% for

Table 2.4 Secondary prevention studies

Study (reference)	Intervention	No. of patients	Sex	Condition	Duration (years)	Reduction (%) TC	CHD
Newcastle [39]	Clofibrate vs. oil	497	M + F	Angina/MI	5	33	21
Edinburgh [40]	Clofibrate vs. oil	717	M + F	Angina/MI	6	21	33
CDP [38]	NA clofibrate placebo	5011	M	MI	5	10 7	4* 7
Stockholm [42]	NA + clofibrate, usual care	555	M + F	MI	5	13	19
FATS [29]	Col + NA or lov, placebo ± col	146	M	↑ Apo B, CHD; family history of CVD	2.5	28†	73
POSCH [30]	Ileal bypass, usual care	838	M + F	↑ TC and/or LDL	5	23	35

NA, nicotinic acid; col, colestipol; lov, lovastatin; CVD, cardiovascular disease; M, male; F, female; TC, total cholesterol.

* An 11% decrease in total mortality was seen in this group at the 15-year follow-up.
† Average for the lovastatin/colestipol and nicotinic acid/colestipol groups.

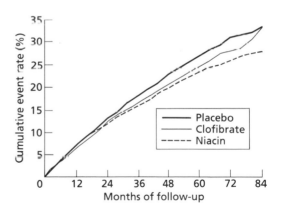

Fig. 2.9 Life-time cumulative event rates for coronary death or definite nonfatal MI in the Coronary Drug Project. *n* denotes total number of patients in clofibrate, niacin, and placebo groups combined, followed through each timepoint. Approximate numbers for individual groups are 2/9, 2/9, and 5/9 times *n* for clofibrate, niacin, and placebo, respectively. (Reproduced from [38].)

niacin), there was no statistically significant benefit compared with placebo for the primary endpoint of total mortality, although a lower rate of definite nonfatal MI was noted for niacin (Fig. 2.9). However, after a mean follow-up of 15 years (nearly 9 years after termination of the treatment), all-cause mortality in the niacin group was 11% lower than in the placebo group, suggesting a late beneficial effect of treatment [41].

Two British trials evaluated the effects of clofibrate in patients with angina and/or previous MI. The first, conducted in the Newcastle upon Tyne region, followed 497 men for 5 years and was associated with a 10% decrease in the serum cholesterol and 22% decrease in triglyceride [39]. The second, a multicenter trial by the Scottish Society of Physicians, followed 717 patients for 6 years and was associated with a 14% decrease in serum cholesterol [40]. In both studies, clofibrate had a beneficial effect in reducing mortality (especially sudden death) and, to a lesser extent, morbidity in patients who presented with angina (with or without previous MI). This effect was independent of initial cholesterol values or the extent of cholesterol reduction. The drug had no significant overall effect on prognosis in patients with MI alone (without angina).

The Stockholm Ischemic Heart Disease Secondary Prevention Study evaluated the effects of combined therapy with niacin and clofibrate in an open, randomized, placebo-controlled trial of 555 male and female survivors of MI [42]. Of these patients 50% had hypertriglyceridemia at baseline, compared to only 13% with hypercholesterolemia. After 5 years of therapy, the treatment group experienced a 13% reduction in cholesterol and a 19% reduction in triglyceride compared to the control group. The CHD mortality was reduced by 36%, and the overall mortality by 26% in the treatment group compared to the control group (Fig. 2.10). This reduction in mortality occurred only in patients with triglyceride levels >1.5 mmol/l (130 mg/dl) and was most pronounced in the group of patients who had a lowering of the serum triglyceride by 30% or more. Since individual lipoproteins were not measured in this study, the relation of CHD to HDL-C changes (which are usually inversely related to triglyceride changes) can only be speculated.

Results of clinical endpoints in the FATS [29] and POSCH [30] studies have already been summarized (see section on angiographic studies).

Meta-analyses of clinical studies

Many of the studies reviewed above found that reducing the serum cholesterol by diet, surgery, and/or drugs reduces the incidence of major coronary events (fatal and nonfatal combined) in men. However, total mortality was usually not decreased. This is generally attributed to several reasons, including the relatively small study population sizes, short follow-up durations, modest cholesterol lowering achieved,

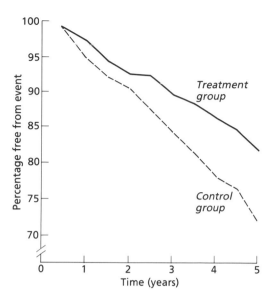

Fig. 2.10 Percentage of patients in the control group and in the treatment group who have not died from ischemic heart disease during the Stockholm Study. All patients who entered into the groups have been considered. (Reproduced from [42].)

and low incidence of cardiovascular events in both the treatment and the control groups. It is important to note that such studies were not designed with the intent to show a decrease in overall mortality, and therefore did not include a sufficiently high statistical power to detect such effect. When the follow-up period was extended beyond the treatment phase in the Coronary Drug Project, a significant decrease in overall mortality was seen in the niacin-treated group compared to the control group [41].

One method of increasing the statistical power is to conduct a quantitative (meta-analytic) evaluation of an aggregate of a number of studies. Such an analysis of six randomized primary prevention trials (nutritional and drug interventions), embracing almost 120 000 person years, was conducted by Muldoon *et al.* [43]. The results of this analysis strengthened the significance of the reduction in CHD mortality, but still did not detect a significant reduction in total mortality. Although the association of increased cancer incidence with lipid lowering, observed in some of the individual studies, was not retained in this meta-analysis, the increased rate of death not related to illness (deaths from accidents, suicide, or violence) was significantly higher in the treatment groups.

A meta-analysis of the results of 22 randomized cholesterol-lowering trials (nine primary prevention and 13 secondary prevention), embracing a total of about 40 000 individuals, was conducted by Yusuf *et al.* [44]. Overall, 8.4% of the subjects in the treatment groups suffered a CHD event compared to 10.7% in the control groups. This represented a

23% risk reduction and was highly significant. The authors note that the risk reduction was directly related to both the degree and the duration of cholesterol lowering; for a standard reduction in cholesterol level of a fixed duration, CHD reduction was similar in drug and dietary intervention trials, in primary and secondary prevention trials, and for fatal and nonfatal events. Mortality from cardiac disease was also significantly reduced; however, overall mortality was not reduced. A more recent meta-analysis of such trials indicates that the efficiency of cholesterol lowering is usually greater in drug trials and in secondary prevention trials, and that a reduction in mortality can be expected only when cholesterol reduction exceeds 8% [45].

Conclusions

The aggregate results of a large number of clinical studies in animals and humans provide convincing evidence that lowering LDL-C levels has a beneficial effect on CHD. This favorable effect has been shown to apply to the rate of progression (and regression) of the anatomic lesion as well as for clinical endpoints in both primary and secondary prevention states. Anatomic regression of lesions has also been demonstrated in femoral arteries [46,47]. In fact, the evidence for treatment benefit in these studies is so strong that a workshop instituted by the American Heart Association in 1989 [48] concluded that "further placebo-controlled intervention trials to test this hypothesis in middle-aged men are not required." Instead, they propose that additional clinical trials are needed to extend the applicability of the LDL hypothesis to other segments of the population, such as people over 60 years of age, women, children, young adults, diabetics, hypertensives, and patients after various cardiac surgical procedures (cardiac transplantation, coronary bypass surgery, and coronary angioplasty). While most studies have excluded women, when women have been included they appear to derive as much benefit from cholesterol lowering as do men [28,30].

Most of the studies have shown that the degree of reduction in atherosclerosis and CHD events is directly related to the degree of reduction of the total and LDL cholesterol, irrespective of the means used to lower these parameters (Fig. 2.11). These studies suggest that for every 1% reduction in LDL-C there is a 2% reduction in CHD events. In fact, it has been argued that the studies underestimate the true effect of cholesterol reduction, due to statistical and methodologic artifacts, and that the true benefit is even higher [45]. The benefit becomes manifest after a latency period of around 2 years, and remains substantial for years after treatment termination. It is conceivable that longer periods of

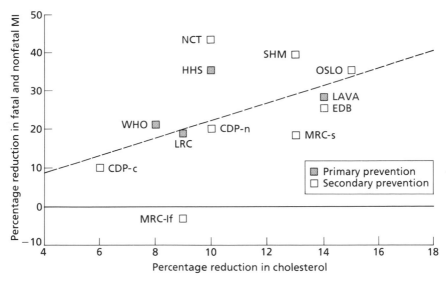

Fig. 2.11 Comparison of the results from 12 randomized cholesterol-lowering trials. Percentage reduction in nonfatal and fatal MI is plotted against the percent reduction in total cholesterol (TC) of treatment group compared with control group. From the regression line, it can be estimated that a reduction in CHD events of approximately 2% can be expected from every 1% reduction in TC, which is similar to the relationship found within the Lipid Research Clinics Coronary Primary Prevention Trial. CDP-c, Coronary Drug Project-clofibrate arm; CDP-n, Coronary Drug Project-niacin arm; EDB, Edinburgh Clofibrate Trial; HHS, Helsinki Heart Study; LAVA, Los Angeles Veterans Administration Trial; LRC, Lipid Research Clinics Coronary Primary Prevention Trial; MRC-lf, Medical Research Council Low-fat Diet Trial; MRC-s, Medical Research Council Soya Oil Diet Trial; NCT, Newcastle Clofibrate Trial, OSLO, Oslo Diet–Heart Study, SHM, Stockholm Study, WHO, World Health Organization Clofibrate Trial.

treatment may further increase the treatment benefit. Concomitant reduction of accompanying risk factors, such as hypertension, smoking, and sedentary lifestyle, may also augment such effects [49]. Small but beneficial changes in risk factors may take many years for complete expression.

As reflected in the FATS [30], clinical benefit from lipoprotein modification can be observed in as short a period as 2 years in patients with established symptomatic CHD. Since this is likely to occur before there is substantial anatomic regression, there may be some merit to cholesterol-lowering regimens that immediately influence clinical disease. Since hypercholesterolemia is associated with abnormalities in the release/response to endothelial-derived relaxing factor (EDRF), and paradoxical coronary vasoconstriction is arrested when hypercholesterolemia is corrected, alteration of the chemical milieu may rapidly improve coronary circulation. Oxidized lipoproteins contribute to this vasoconstrictive response.

The value of modification of other lipoproteins remains controversial. Despite epidemiologic evidence relating HDL-C to protection from CHD, no trial to date has been conducted to directly test the benefit of raising isolated low HDL-C. However, several studies addressed this point indirectly. Two dietary angiographic studies found that changes in the HDL:total cholesterol and HDL:LDL cholesterol ratios predicted lesion growth better than the LDL-C alone [18,24]. The Helsinki Heart Study [36] found that changes in LDL-C and HDL-C levels were independently associated with CHD reduction, and similar effects were observed in the LRC-CPPT and the NHLBI studies [25,35]. Thus, although these studies involved mostly hyperlipidemic men, the value of raising HDL-C in subjects with low HDL-C levels is strongly implicated.

On the other hand, the evidence for a beneficial effect of lowering triglyceride is less clear. Although the Stockholm Study showed that the decreased mortality was strongly related to the reduction in triglyceride [42], other studies did not find such relationships. These results may be partly confounded by the inverse relationship between triglyceride levels and HDL-C levels, as well as by the great intraindividual and laboratory variability in triglyceride measurements [50]. Since epidemiologic studies suggest that elevated triglycerides may be more atherogenic in women than in men, the fact that most of the intervention studies included male subjects only may also contribute to these results.

Finally, one cannot ignore the controversial issue relating to the fact that, with the exception of two studies (the Coronary Drug Project 15-year follow-up study [39] and the Stockholm Study [42]), the overall mortality was not significantly reduced despite a reduction in cardiovascular mortality. The increase in noncardiovascular mortality in the treatment groups followed no consistent pattern (cancer in some studies, violence and suicide in others) and was unrelated to the degree or duration of cholesterol lowering. Furthermore, individual examinations of the homicides, suicides, and accidental deaths in the active treatment arms of the Helsinki Heart Study and the LRC-CPPT found no evidence to support the causal association between the use of lipid-lowering drugs and these deaths [51]. However, insufficient data exist on the effect of cholesterol lowering on behavior patterns and psychologic status, and future studies will have to assess these issues.

In summary, the clinical studies performed to date provide unequivocal evidence that modification of the serum lipoproteins substantially protects against CHD. These exciting findings have already been translated into practical guidelines for management of dyslipidemia

Table 2.5 Treatment of dyslipidemia and CHD: issues to be resolved

Do women respond as well to lipid-modifying therapy as men?

Do blacks and other minority groups respond as well to lipid-modifying therapy as whites?

Do the elderly derive benefit from lipid modification?

Is correction of isolated low HDL-C beneficial?

Does correction of hypertriglyceridemia, alone or in combination with low HDL-C, protect against CHD?

Does reduction of elevated levels of lipoprotein(a) influence atherosclerosis?

Does treatment of lipid disturbances in patients with diabetes mellitus, chronic renal failure, or the nephrotic syndrome influence the natural history of CHD?

Does treatment of lipid disturbances in patients that have undergone coronary bypass grafting, angioplasty, or cardiac transplantation reduce the frequency of stenosis/restenosis?

Do individuals with existing CHD and "normal" lipoprotein levels derive benefit from further modification of their lipoproteins?

How long should treatment for lipid disorders be instituted, and what are the optimal goals of therapy for different clinical conditions?

How early should treatment be initiated in order to be protective in asymptomatic but high-risk individuals?

in several countries. However, many debatable issues concerning the treatment of dyslipidemia still exist (Table 2.5), and further studies are needed to resolve them. It is conceivable that many of these dilemmas will be resolved within the next decade or two, and that the medical treatment of atherosclerosis will have a notable effect on the quality and length of life.

References

1 Rossouw JE, Rifkind BM. Does lowering serum cholesterol levels lower coronary heart disease risk? *Endocrinol Metab Clin North Am* 1990;19:279–97.
2 Munro JM, Cotran RS. Biology of disease. The pathogenesis of atherosclerosis: atherogenesis and inflammation. *Lab Invest* 1988;58:249–61.
3 St Clair RW. Atherosclerosis regression in animal models: Current concepts of cellular and biochemical mechanisms. *Prog Cardiovasc Dis* 1983;26:109–32.
4 Blankenhorn BH, Kramsch DM. Reversal of atherosis and sclerosis. The two components of atherosclerosis. *Circulation* 1989;79:1–6.
5 Wissler RW. Evidence for regression of advanced atherosclerotic plaques. *Artery* 1979;5:398–408.
6 Clarkson TB, Bond MG, Bullock BC, McLaughlin KJ, Sawyer JK. A study of atherosclerosis regression in *Macaca mulatta*. V. Changes in abdominal aorta and carotid and coronary arteries from animals with atherosclerosis induced for 38 months and

then regressed for 24 or 48 months at plasma cholesterol concentrations of 300 or 200 mg/dl. *Exp Mol Pathol* 1984;41:96−118.

7 Hollander W, Kirkpatrick B, Paddock JL *et al.* Studies on the progression and regression of coronary and peripheral atherosclerosis in the cynomolgous monkey. I. Effects of dipyridamole and aspirin. *Exp Mol Pathol* 1979;30:55−73.

8 Waters DD, Lespèrance J. Regression of coronary athero-sclerosis. Angiographic perspective. *Drugs* 1988;36:37−42.

9 Malinow MR. Atherosclerosis: progression, regression and resolution. *Am Heart J* 1984;108:1523−37.

10 Detre KM, Kelsey SF, Passamani ER *et al.* Reliability of assessing change with sequential coronary arteriography. *Am Heart J* 1982;104:816−23.

11 Reiber JHC, Serruys PW, Kooijman CJ *et al.* Assessment of short-, medium- and long-term variations in arterial dimensions from computer-assisted quantitation of coronary cineangiograms. *Circulation* 1985;71:280−8.

12 Superko RH, Wood PD, Haskell WL. Coronary heart disease and risk factor modification: is there a threshold? *Am J Med* 1985;78:826−38.

13 Knight L, Scheibel R, Amplatz K, Varco R, Buchwald H. Radiographic appraisal of the Minnesota partial ileal bypass study. *Surg Forum* 1972;23:141−2.

14 Buchwald H, Moore RB, Varco RL. Clinical status of the partial ileal bypass operation. *Circulation* 1972;49(Suppl 1):I22−I37.

15 Buchwald H, Moore RB, Rucker RD *et al.* Clinical angiographic regression of atherosclerosis after partial ileal bypass. *Atherosclerosis* 1983;46:117−28.

16 Starzl TE, Chase PH, Putnam CW, Nora JJ. Follow-up of patient with portacaval shunt for the treatment of hyperlipidemia. *Lancet* 1974;ii:714−15.

17 Thompson GR, Myant MB. Regression of atherosclerosis. *Atherosclerosis* 1980;35:347−8.

18 Arntzenius AC, Kromhout D, Barth JD *et al.* Diet lipoproteins and the progression of coronary atherosclerosis: The Leiden Intervention Trial. *N Engl J Med* 1985;312:805−11.

19 Ost CR, Stenson S. Regression of peripheral atherosclerosis during therapy with high doses of nicotinic acid. *Scand J Clin Lab Invest* 1967;19(Suppl 93):241−5.

20 Basta LL, Williams C, Kioschos J, Spector AA. Regression of atherosclerosis stenosing lesions of the renal arteries and spontaneous cure of systemic hypertension through control of hyperlipidemia. *Am J Med* 1976;61:420−3.

21 Brandt R, Blankenhorn DH, Crawford DW, Brooks SH. Regression and progression of early femoral atherosclerosis in treated hyperlipoproteinemic patients. *Ann Intern Med* 1977;86:139−46.

22 Nikkila EA, Viikinkoski P, Valle M. Effect of lipid lowering treatment on progression of coronary atherosclerosis assessed by angiography (abstract). *Circulation* 1978;57(Suppl II):II50.

23 Kuo PT, Hayase K, Kostis JB, Moreyra AB. Use of combined diet and colestipol in long-term treatment of patients with type II hyperlipoproteinemia. *Circulation* 1979;59:199−211.

24 Nikkila EA, Viikinkoski P, Valle M *et al.* Prevention of progression of coronary atherosclerosis by treatment of hyperlipidemia: a seven year prospective angiographic study. *Br Med J* 1984;289:220−3.

25 Brensike JF, Levy RI, Kelsby SF *et al.* Effects of therapy with cholestyramine on progression of arteriosclerosis. Results of the NHLBI Type II Coronary Intervention Study. *Circulation* 1984;69:313.

26 Blakenhorn DH, Nessim SA, Johnson RL *et al.* Beneficial effects of combined colestipol−niacin therapy on coronary atherosclerosis and coronary venous bypass grafts. *JAMA* 1987;257:3233−40.

27 Cashin-Hemphill L, Mack WJ, Pogoda JM *et al.* Beneficial effects of colestipol−niacin on coronary atherosclerosis. A 4-year follow-up. *JAMA* 1990;264:3013−17.

28 Kane JP, Malloy MJ, Ports TA. Regression of coronary atherosclerosis during treatment of familial hypercholesterolemia with combined drug regimens. *JAMA* 1990;264:3007–12.

29 Brown G, Albers JJ, Fisher LD *et al*. Regression of coronary artery disease as a result of intensive lipid-lowering therapy in men with high levels of apolipoprotein B. *N Engl J Med* 1990;323:1289–98.

30 Buchwald H, Varco RL, Matts JP *et al*. Effect of partial ileal bypass surgery on mortality and morbidity from coronary heart disease in patients with hypercholesterolemia. Report of the Program on the Surgical Control of the Hyperlipidemias (POSCH). *N Engl J Med* 1990;323:946–55.

31 Dayton S, Pearce MI, Hashimoto S *et al*. A controlled clinical trial of a diet high in unsaturated fat in preventing complications of atherosclerosis. *Circulation* 1969;40(Suppl 2):1–63.

32 Miettinen M, Turpeinen O, Karvonen MJ, Elosuo R, Paavilainen E. Effect of cholesterol-lowering diet on mortality from coronary heart disease and other causes: a twelve-year clinical trial in men and women. *Lancet* 1972;ii:835–8.

33 Frantz ID, Dawson EA, Ashman PL *et al*. Test effect of lipid lowering by diet on cardiovascular risk. The Minnesota Coronary Survey. *Arteriosclerosis* 1989;9:129–35.

34 Committee of Principle Investigators, WHO Clofibrate Trial. A cooperate trial in the primary prevention of ischemic heart disease using clofibrate. *Br Heart J* 1978;40:1069–118.

35 The Lipid Research Clinics Coronary Primary Prevention Trial results. I. Reduction in incidence of coronary heart disease. *JAMA* 1984;251:351–62.

36 Frick MH, Elo O, Happa K *et al*. Helsinki heart study: primary-prevention trial with gemfibrozil in middle-aged men with dyslipidemia, safety of treatment, changes in risk factors and incidence of heart disease. *N Engl J Med* 1987;317:1237–45.

37 Rossouw JE, Lewis B, Rifkind BM. The value of lowering cholesterol after myocardial infarction. *N Engl J Med* 1990;323:1112–19.

38 Coronary Drug Project Research Group: Clofibrate and niacin in coronary heart disease. *JAMA* 1975;231:360–80.

39 Canner Pl, Berge KG, Wegner K *et al*. Fifteen year mortality in the Coronary Drug Project; Long-term benefit with niacin. *J Am Coll Cardiol* 1986;8:1245–55.

40 Group of physicians of the Newcastle upon Tyne Region. Trial of clofibrate in the treatment of ischemic heart disease . *Br Med J* 1971;4:767–75.

41 Research Committee of the Scottish Society of Physicians. Ischemic heart disease: a secondary prevention trial using clofibrate. *Br Med J* 1971;4:775–84.

42 Carlson LA, Rosenhamer G. Reduction of mortality in the Stockholm Ischemic Heart Disease Secondary Prevention Study by combined treatment with clofibrate and nicotinic acid. *Acta Med Scand* 1988;223:405–18.

43 Muldoon M, Manuck SB, Matthews KA. Lowering cholesterol concentrations and mortality: a quantitative review of primary prevention trials. *Br Med J* 1990;301:309–14.

44 Yusuf S, Wittes J, Friedman L. Overview of results of randomized clinical trials in heart disease. II. Unstable angina, heart failure, primary prevention with aspirin and risk factor modification. *JAMA* 1989;260:2259–63.

45 Holme I. An analysis of randomized trials evaluating the effect of cholesterol reduction on total mortality and coronary heart disease incidence. *Circulation* 1990;82:1916–24.

46 Duffield RGM, Miller NE, Brunt JNH *et al*. Treatment of hyperlipidemia retards progression of symptomatic femoral atherosclerosis. A randomized controlled trial. *Lancet* 1983;ii:639–42.

47 Blankenhorn DH, Azen SP, Crawford DW *et al*. Effects of colestipol–niacin therapy on human femoral atherosclerosis. *Circulation* 1991;83:438–47.

48 Levi RI, Blankenhorn DH, Davis E *et al*. Workshop V: Intervention studies. *Circulation* 1989;80:739–43.

49 Kannel WB, for the MRFIT Research Group. Overall and coronary heart disease mortality rates in relation to major risk factors in 325 348 men screened for the MRFIT. *Am Heart J* 1986;112:825–36.

50 Austin MA. Plasma triglyceride and coronary heart disease. *Arterioscler Thromb* 1991; 11:2–14.

51 Wysowski DK, Gross TP. Deaths due to accidents and violence in two recent trials of cholesterol-lowering drugs. *Arch Intern Med* 1990;150:2169–72.

52 Oberman A, Kreisberg RA, Henkin Y. *The Principles and Management of Lipid Disorders: A Primary Care Approach.* Baltimore: Williams & Wilkins.

53 Coronary Heart Disease Seminar Series: Lipid regulation and risk prevention. Parke-Davis, Division of Warner-Lambert Co., 1991.

Section II
Current Concepts of the Atherogenicity of Lipoproteins

Chapter 3 ⸺⸺⸺⸺⸺⸺⸺⸺⸺⸺
Structure and Metabolism of the Plasma Lipoproteins

DONALD M. SMALL

Introduction

The purpose of this chapter is to review briefly the general structure and metabolism of the plasma lipoproteins. Subsequent chapters will deal more specifically with certain classes of lipoproteins such as low-density lipoproteins (LDL), triglyceride-rich lipoproteins, and high-density lipoproteins (HDL), their structure, heterogeneity, and metabolism. A number of previous reviews have appeared on the structure of lipoproteins [1–5] and many on their metabolism (e.g., [5–13]). The present review will summarize the general field and concentrate on some recent advances. The reader is referred to the reviews mentioned above for further details and for older but important work.

In the field of lipoprotein structure the past few years have seen major advances in two specific areas. First, the determination of the primary structure of apolipoprotein B (apo B) in 1986 by several separate laboratories [14–18] marked a fundamental breakthrough in the understanding of apo B-containing lipoproteins and the functions of apo B. However, the enormity of the primary structure alone created a whole new galaxy of questions relating to its secondary and tertiary structure, its accommodation with lipids, its conformational flexibility, the relation of structure to function (e.g., the structure of its liganding and heparin-binding sites), and so on. While much speculation exists concerning putative structures of apo B and its fragments, there is not yet much hard data to discuss in terms of specific structures of apo B on LDL or on triglyceride-rich lipoproteins. Nevertheless, there are some recent works linking the primary structure to properties of different parts of apo B and their changes with lipid structure.

The second breakthrough deals with exchangeable, HDL-like apoproteins. In 1991 the first crystallographic three-dimensional structures of apolipoproteins were reported: apolipophorin III from the locust [19] and the 22-kDa fragment of human apo E-III containing the liganding site for the LDL receptor [20]. Both structures have many of the characteristics which had been predicted for exchangeable apolipoproteins using indirect methods and modeling. Both contain large amounts of amphipathic α-helix packed in bundles with the hydrophobic part of the helix towards the center of the protein monomer. However some surprises were found in the structure as will be discussed later (see pp. 62–68).

Table 3.1 The apoproteins*

Protein	Number of amino acids	Molecular weight	Anhydrous molecular volume (Å^3) ($\bar{V} = 0.73\,\text{cm}^3/\text{g}$)	Approximate hydrophobic surface area (Å^2)[†]	Function/cofactor[‡]
Nonexchangeable					
B$_{100}$	4536	513 000	617 193	61 719	Ligand for LDL receptor (Mediates VLDL assembly and exocytosis from hepatocyte)
B$_{48}$	2152	246 000	295 964	29 596	(Mediates chylomicron assembly and exocytosis from enterocytes)
Exchangeable—soluble					
A-I	243	28 100	33 808	3 381	Specific LCAT activator
A-II	77	17 400[§]	20 934[§]	2 093[§]	
A-IV	391	42 500	51 132	5 113	Nonspecific LCAT activator
C-I	57	6 605	7 946	795	Inhibits chylomicron uptake (also C-II and C-III)
C-II	79	8 824	10 616	1 062	LPL activator
C-III	79	8 750	10 527	1 053	(Inhibits LPL)
D	—	~20 000	24 061	2 406	(Involved CE transfer)
E	299	34 200	41 145	4 115	Ligand for LDL receptor and chylomicron receptor on hepatocytes

* Revised from [2]. Data for B$_{100}$ and B$_{48}$ are taken from [14–18].
† Assuming an average anhydrous protein thickness of about 10 Å.
‡ Tentative functions are indicated in parentheses.
§ Calculated as a disulfide-linked dimer of two 77 amino acid monomers.

Progress in the area of metabolism has been directed more towards the complexity of lipoprotein metabolism and in particular the compositional complexity of lipoprotein species within a given class and their differing metabolism.

Lipoprotein structure: general considerations

All lipoproteins are macromolecular assemblies of specific apoproteins (see Table 3.1) and lipids held together by noncovalent forces [1,2]. Two general structural categories (Fig. 3.1) may be described: (i) lipoproteins that are emulsion or microemulsion particles containing a core of relatively nonpolar lipid surrounded by a surface of polar lipids and apoproteins; and (ii) lipoproteins which do not contain a nonpolar core but are made up of polar lipids generally in a bilayered conformation. Discoidal lipoproteins and closed vesicles make up the bilayered category. Chylomicrons, large very low-density lipoproteins (VLDL) and some of their remnants (i.e., particles greater than 50.0 nm diameter) belong to the class of emulsions, whereas particles less than 50.0 nm (small VLDL, intermediate-density lipoproteins (IDL), LDL, and the quasispherical HDL particles like HDL_2 and HDL_3) are microemulsions. All have cores of triglyceride and/or cholesterol esters and a surface stabilized by different apoproteins and phospholipids. Some of the particles in the complex class of lipoproteins called the "HDL system" are discoidal and do not have core lipids. Further, some very small $IIDL_3$-like particles may also be largely devoid of core lipids, but their precise structure is not known. They may be very small disks or globules. These will be discussed later in the metabolism section (see pp. 77–84). During the hydrolysis of chylomicrons and VLDL, some surface remnants are also formed [21–24] which consist of vesicles of phospholipid and adsorbed exchangeable apolipoproteins. These appear to enter the HDL system and act as a source of phospholipid for that system [21–23]. Chylomicrons are the largest of the triglyceride-rich emulsion particles and are formed in the intestine during the absorption of fat. The core contains mainly triacylglycerols, a very small amount of cholesterol ester, and a few of other nonpolar molecules [1,25]. The surface contains apo B_{48} and apo As, principally apo A-I and apo A-IV. The great majority of the surface, perhaps for 80–85%, is made up of phospholipid of which most is phosphatidylcholine [26]. The surface and cores of the chylomicron contain very little free cholesterol [1,25].

VLDL is a term used here to describe nascent particles secreted by the liver, the original definition being based on the flotation characteristics. However, particles floating in VLDL density range can also come from

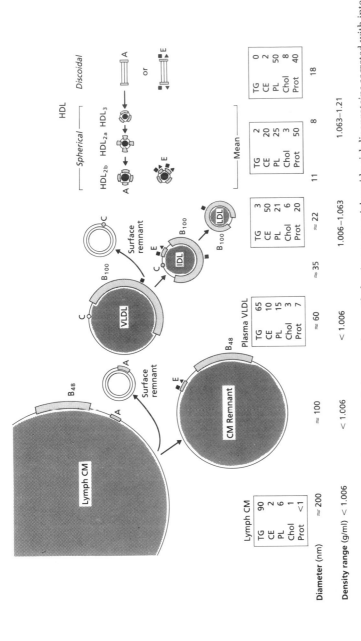

| Diameter (nm) | ≈ 200 | ≈ 100 | ≈ 60 | ≈ 35 | ≈ 22 | 11 | 8 | 18 |
| Density range (g/ml) | < 1.006 | < 1.006 | < 1.006 | 1.006–1.063 | 1.006–1.063 | | 1.063–1.21 | |

Lymph CM

TG	90
CE	2
PL	6
Chol	1
Prot	<1

Plasma VLDL

TG	65
CE	10
PL	15
Chol	3
Prot	7

TG	3
CE	50
PL	21
Chol	6
Prot	20

TG	2
CE	20
PL	25
Chol	3
Prot	50

TG	0
CE	2
PL	50
Chol	8
Prot	40

Fig. 3.1 Structure and composition of the major lipoproteins in human plasma. Chylomicrons are triglyceride-rich lipoproteins secreted with intestinal apo B (B$_{48}$) and apo A (A). In plasma they are catabolized by lipoprotein lipase to a B$_{48}$ core remnant and surface remnants that contain phospholipids, cholesterol, and some of the soluble apoproteins (A, etc.). VLDLs are also triglyceride-rich particles secreted from the liver with apo B$_{100}$ and other soluble apoproteins. In plasma they are converted to VLDL remnants, IDL, and finally to LDL, a cholesterol ester-rich microemulsion-sized particle that contains almost exclusively apo B$_{100}$. HDL is a heterogeneous group of both spherical and discoidal particles. Exchangeable apolipoprotein classes (A, E, and C) are present in HDL. The mean composition of spherical HDL shows that it is cholesterol ester, phospholipid-rich microemulsion with about 50% by weight apoprotein. Discoidal HDLs are 15.0–18.0 nm in diameter and are one bilayer thick (~5.0 nm) and contain almost no core lipids (TG and CE). The mean estimates of diameter and density range are given below the particles.

The small black square on apo B$_{100}$ and on apo E is the liganding region for the LDL receptor and the black triangle on apo E represents the chylomicron receptor ligand. For further discussion see text. (Modified from [2].)

the intestine. Nascent VLDL secreted from the liver contain apo B_{100} and probably some of the smaller apoproteins (apo C, apo E, apo A-I). The core consists mainly of triacylglycerols but depending upon input of cholesterol to the liver varying amounts of cholesterol ester may also be present. The surface is made up largely of phosphatidylcholine, small amounts of cholesterol, apo B_{100}, and some smaller exchangeable apolipoproteins. Up to 70% of the surface is made up of lipids and the rest of apoproteins. Both apo B_{100} and apo B_{48} are nonexchangeable apolipoproteins and remain with the core particle from secretion to cellular uptake and catabolism. On the other hand, all of the rest of the apolipoproteins are more or less exchangeable between different fractions and subfractions of lipoproteins.

The HDL system is a complex group of globular and discoidal particles generally having a density between 1.063 and 1.21 g/ml. The apoproteins are all of the exchangeable type (A,C,D,E) and the major lipids are phospholipids, cholesterol esters, cholesterol, and triacylglycerols, respectively. The major HDLs in human plasma are HDL_3 and HDL_2. The primary structure of all of the major apolipoproteins has been determined and their putative structures estimated [3,4]. Table 3.1 gives the number of amino acids, molecular weight and volume, the estimated hydrophobic surface area, and the known functions.

HDL and the exchangeable apolipoproteins

As first proposed by Segrest et al. [27] the exchangeable apolipoproteins contain amphipathic α-helices in 22-residue repeats. When the amino acid sequence is wound up in a helical wheel [28] it becomes quite clear that one side of the α-helix is hydrophobic and the other hydrophilic. This structure suggested to this author many years ago that amphipathic helices in apoproteins might act like a string of connected planar detergent molecules, for instance, like a necklace of bile salts, which could act to form discoidal aggregates with phospholipids and cholesterol [29]. In the last 10 years many reviews and theoretical discussions of the amphipathic helix and the potential structures of apolipoproteins have been put forward (for instance [3,4,30−33]). The two recent crystalline structures unambiguously prove the presence of amphipathic helices in apolipophorin III (apoLP-III, [19]) and in the 22-kDa fragment of apo E [20].

Segrest et al. have classified the amphipathic helices into at least seven different categories [3,4]. The category most typical of apolipoproteins is called class A. These amphipathic helices have roughly equal polar and nonpolar interfaces. The polar face has negatively charged

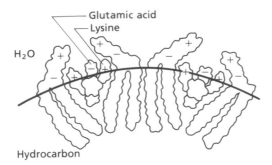

H₂O ... Glutamic acid / Lysine ... Hydrocarbon

Fig. 3.2 Schematic diagram of a snorkel model of amphipathic helices of class A motif, as described by Segrest *et al.* [4], showing postulated insertion into phospholipid monolayer of an HDL particle. The long axis of the amphipathic helix runs in the plane of the surface of the HDL particle. The dimensions are approximately to scale. Note the snorkeling of the lysine residues and the negatively charged residue in the center of the polar face. These helices form a wedge-shaped structure which would aid in maintaining the sharp curvature of the HDL surface. (We thank Dr Segrest for permitting us to redraw his figure [4] so that it conforms to a curved surface.)

amino acids in the middle, for instance glutamic acid, and two positively charged amino acids at the interface between polar and hydrophobic faces. The latter are usually lysines which protrude from the helix with a short hydrophobic neck ending in a positive charge ($-CH_2-CH_2-CH_2-CH_2-NH_3^+$). These have been called snorkels, as the hydrophobic bottom can interact with the hydrophobic surface of the lipid and a charged top can interact with the water interface. While class A amphipathic helices can stabilize phospholipid disks, they also fit particularly well into a sharply curved surface as would occur on HDL_3, as shown in Fig. 3.2. Many of the apolipoproteins contain other types of amphipathic helices, and in fact the helices described in the two crystalline structures [19,20] are not typical class A amphipathic helices. Some of these helices do not interact well with lipoprotein surfaces but many interact with phospholipids; this may be because they lack the class A motif [4].

APOLP-III

The first crystalline structure described, interestingly, was not of a human apolipoprotein but one from a rather unlikely source, the migratory locust. The authors of this report [19] stated that, "The major function of apoLP-III is to assist in the delivery of lipid from the fat body to flight muscles during prolonged flight." ApoLP-III can exist as a free monomer in hemolymph and then bind to large lipoprotein particles as

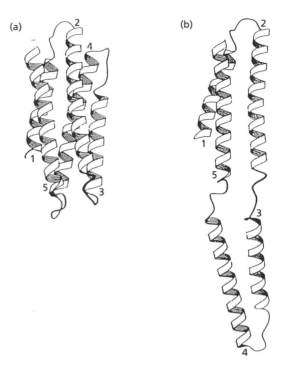

Fig. 3.3 Ribbon drawings of the apoLP-III structure in folded and unfolded form. (a) A ribbon drawing representing the apoLP-III structure as seen in the crystalline state. Each helix is labeled by number starting with 1 at the NH₂ terminal to 5 at the COOH terminal. (b) A ribbon drawing of the putative unfolded form of the apoLP-III structure as it binds to the lipophorin particle. Again, each helix is labeled as described. (Reproduced with permission from [19].)

they leave the fat body. Since it could be found as a free monomer in hemolymph the authors thought it was a good candidate for crystallization [19]. Further, the amino acid sequence of this apolipoprotein showed many similarities to the sequences of human exchangeable apolipoproteins and the regions of potential amphipathic helix were identified [34]. The protein crystals were grown without detergent [35], isomorphous heavy metals substituted using standard soaking techniques, and the crystalline structure solved and refined to 0.25 nm [19]. A ribbon structure is shown in Fig. 3.3a. Although the molecule consists of 161 amino acids the first six N terminal and the last five C-terminal amino acids were disordered and could not be identified. The approximate overall length of the crystal is 5.3 nm and the width is about 2.2 nm. The structure has five α-helices connected by loops of varying lengths. The five α-helices (1, residues 7−32; 2, residues 35−66; 3, residues 70−86; 4, residues 95−121; 5, residues 129−156) all have amphipathic characteristics. They form a tight up and down helical bundle [36] with the hydrophobic faces pointing towards the interior and the hydrophilic faces pointing towards the exterior. Four observable prolines either terminate helices (residues 35, 95, 129) or are present in turns (residue 33). Two however, at positions 118 and 120, are part of an amphipathic helix. Since all but three hydrophobic residues are in the central hydrophobic area in the crystal and involved in hydrophobic interactions with each other it is unlikely that this apoLP-III would associate with lipid in its crystalline conformation. It was suggested that the three hydrophobic amino acids which point toward the outside or solvent side (residues 20, 30, 122) may be important in initiating binding to the lipophorin lipid particle [19]. It had been noted previously [37,38] that apoLP-III unfolds at an air–water interface to cover much more area than the crystal could. With the crystalline conformation the area occupied at an interface would be about $1200 \, \text{Å}^2$, whereas the area estimated at an air–water interface was about $3400 \, \text{Å}^2$ [37,38]. It was therefore argued that the molecule must undergo a marked conformational change and suggested (Fig. 3.3b) that the regions between helix 2 and 3 and between 4 and 5 undergo a conformational change to expose an elongated molecule in which the hydrophobic parts would be on one face and the hydrophilic on the other face. Our early studies [29,37–41] on the conformational flexibility of apo A-I in the presence [37,39–41] and absence [37,38] of lipid indicated that such changes were possible and indeed to be predicted on an energetic basis. Therefore this crystalline structure clearly demonstrated the existence of α-helices in the crystal in which the hydrophobic regions associate to form relatively globular protein. The physical–chemical evidence suggests that, in the presence of lipid, hinge areas exist within the turns of the apolipoprotein which allow it to open up, expose its hydrophobic faces to lipid and thus bind. It is gratifying to all of us who have attempted to understand apolipoprotein and lipoprotein structure in the absence of crystallographic structures that many of the predictions made have been borne out by this structure.

THE 22-kDa FRAGMENT OF APO E-III

Investigators have been attempting, without success, to crystallize human apolipoproteins for the past 20 years. However, the fact that human apolipoproteins tend to aggregate in solution in the absence of lipids, are often heterogeneous, and are usually glycosylated with complex carbohydrate chains has frustrated attempts to crystallize them. In 1988, Wetterau and Aggerbeck and their colleagues at the Gladstone Foundation [42,43] found that apo E, a 299-residue protein (with a relative molecular weight of 34 200) appeared to be made up of two independently folded domains. A 22-kDa domain behaved like a globular protein, had a high free energy of stabilization, and did not aggregate, while the other part ($\sim$12 kDa) behaved like apo A-I and

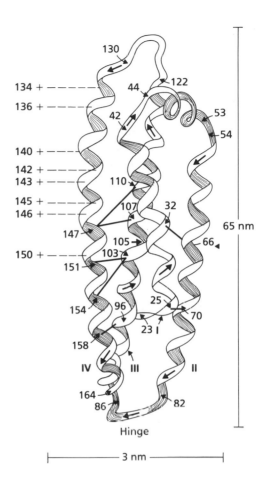

Fig. 3.4 Ribbon diagram of the NH₂ terminal 22-kDa fragment of apo E-III. The positions of key residues are indicated. The helices are numbered I–IV. The positions of the interhelix salt bridges between antiparallel helices I and II and between III and IV are indicated by the solid lines. The liganding region involves the positively charged region between residue 134 and 150 on helix IV. (Redrawn with permission from [20].)

other small apoproteins. It aggregated, bound lipid avidly, and had a low free energy of stabilization. The N-terminal 22-kDa fragment (residues 1–191) also contained the ligand-binding site for the LDL receptor and the putative chylomicron receptor. Because of its physical properties it became a good prospect for crystallization. Crystallization was induced by raising the pH from 4.5 to 5.3 in a solution containing 15% polyethylene glycol (PEG), 0.2% β-n-octylglucopyranoside, acetate buffer, and 0.1% mercaptoethanol. The structure determined to 0.25 nm [20] shows a four-helix bundle (Fig. 3.4) rather similar to the five-helix bundle shown for apoLP-III (Fig. 3.3). The key amino acids are shown as well as the liganding region from arginine 134 to arginine 150. The first 22 and the last 27 amino acids are not seen. An interesting surprise is the particularly long helical bundle. Helix III and helix IV are 36 and 35 amino acids long, respectively. As in the apoLP-III structure, subsequent helices are antiparallel and are connected by short loops except helices I and II which are connected by a short α-helix (residues 44–53). While much of the previous speculations concerning amphipathic helix structure focused on the 11/22 amino acid repeats, and indicated in general that turns or loops separated the 22 amino acid repeats, this structure shows that two 22 amino acid repeats are linked together in both helix III and helix IV to form two very long (~6.0 nm) helices. There appear to be two rather striking helical interactions which were not noted in apoLP-III. The first involves interhelical salt bridges between helices I and II (two salt bridges) and between helices III and IV (five salt bridges). These salt bridges stabilize the I and II helices and the III and IV helices into two domains each consisting of two helices with a hydrophobic side of both pointing in the same direction. Helices I and II abut helices III and IV in the crystal so that most of the hydrophobic amino acids are in the interior of the crystal. Second, a hydrophobic packing motif was noted between helices I and IV, and between helices II and III. This motif is a leucine zipper type of interaction which stabilizes the hydrophobic interactions between these apposed helices. It is conceivable that the leucine zipper simply forms because of the availability of leucines, but it might have some significance in the conformation of the liganding region. It should be noted that the entire hydrophobic side of the liganding region on helix IV is involved in the leucine zipper interaction between helix IV and helix I. In the liganding region on helix IV there are nine basic residues which produces "a large region of positive electrostatic potential extending 1.5 nm out of the protein" [20]. Even though the liganding area has a very large positive potential and protrudes into the solvent, the free 22-kDa fragment does not bind particularly strongly to the LDL receptor. The 22-kDa fragment binds poorly to plasma lipoproteins but binds quite well to dimyristoyl phosphatidylcholine (DMPC) to form discoidal aggregates [44]. The affinity for the LDL receptor of the 22-kDa fragment on the discoidal DMPC aggregates appears to be 500× greater than the free protein [20]. This clearly suggests a major conformational change in the liganding region upon binding to lipid.

In the crystalline structure the hydrophobic region is mostly hidden from access to the aqueous phase. Thus, on lipid binding major changes must occur. The internal hydrophobic interactions must be replaced with interaction of the hydrophobic side of the amphipathic helices with lipid. This could be easily accomplished by considering residues 82–86 as a hinge. This region was not well differentiated in the structure [20] suggesting that it is conformationally labile. Opening the structure to produce one analogous to that suggested for apoLP-III (see Fig. 3.3b)

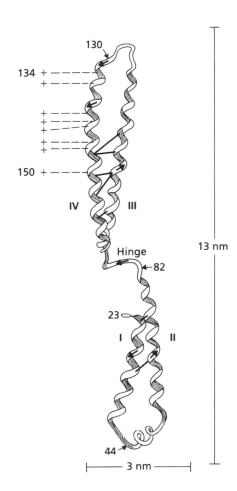

Fig. 3.5 Possible structure of 22-kDa fragment of apo E-III on a phospholipid disk. The putative hinge region between residues 82 and 86 could allow the molecule to open into an elongated structure with all the hydrophobic residues on one face and the hydrophilic residues on the opposite face. Such a structure could wrap around the perimeter of a disk of DMPC to cover the hydrocarbon acyl chains. The estimated hydrophobic surface area would be about 31 nm² (3100 Å²) (see text).

would be particularly effective if the salt bonds connecting helices I and II, and III and IV were maintained. Considering that most of the hydrophobic amino acids are hidden in the crystal it is unlikely that it would bind to lipid without conformational change. If the structure were opened up (as shown in Fig. 3.5) then all of the hydrophobic faces would face the same surface. Assuming that the total structure is about 13.0 nm (130 Å) long and each helix is about 1.2 nm (12 Å) wide, then the total hydrophobic surface is $2 \times 12 \times 130 = 3100$ Å². Side-by-side helices (e.g., I and II or III and IV) would be about 24 Å wide, which is just about the width of the hydrophobic part of a DMPC bilayer [45,46]. Thus, the helices could wrap around the surface of the bilayer with the axis of the helix parallel to the plane of the bilayer and perpendicular to the phospholipid chains and easily form discoidal aggregates. The side-by-side helix pair might not easily bind to a small, globular-shaped lipoprotein (see Fig. 3.2) since single helices are required. This discoidal protein orientation is not the same as that predicted for apo A-I phosphatidylcholine interaction [47,48]. Using polarized Fourier transform infrared spectroscopy this group has suggested that the axes of the amphipathic helices lie parallel to the phospholipid chains and not perpendicular. To realize an apo A-I-like structure with the 22-kDa fragment of apo E one would have to break the salt bonds and create turns in midhelical regions within helices II, III, and IV.

Another possible structure involving the hinge at 82–86 would be simply to open the structure like two pages in a book so that four helices all lay side by side with the hydrophobic faces all facing the same surface. Four helices would have a width of about 4.8 nm (48 Å), which is more than necessary to cover the hydrophobic surface of the discoidal lipoprotein.

Apo B-containing lipoproteins

A major breakthrough in understanding apo B-containing lipoproteins came with the determination of the primary amino acid sequence of apo B by several groups in 1986 [14–18]. These studies showed that apo B was a peptide chain made up of 4563 amino acids with a predicted molecular mass of about 512 kDa. The protein has 19 potential glycosylation sites of which 16 are glycosylated, and 25 cysteines of which most are linked in disulfide bonds [49,50]. Computer estimates of secondary structure showed fairly large amounts of β-sheet and α-helix [17] consistent with studies of secondary structure of apo B [51–53]. It is hard to comprehend what the atomic structure of such a large protein might be. Certainly crystallization of apo B and the determination of its three-dimensional structure presents a formidable challenge. From spectroscopy, primarily circular dichroism and ultraviolet, we know that there are considerable amounts of β-sheet and α-helix in the structure of apo B on LDL [52]. Apo B inserted into vesicles [51], solubilized in bile salt [51,52], and bound to microemulsion particles [53] also contains considerable secondary structure but somewhat different from that of apo B on LDL. Attempts have been made to determine the physical domains in apo B, by microcalorimetry [52], electron microscopic studies [54–57], immunoelectron microscopic studies [58], and limited proteolysis. Local conformational changes have been monitored by chemical studies using enzymes to clip apo B at susceptible positions [15,49,50,59–65], by monoclonal antibody binding [65–68], and by molecular biologic techniques [69,70].

Using low precision calorimetry it was shown more than 16 years ago that LDL underwent at least two thermal transitions on heating [71]. The first was the order−disorder transition of the cholesterol esters in the core of the particle and the second at higher temperatures was a complex transition involving protein denaturation and particle disruption [71,72]. More recently, utilizing highly sensitive microcalorimetry, it has been shown that the protein transition in LDL consists of at least two separate transitions [52]. The first, occurring between about 45 and 57°C, is a reversible, low enthalpy transition involving the reorganization of apo B on LDL. In this transition range no changes in secondary structure occur indicating that this is a cooperative reversible conformational change in tertiary structure [52]. The second transition is similar to those described previously [71,72] and involves the unfolding denaturation and disruption of apo B on LDL between 65 and 80°C.

The behavior of apo B solubilized in the bile salt, sodium deoxycholate, however, is more informative. Using deconvolution procedures, five separate reversible transitions occur with peak temperatures between 45 and 55°C. In addition a higher temperature denaturation transition occurs at about 65°C. The five separate reversible transitions have roughly similar enthalpy. The lowest transition, at 45°C, accounts for about 28% of the total enthalpy while the other four transitions account for about 16−20% each of the total enthalpy. Changes in secondary structure occur during these transitions. These studies indicate that the apo B, solubilized in sodium deoxycholate, has five domains undergoing independent thermal transitions. One can speculate that one domain has almost 30% of the protein mass while the other domains are somewhat smaller being slightly less than 20% each. Attempts at deconvoluting the calorimetric transitions for apo B on intact LDL to look for separate domains have been unsuccessful.

Recent cryoelectron microscopic studies utilizing unstained frozen LDL in vitreous ice appear to indicate that the protein is fairly broadly spread over the surface of the LDL particle [56]. However, there appear to be five clumps of electron density which could correspond to five independent domains of apo B. Immunoelectron microscopy of LDL stuck on grids also appears to indicate that different epitopes are widely spread over the surface of the LDL particle [58].

A number of chemical studies on LDL have been carried out utilizing proteases. Yang et al. [15,49,50] utilized trypsin to produce fragments which remain bound to LDL (trypsin-nonreleasable (TN)), fragments which were released to the aqueous phase (trypsin-releasable (TR)), and fragments found in both (TN−TR): 31% of apo B was TN, 34% TR, 24% TN−TR, and 11% was not identified. The peptides were separated,

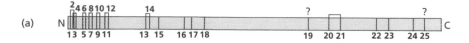

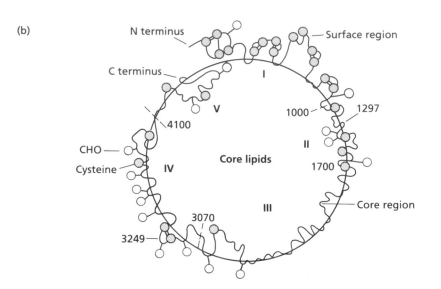

Fig. 3.6 Schematic representation of cysteines (a) and apo B$_{100}$ structure (b) on low-density lipoprotein (LDL). For simplicity, the trypsin-releasable regions are shown outside, and the trypsin-nonreleasable regions inside, the core of the LDL particle. Relative lengths of peptides are not drawn to scale and the surface–core orientation is presented to allow easy visualization of trypsin releasability. It does not imply that the different parts of apo B$_{100}$ are physically on the surface or buried inside the lipoprotein particle. The five hypothetical domains are separated by dashed lines. The thrombin cleavage sites at residues 1297 and 3249 are marked. The locations of the 16 identified N-glycosylated carbohydrates are indicated by (○). Locations of the apo B$_{100}$ disulfide and sulfhydryl peptides are shown in (a). Positions of cysteine amino acids on apo B$_{100}$ were numbered from N to C terminus. There are a total of 25 cysteines. Cysteine residues are indicated by (☺) and disulfide bridges are indicated by (=). (Reproduced with permission from [49].)

isolated, and sequenced, and then related to the primary structure. Yang *et al.* [15,50] describe five roughly equal domains as shown in Fig. 3.6. Domain 1, the amino-terminal 1000 amino acids, consists mainly of TR fragments and contains only a few lipid-bound TN peptides. Domain 2, 1001–1700, has alternating TR and TN areas. Domain 3, 1701–3070, is a large domain consisting largely of lipid-bound TN peptides. Domain 4, 3071–4100, is another mixed domain. Domain 5, the smallest domain 4101–4536, is made up of TN peptides. The relation of tryptic action and protein structure is not clear. However, it is reasonable to assume that the region cleaved by the enzyme is not buried in the lipid part of the lipoprotein but accessible on the surface to the enzyme. If a peptide is released into the aqueous phase it either was not firmly bound to lipid in the native state, or it underwent a conformational change which allowed it to separate from the lipoprotein. If the peptide remains attached to the lipoprotein then it was either bound in the native state (most likely) or underwent a conformational change which allowed it to attach. Since some fragments are found in both TN and TR fractions they must at least have the capacity to bind under the right condition. Assuming that the bound or nonbound state of the peptide reflects the native state then at least 60% of the protein has the capacity to bind LDL lipid. There are 25 cysteines present and 16 are involved in disulfide bonds [49] (Fig. 3.6). All disulfide links are in TR regions [49]. Of 19 potential glycosylation sites 16 are glycosylated. Most, but not all, are on TR peptides [50]; four are on TN peptides.

The composition of releasable water-soluble peptides is not easily explained by increased charge density or an overall increase in the proportion of water-soluble amino acids or even glycosylation. In fact the average hydrophobicity of domains 1–4 is very similar to that of the total protein. Domain 5 which has the greatest abundance of TN peptides is however more hydrophobic. In comparing estimates of hydrophobic moment or hydrophobicity with the isolated peptides, it does appear that those which remain with the particle may be slightly more hydrophobic, but many exceptions occur and the tendency to remain with the particle or be released into the aqueous environment certainly does not solely depend on the presence of a large number of hydrophobic amino acids. When a different series of proteases was used to produce apo B digestion some 26 lipophilic peptides were found and were more or less distributed throughout the protein [73]. Thus, in a gross sense it would appear that regions throughout apo B have the capacity to bind to LDL even though domain 1 would appear to be largely hydrophilic as compared to domain 5.

The deduced low hydrophobicity of domain 1 becomes a more complicated issue when looked at using different lipid substrates When the N-terminal 17% of the apo B gene was transfected into cells which do not make apo B, the B_{17} peptide (amino acids 1–782) was expressed and secreted as a lipid-free peptide [74]. If cells producing B_{17} were supplemented with oleic acid to increase the production of triacylglycerols some B_{17} floated with secreted triacylglycerol particles. The lipid-free B_{17} readily bound to multilamellar liposomes converting them into 23.9 nm discoidal aggregates of relatively fixed size containing about two B_{17} peptides and 2250 phospholipids [74]. From the stoichiometry and size of the disks it was estimated that approximately 70% of the amino acids in B_{17} must bind directly to lipid in order to produce the discoidal aggregates noted. An estimation of the secondary structure of this region of apo B_{17} predicts many amphipathic helices and amphipathic β-sheets. Spectroscopy of B_{17} on disks gave 39% α-helix and 36% β-sheet [74]. Presumably most of these bind to lipid. In a series of unpublished experiments B_{17} also binds to emulsion particles consisting of phospholipid, cholesterol, and triolein. Thus, the physical description of domains produced using proteolytic enzymes on apo B and on LDL are somewhat arbitrary. Domain 1 clearly has a high capacity to bind certain kinds of lipids, although it has a very limited number of peptides associated with LDL after trypsin treatment. The complexity of the structure of apo B will keep many investigators busy for a long time.

As judged by enzyme hydrolytic susceptibility and monoclonal antibody binding, apo B undergoes conformational changes related to the size of the particle and to its lipid composition. Some epitopes present on apo B in LDL are covered in VLDL [75] and vice versa; furthermore, the receptor domain appears to bind far less well to the LDL receptor in VLDL compared to LDL. Finally, in a recent study using very limited proteolysis two susceptible sites were found, 1280–1320 and 3280–3380, which when cleaved gave three large domains [76]. In VLDL the first site is protected and only two large domains are produced. To attempt to study particles of similar size but different lipid composition, triglyceride-rich, Tangier LDL was compared to normal LDL. Epitopes and enzyme cleavage sites were different from normal LDL but were restored when Tangier LDL triglycerol was exchanged for cholesterol ester so that its composition resembled normal LDL [77]. Thus, as with many other apoproteins, conformational flexibility is present in apo B which allows it to adapt to different curvatures, and different surface and core of lipid compositions.

Lipoprotein metabolism

The knowledge of lipoprotein metabolism has moved a long way from the static billiard ball concepts of 40 years ago [78]. The general outlines were well in place by the late 1970s [79] but a number of modifications and complexities, particularly in compositional heterogeneity [80], have been reported since then. It is now quite apparent that VLDL and LDL come in different sizes and compositions and that some large VLDL behave like chylomicrons and produce remnants which are taken up rapidly by the liver. Therefore not all apo B_{100} ends up in LDL. Furthermore, the roles of cholesteryl ester transfer protein (CETP) [11,12,81] and lipoprotein lipase [82–84] are becoming clearer. The metabolism of lipoproteins can be conveniently divided into two general domains: (i) the metabolism of apo B-containing lipoproteins; and (ii) the metabolism of HDL lipoproteins. The division is necessarily arbitrary since the two are linked together through both the exchangeable apolipoproteins and lipids, and transfer proteins and enzymes.

The metabolism of apo B-containing lipoproteins

Figure 3.7 gives a general summary of the metabolism of apo B-containing lipoproteins.

Step 1. Dietary lipids and cholesterol are emulsified in the stomach and acted on by gastric and lingual lipase (for reviews see [85,86]). This liberates some fatty acid to produce emulsions which contain some free fatty acid and diacylglycerols as well as triacylglycerols and cholesterol. Most of the cholesterol taken in the diet is in the form of free cholesterol in the membranes of cells and not in the form of cholesterol ester. Free fatty acids and amino acids stimulate release of secretagogues (cholecystokinin and pancreozymin) which cause the pancreas to release lipases and the liver to release bile. Secretin stimulates the release of bicarbonate-rich, high-pH fluid which increases the very acidic pH of the stomach contents to near neutral in the upper intestine. A number of lipases hydrolyze the remaining triglyceride to 2-monoacylglycerol and fatty acids [86], which are solubilized in bile salt mixed micelles, transported to the intestinal epithelium, and absorbed.

Step 2. Once in the enterocyte much of the 2-monoglyceride is reacylated into triacylglycerols [86], some of the cholesterol is esterified, and these lipids are packed into nascent chylomicrons in the endoplasmic reticulum and Golgi apparatus. Apo B_{48}, and in some species apo B_{100}, is added during the assembly process and is a key factor in the release of the nascent chylomicron into the extracellular space outside the basolateral surface of the enterocyte. Without apo B, chylomicrons are not released and triglyceride is stored in the cell [86]. The chylomicron appears to be secreted with apo B_{48} and apo A-I and apo A-IV on the surface. Once released, chylomicrons enter the lymph from the extracellular space and pass into the systemic circulation from the thoracic duct.

Step 3. In the lymph and in the systemic circulation a number of physical changes occur ([1] and references therein). First, exchangeable apoproteins, primarily apo Cs and some apo E, adsorb to the surface. Apo A-IV and some apo A-I appear to be pushed off the surface to enter

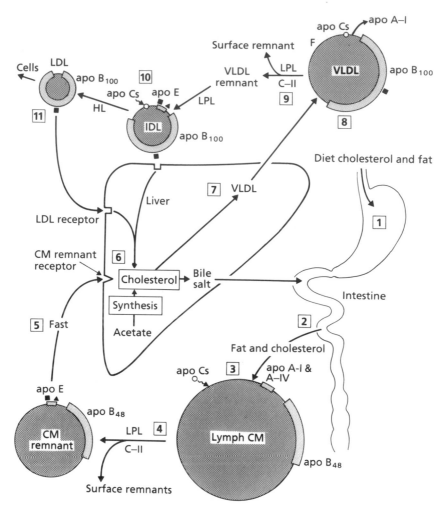

Fig. 3.7 Schematic representation of the major features of apo B lipoprotein metabolism. *Step 1*: Digestion absorption of fat (triglycerides) and cholesterol. *Step 2*: Assembly and secretion of dietary fat and cholesterol into chylomicrons. *Step 3*: Physical change in chylomicrons on release into lymph and blood. *Step 4*: Lipolysis by lipoprotein lipase (LPL) to produce core and surface remnants. *Step 5*: Rapid receptor mediated endocytosis into liver. *Step 6*: Catabolism of chylomicron core remnants and redistribution of the breakdown products, cholesterol and fatty acids. Bile salt and cholesterol excretion into bile. *Step 7*: VLDL assembly and secretion. *Step 8*: Physical change in VLDL in blood. *Step 9*: Hydrolysis of VLDL to form core and surface remnants. *Step 10*: Remodeling of VLDL remnants and IDL to LDL. *Step 11*: Uptake of LDL. Symbols and abbreviations are the same as in Figure 3.1.

both the HDL fraction and the fraction more dense than 1.21 g/ml. Since the concentration of free cholesterol is very low in the surface and core of chylomicrons, free cholesterol at a higher chemical potential in the membranes of blood cells, endothelium, and circulating lipoproteins moves into nascent chylomicrons. At the same time some phospholipid comes off the surface and is probably transferred to the HDL fraction.

Step 4.   Chylomicrons then circulate to capillaries, the lung being the first capillary bed. They bind through heparin-binding sites to the capillary endothelium where lipoprotein lipase and its cofactor apo C-II hydrolyze triacylglycerol [82–84]. Surface orientated triacylglycerol is probably the substrate [88]. During this process large amounts of free fatty acids and 2-monoacylglycerols are formed. Since these partition mainly to the surface of the chylomicron [89–91] they cause surface redundancies along with the excessive phospholipid. Much of the fatty acid and probably some of the monoacylglycerol is removed by albumin or partitions into the membranes of the capillary cells [92]. The phospholipid, however, appears to come off as sheets or vesicles and enter the HDL fraction [1,21–24]. There it acts as a source of new phospholipid which can be utilized in forming phospholipid-rich HDL and become a substrate for lecithin cholesterol acyltransferase (LCAT). During this process the core remnant becomes relatively enriched in free cholesterol such that the surface concentration increases from about one cholesterol to seven phospholipids in the nascent particle to one cholesterol to two phospholipids [1,25].

Step 5.   When the core remnant is released back into the circulation apo E remains bound to the surface and the remnant is rapidly recognized by the putative chylomicron remnant receptor [93], perhaps the "LDL receptor related protein" (LRP) [94,95], and taken up into the liver by receptor mediated endocytosis [96,97]. In the liver it is processed through endosomes to lysosomes and ultimately the lipid is broken down into fatty acids, free cholesterol, amino acids, etc., which enter the cellular pool [98–101]. The released fatty acid can be catabolized and used for energy, utilized for VLDL triglyceride and phospholipid synthesis, or stored as triacylglycerol droplets in the liver. Most of the cholesterol in the diet which is absorbed into the chylomicrons is transported to the liver. In fact, since the net amount of cholesterol in the nascent chylomicron may be less than the net amount in its remnant [1] some cholesterol which was present in cell membranes and other lipoproteins may end up being transported to the liver in remnants.

Step 6.   The cholesterol enters the cellular pool where it controls cholesterol synthesis, receptor expression [102], and probably, at least to some extent, bile salt synthesis. Ultimately, cholesterol in the liver may be lost through catabolism into bile salts, secretion into bile, or resecretion in nascent VLDL.

Step 7.   VLDL appears to be assembled in a particular region of the endoplasmic reticulum and in the *trans* Golgi cisternae [104–107] in a fashion similar to chylomicron synthesis in the intestine. An appreciable fraction of newly synthesized apo B appears to be destroyed in the liver. However, apo B secretion does in part depend upon the influx of remnants and fatty acids. When influx of fatty acid is high more apo B is secreted in VLDL and less broken down [108]. The mechanisms for chylomicron and VLDL synthesis, assembly, and secretion are in an active state of research at the present time [108–111] but are outside the scope of this review. Rat Golgi VLDL have now been isolated and appear to contain very little cholesterol and more phospholipid than plasma VLDL. They have only one cholesterol for 19 phospholipids [111]. They also contain apo B, apo E, apo A-I, and a few apo Cs. When mixed with plasma they gain cholesterol, lose phospholipids, gain apo Cs, and lose apo A-I. These changes are rather similar to those of nascent chylomicrons when they enter blood [1,21,24].

Step 8.   Nascent VLDL is exocytosed into the space of Disse and enters the plasma compartment. It has a surface composition of lipids very similar to chylomicrons, being very low in free cholesterol [1]. Apo B is an obligatory part of the secretion process. In the absence of apo B_{100} no apo B_{100}–VLDL are secreted and no apo B_{100}–VLDL or LDL are present in plasma [113,114]. VLDL is therefore secreted with apo B_{100}, apo E, apo A-I, and probably some apo Cs attached to the surface. Apo A-I is rapidly lost [111]. Once in plasma, other apoproteins adsorb to the surface; cholesterol also is adsorbed as in the chylomicrons.

Step 9.   VLDL is hydrolyzed in a fashion analogous to chylomicrons by lipoprotein lipase and its cofactor apo C-II to produce VLDL core remnants and some surface phospholipid remnants which enter the HDL fraction [114]. The large core remnants of VLDL appear to be taken up, like chylomicron remnants, by the liver. Smaller VLDL produce smaller core remnants which may ultimately end up as IDL or LDL.

Step 10.   Small core remnants and IDL appear to be acted on by the liver to remove excess triacylglycerol and phospholipid. The particle becomes smaller, and the adsorbed apo E and apo C appear to leave the particle giving rise to a small final remnant, the LDL particle. Whether the small VLDL remnants and IDL are actually taken up by the liver, acted on by enzymes, and resecreted as LDL is not yet clear, but hepatic lipase appears to play an important role in this remodeling process. Under normal physiologic conditions the remodeling of VLDL remnants to LDL is apparently fairly rapid.

Step 11. Circulating LDL can be taken up by cells which need lipids and cholesterol and express the LDL receptor, i.e., cells which turn over rapidly or cells which have been injured. That not removed by peripheral cells is taken up by the liver. About half of the LDL cholesterol is probably taken up by the liver.

During these processes phospholipids and cholesterol exchange between particles. Free cholesterol tends to move towards an equilibrium. Thus, nascent particles gain and resident particles and cell membranes lose cholesterol. In species with active CETP, cholesterol ester transfers from particles which are rich in cholesteryl ester to those which are poor, for instance from LDL to triglyceride-rich HDL or from cholesterol ester-rich HDL to chylomicrons and VLDL. Thus the system is in a constant state of flux with respect to lipid and exchangeable apolipoproteins. Apo B appears to stay attached to the core from secretion to uptake and is therefore a marker for the core remnant.

The HDL system

Since our earlier discussions of HDL metabolism [2,22,23,29] the complexity of lipoprotein particles within HDL has become staggering. A large number of techniques, some new and some old, ranging from immunoadsorption [115] to isotachophoresis [116] have been employed. Even two-dimensional gels have been used [117] to demonstrate a large variety of different HDL sizes and compositions. However, without complete lipid and protein compositions of each of the individual unique particles it is difficult to know how fractions isolated by an electrophoretic method compared to those isolated by an immunoadsorptive column. Therefore, until the situation becomes somewhat more unified the author will concentrate on the general features of the HDL system and try to bring into play some of the important new findings.

Figure 3.8 shows the general scheme of the HDL system.

Step 1. HDL can come from at least three sources, the liver, the small intestine, and probably from certain cells. In the liver it has been shown that both small HDL$_3$-like particles containing apo A-I, phospholipid and a small amount of cholesterol ester are secreted. Discoidal lipoproteins,

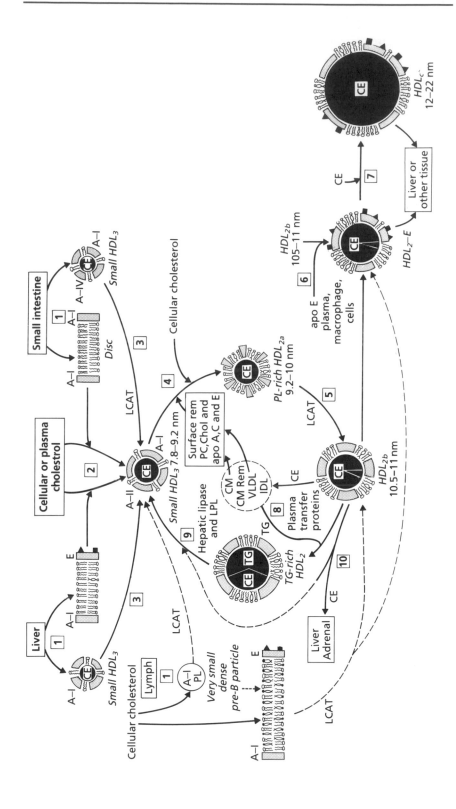

Fig. 3.8 The HDL system. General metabolism of HDL and how it relates to some of the various kinds of HDL that can be isolated from plasma. The sizes of the molecules [cholesterol ( ) and phospholipid ( )] and the particles are drawn approximately to scale. Several processes may occur simultaneously but have been divided into 10 steps. *Step 1:* Newly synthesized nascent particles are secreted from both the liver and the small intestine. The major apoproteins from the liver are apo A-I and apo E, whereas in the intestine apo A-I and apo A-IV predominate. Nascent particles also probably originate in extracellular fluid and lymph. *Step 2:* Discoidal nascent HDL pick up a net amount of free cholesterol, and LCAT converts these to small spherical HDL_3 particles. *Step 3:* The small nascent quasispherical HDL_3-like particles are presumed to enter the plasma to contribute part of the small HDL_3 fraction. *Step 4:* During lipolysis of VLDLs and chylomicrons, surface remnants of phospholipid, cholesterol, and exchangeable apolipoproteins fuse with small HDL_3 to produce a larger phospholipid-rich HDL_{2a}. This lipoprotein can take up cholesterol from cells or plasma. The conformation of apo A-I is probably different from that on the small HDL_3 particle. This difference is indicated by the change in shape of the protein moiety. *Step 5:* LCAT reacts with HDL_{2a} to produce cholesterol ester, which enlarges the core and decreases the relative amount of phospholipid and free cholesterol in the surface to produce HDL_{2b}. *Step 6:* Apo E may be transferred to HDL_{2b} from plasma, which may be taken up by the liver or by the B/E receptor in tissues that require cholesterol. *Step 7:* Under special conditions (cholesterol feeding, CETP deficiency) increasing amounts of cholesterol ester may be incorporated into HDL_2 to make a larger cholesterol ester-rich HDL (HDL_c). This particle contains apo E and may be rapidly taken up by the liver or other tissues. *Step 8:* As an ongoing process, cholesterol ester is transferred out of the cholesterol ester-rich HDL_2 into cholesterol ester-poor chylomicrons, VLDLs, and their remnants in exchange for triacylglycerols. This transfer results in a particle with a core potentially rich in triglyceride, the "TG-rich HDL_2." *Step 9:* As the process described in step 8 ensues, triacylglycerol and some of the phospholipid are hydrolyzed by hepatic lipase and perhaps lipoprotein lipase. This step reduces both surface and core of the particle and converts it back to a small HDL_3-like particle. Thus, the HDL_3—HDL_2—HDL_2—HDL_3 cycle is completed. *Step 10:* In specific tissues, e.g., adrenal and liver, cholesterol ester appears to be selectively extracted from HDL_2, leaving a cholesterol ester-depleted particle which probably reenters the cycle. (Modified from [2].)

mainly phospholipids and apo A-I and/or apo E, are also secreted [118, 119]. Similar small HDL particles and disks appear to arise from the intestine although apo A-IV is a major apolipoprotein and apo E is absent [120–122]. Finally, large discoidal lipoproteins containing apo E and some apo A-I are found in lymph [123–129]. The apo E, but probably not the apo A-I, appears to be synthesized by cells in the tissue space [130]. These large discoidal particles are rich in free cholesterol and they are not generally recognized in plasma. They therefore may be thought of as HDL generated by cells and secreted or assembled in the extracellular space. Small, very dense pre-β-particles are also present in the lymph (P. Roheim, personal communication, 1991). These contain apo A-I and perhaps some phospholipid, and are probably generated by the dissociation of larger HDL particles from plasma. Both of these particles are good substrates for LCAT. Small particles probably give rise to small HDL$_3$ and the large apo E-containing particles probably give rise to apo E-containing HDL$_2$ in the presence of LCAT.

Steps 2 and 3. These steps involve the removal of cholesterol from cell membranes (or other plasma lipoproteins) into acceptor particles (probably nascent particles), its conversion to cholesterol esters by LCAT, and the formation of plasma HDL$_3$. The process of removal of cholesterol from cultured skin fibroblasts into the HDL system has been studied [117, 131, 132] using a rapid separation technique and applying two-dimensional electrophoresis to separate HDL species. These authors have been able to identify the path of radioactive cellular cholesterol as it is removed from cells and progresses through a series of HDL particles (Fig. 3.9). Agarose gel electrophoresis was carried out in the horizontal mode and is polyacrylamide gel electrophoresis in a vertical mode. Antibody stains for apoproteins were used to identify HDL species. The studies confirm that the vast majority of the HDL has α-mobility corresponding to HDL$_3$ and HDL$_2$ (see Fig. 3.9a). However, several minor species of HDL were found in the pre-β-region and these were called pre-β$_1$-, pre-β$_2$-, and pre-β$_3$-A-I containing HDL. Using a modification of the pulse-chase protocol, labeled cellular cholesterol was shown to transfer first to pre-β$_1$, to pre-β$_2$, to pre-β$_3$ and finally into α-migrating HDL, primarily as cholesterol ester (Fig. 3.9). Using the reported lipoprotein's size and composition [130–132] one can speculate about the structure (Fig. 3.10). Pre-β$_1$ appears to have one apo A-I molecule, 14 free cholesterols, and no cholesteryl ester. Since its reported molecular mass is about 71 kDa [130] it should contain about 48 phospholipids or less depending on hydration. This is apparently the initial acceptor for free cholesterol. It could form a very small disk of approxi-

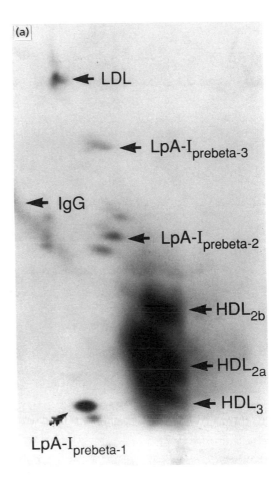

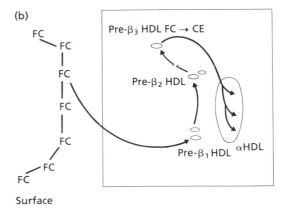

Fig. 3.9 The genesis of HDL in plasma from cell-derived cholesterol. (a) Two-dimensional electrophoresis stained for apo A-I. (b) The box represents the two-dimensional electrophoresis plate showing the positions of pre-β and α-HDL species. The arrows indicate the path of movement of radiolabeled cholesterol from cells through pre-β to α-HDL. (Photo for (a) was kindly provided by Dr Christopher Fielding and reproduced with his permission. (b) Reproduced with permission from [131].)

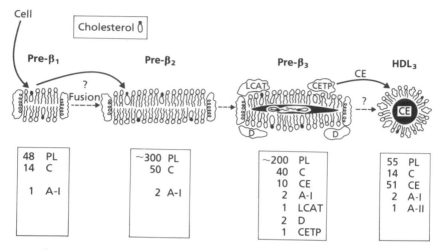

Fig. 3.10 Possible structures of pre-β cholesterol acceptors and reaction complex (pre-β₃) HDLs. Compositional data taken from [130–132].

mately 6.0 nm in diameter (as shown in Fig. 3.10) consisting of one apo A-I and its eight α-helices wound around a very small discoidal bilayer of phospholipid and free cholesterol. It could also form a globular structure. Free labeled cholesterol then passes from the pre-β₁ to pre-β₂, a much larger, clearly discoidal particle containing two apo A-Is, approximately 300 phospholipids, and 50 cholesterols. While cholesterol could diffuse from pre-β₁ to pre-β₂ it is more likely that it forms from fusion of pre-β₁-particles to form a larger disk. At least four to six pre-β₁-particles would need to fuse to form a pre-β₂-particle and therefore approximately two to four apo A-Is would have to be lost during the process. An alternative process could have two pre-β₁-particles fusing with some phospholipid-cholesterol bilayers arising from some other source. Pre-β₃ is a very minor particle and appears to be the particle in which active synthesis of cholesterol ester by LCAT occurs and perhaps the particle from which the cholesterol ester is also removed. The particle is similar to pre-β₂ but has more proteins including an LCAT molecule, a CETP and two apo Ds. A large but dense bilayered particle would be expected. This particle contains a small amount of cholesteryl ester. From the stoichiometry the cholesterol ester would be beginning to form a lens between the hydrocarbon ends of the phospholipid. Labeled cholesteryl ester in pre-β₃ finally ends up in α-migrating HDL₃. It could get there by being transported by CETP to HDL₃ or the particle could be acted on extensively by LCAT converting the discoidal particle to a sphere like HDL. During this process CETP and apo D would be lost and apo A-II added. In any event, it appears that within this isolated tissue culture system radioactive-free cholesterol is transported from cell membranes down a cascade of particles, one of which contains LCAT and CETP where cholesterol is esterified and then transfused into classical α-migrating HDL. It is not known if this system occurs *in vivo*. It is also not certain that the small nascent HDL_3-like particle secreted from the liver and the small intestine, and also found in lymph as a small pre-β-particle, are the same as the pre-$β_1$ described in this system. Furthermore, it is not clear what relation this system has to lipoproteins isolated by other techniques, for example isotachophoresis in which an apo A-I–apo A-IV-containing particle appeared to be a very good substrate for LCAT [116]. Future studies should integrate these findings over the next several years to give us a clearer picture of the transport and metabolism of cholesterol from cells to the HDL system.

Step 4. This step involves the enrichment of the surface of HDL_3-like particles with phospholipid and free cholesterol. Phospholipid can come from a variety of sources but one major source is the surface remnants produced during lipolysis of chylomicrons and VLDL. These surface remnants contain very low free cholesterol and therefore phospholipid-rich HDL_{2a}-like particles are good acceptors for free cholesterol and good substrates for LCAT. Since surface is added some apoproteins may be lost or be required to change conformation to fill in the surface.

Step 5. LCAT uses 1 mole of phospholipid and 1 mole of cholesterol to produce 1 mole of cholesterol ester and 1 mole of lysolecithin [133]. The lysolecithin is removed by albumin. Since surface components are reduced and core cholesterol esters are increased, these particles, HDL_{2b}, would require surface stabilization. This probably occurs by conformational changes in the apoproteins, especially apo A-I [134, 135], or by addition of more surface active molecules (apoproteins or phospholipids).

Step 6. Through exchange of apo E for apo A-I or the conversion of large, lymphatic, apo E-containing disks by LCAT to form HDL_2-like particles, apo E-containing HDL_2 are formed. These particles can be rapidly taken up by the liver or other tissues expressing the LDL receptor [136]. In the presence of hypercholesterolemia such particles (*Step* 7) can be converted into HDL_c, large HDL particles containing many molecules of cholesteryl ester which are also rapidly cleared by the liver [136].

Step 8. The plasma contains some proteins that enhance the movement of lipids between lipoproteins [11,12]. Perhaps the most important is

CETP, which is active in some species, in particular humans and rabbits and essentially absent in mice and rats. CETP catalyzes the net movement of cholesteryl esters from HDL, particularly from HDL_2 to triglyceride-rich lipoproteins. In exchange, triacylglycerols are returned to the HDL to enrich their content of triacylglycerol. In fact, in the presence of hypertriglyceridemia all major classes of HDL are enriched in triglycerides. This may be one of the mechanisms by which cholesteryl ester is returned to the liver, i.e., cholesteryl ester formed by LCAT reactions in the HDL system is transferred to triglyceride-rich lipoproteins which are converted to remnants and returned to the liver. In the genetic absence of CETP, affected humans have high levels of HDL, especially large apo A-I rich HDL, and apo E-rich HDL_c [137]. However, the transfer process is more complicated. It has now been shown [138] that LDL can transfer cholesteryl esters to HDL in exchange for triglyceride. Thus, some LDL cholesteryl ester may be transferred via HDL into apo B remnants and returned to the liver.

Step 9.   Triglyceride-rich HDL_2 particles can be acted upon by hepatic lipase to reduce the content of triacylglycerol and phospholipids, particularly phosphatidylethanolamine [139]. This reduces both the core and surface size of the particle and therefore would convert an HDL_2 particle back into an HDL_3 particle. In the presence of chronic hypertriglyceridemia a large fraction of HDL_2 is connected to HDL_3. This could explain the decreased levels of HDL_2 in these patients. Thus, in plasma there is a cycle in which HDL_3 enlarges to HDL_2, becomes enriched in triglycerides, and is reduced in size by lipases back to HDL_3.

Step 10.   It has been shown recently that some cholesteryl ester can be selectively taken up by the liver and the adrenal without taking up the apolipoproteins of the HDL particle [140]. This implies that cholesteryl esters are simply transferred out of the core converting larger particles to smaller particles. The cholesterol ester taken up in this fashion appears to follow a different cellular path than that taken up by receptor-mediated endocytosis [141].

The HDL system is an extremely complex system of particles and interactions. Certainly, minor species of HDL particles not recognized readily in the past may be the primary acceptors in cholesterol from tissue and may be the metabolic centers for the conversion of cholesteryl esters in their transport to other common particles. The interaction of surface remnants from triglyceride-rich lipoproteins and HDL remains to be defined more clearly. Finally, the different techniques for isolation of

HDL need to be compared and understood so that a general consensus concerning particle structure, metabolism, interactions, and remodeling can be better defined.

Acknowledgments

The author wishes to acknowledge Irene Miller and Margaret Gibbons for preparation of the manuscript. He also wishes to thank Karl Weisgraber for providing pictures of the crystallographic of the 22 kDa-fragment of apo E-3, C-Y Yang for the picture of apo B, and Chris Fielding for the picture of the two-dimensional gel stained for apo A-I. Supported by NIH Grant HL26335 (D.M. Small, P.I.).

References

1   Miller KW, Small DM. Structure of triglyceride-rich lipoproteins: An analysis of core and surface phases. In *Plasma Lipoproteins. New Comprehensive Biochemistry*, Vol. 14 (ed. AM Gotto Jr). Amsterdam: Elsevier, 1987:1–75.
2   Atkinson D, Small DM. Recombinant lipoproteins. Implications for structure and assembly of native lipoproteins. *Annu Rev Biophys Biophys Chem* 1986;15:403–56.
3   Segrest JP, De Loof H, Dohlman JG, Broluillette CG, Anantharamaiah GM. Amphipathic helix motif: Classes and properties. *Proteins* 1990;8:103–17.
4   Segrest JP, Jones MK, De Loof H, Broluillette CG, Venkatachalapathi YV, Anantharamaiah GM. *J Lipid Res* 1992;33:141–66.
5   Scanu AM, Landsberger FR. Lipoprotein structure. *Ann NY Acad Sci* 1980·348:1–436.
6   Havel RJ, Kane JP. Introduction: Structure and metabolism of plasma lipoproteins. In *Lipoprotein and Lipid Metabolism Disorders. The Metabolic Basis of Inherited Disease*, 6th edn, Vol. 1, Part 7 (ed. CR Scriver, AL Beaudet, WS Sly, D Valle). New York: McGraw-Hill, 1989:1129–38.
7   Gotto AM Jr (ed.). *Plasma Lipoproteins. New Comprehensive Biochemistry*, Vol. 14. Amsterdam: Elsevier, 1987.
8   Segrest JP, Albers JJ. *Plasma Lipoproteins, Part A. Preparation, Structure, and Molecular Biology. Methods in Enzymology*, Vol. 128. Orlando: Academic Press, 1986.
9   Albers JJ, Segrest JP. *Plasma Lipoproteins, Part B. Characterization, Cell Biology, and Metabolism. Methods in Enzymology*, Vol. 129. Orlando: Academic Press, 1986.
10 Catapano AL, Salvioli G, Cergami C. *High-Density Lipoproteins: Physiopathological Aspects and Clinical Significance. Atherosclerosis Reviews*, Vol. 16. New York: Raven Press, 1987.
11 Quig DW, Zilversmit DB. Plasma lipid transfer activities. *Annu Rev Nutr* 1990;10: 169–93.
12 Tall AR. Plasma high density lipoproteins. Metabolism and relationship to atherogenesis. *J Clin Invest* 1990;86:379–84.
13 Grundy SM, Denke MA. Dietary influences on serum lipids and lipoproteins. *J Lipid Res* 1990;31:1149–72.
14 Knott TJ, Pease RJ, Powell LM *et al*. Complete protein sequence and identification of structural domains of human apolipoprotein B. *Nature* 1986;323:734–8.
15 Yang C-Y, Chen S-H, Gianturco S *et al*. Sequence, structure, receptor-binding domains and internal repeats of human apolipoprotein B-100. *Nature* 1986;323: 738–42.
16 Chen S-H, Yang C-Y, Chen P-F *et al*. The complete cDNA and amino acid sequence of human apolipoprotein B-100. *J Biol Chem* 1986;261:12918–21.

17 Cladaras C, Hadzopoulou-Cladaras M, Nolte RT, Atkinson D, Zannis VI. The complete sequence and structural analysis of human apolipoprotein B-100: relationship between apoB-100 and apoB-48 forms. *EMBO J* 1986;5:3495–507.

18 Law SW, Grant SM, Higuchi K *et al.* Human liver apolipoprotein B-100 cDNA: complete nucleic acid and derived amino acid sequence. *Proc Natl Acad Sci USA* 1986;83:8142–6.

19 Breiter DR, Kanost MR, Benning MM *et al.* Molecular structure of an apolipoprotein determined at 2.5-Å resolution. *Biochemistry* 1991;30:603–8.

20 Wilson C, Wardell MR, Weisgraber KH, Mahley RW, Agard DA. Three-dimensional structure of the LDL receptor-binding domain of human apolipoprotein E. *Science* 1991;252:1817–22.

21 Redgrave TG, Small DM. Quantitation of the transfer of surface components of chylomicrons to the high density lipoprotein fraction density during the catabolism of chylomicrons in the rat. *J Clin Invest* 1976;64:162–71.

22 Tall AR, Small DM. Plasma high density lipoproteins. *N Engl J Med* 1978;299:1232–6.

23 Tall AR, Small DM. Body cholesterol removal: Role of plasma high density lipoproteins. *Adv Lipid Res* 1980;17:1–51.

24 Mjøs OD, Faergeman O, Hamilton RL, Havel RJ. Characterization of remnants produced during the metabolism of triglyceride-rich lipoproteins of blood plasma and intestinal lymph in the rat. *J Clin Invest* 1975;56:603–15.

25 Miller KW, Small DM. Surface-to-core and interparticle equilibrium distributions of triglyceride-rich lipoprotein lipids. *J Biol Chem* 1983;258:13772–84.

26 Patton GM, Bennett Clark S, Fasulo JM, Robins SJ. Utilization of individual lecithins in intestinal lipoprotein formation. *J Clin Invest* 1984;73:231–40.

27 Segrest JP, Jackson RL, Morrisett JD, Gotto AM Jr. A molecular theory of lipid–protein interactions in the plasma lipoproteins. *FEBS Lett* 1974;38:247–53.

28 Shiffer J, Edmundson AB. Use of helical wheels to represent the structures of proteins and to identify segments with helical potential. *Biophys J* 1967;7:121–35.

29 Small DM. The Eppinger Prize Lecture. Bile salts of the blood. High density lipoprotein systems and cholesterol removal. In *Liver and Bile* (eds L Bianchi, W Gerok, K Sickinger). Lancaster: MTP Press, 1977:89–100.

30 Boguski MS, Elshourbagy NA, Taylor JM, Gordon JI. Comparative analysis of the repeated sequences in rat apolipoprotein A-I, A-IV and E. *Proc Natl Acad Sci USA* 1985;82:992–6.

31 Kaiser ET, Kezdy FJ. Secondary structures of proteins and peptides in amphiphilic environments. *Proc Natl Acad Sci USA* 1983;80:1137–40.

32 Eisenberg D, Weiss RM, Terwilliger TC. The helical hydrophobic moment: a measure of the amphipathicity of a helix. *Nature* 1982;299:371–4.

33 Eisenberg D, Weiss RM, Ferwilliger TC. The hydrophobic moment detects periodicity in protein hydrophobicity. *Proc Nat Acad Sci USA* 1984;81:140–4.

34 Kanost MR, Boguski MS, Freeman M *et al.* Primary structure of apolipophorin-III from the migratory locust, *Locusta migratoria. J Biol Chem* 1988;263:10568–73.

35 Holden HM, Kanost MR, Law JH, Rayment I, Wells MA. Crystallization and preliminary analysis of crystals of apolipophorin III isolated from *Locusta migratoria. J Biol Chem* 1988;263:3960–2.

36 Richardson JS. The anatomy and taxonomy of protein structure. *Adv Protein Chem* 1981;34:167–339.

37 Tall AR, Small DM, Shipley GG, Lees RS. Apoprotein stability and lipid–protein interaction in human plasma high density lipoproteins. *Proc Natl Acad Sci USA* 1975;72:4940–2.

38 Tall AR, Shipley GG, Small DM. Conformational and thermodynamic properties of apoA-I from human plasma high density lipoproteins. *J Biol Chem* 1976;251:3749–55.

39 Tall AR, Small DM. Solubilization of phospholipid membranes by human plasma high density lipoproteins. *Nature* 1977;265:163–4.

40 Tall AR, Deckelbaum RJ, Small DM, Shipley GG. Thermal behavior of human plasma high density lipoprotein. *Biochim Biophys Acta* 1977;487:145–53.

41 Tall AR, Small DM, Deckelbaum RJ, Shipley GG. Structure and thermodynamic properties of high density lipoprotein recombinants. *J Biol Chem* 1977;252:4701–17.

42 Wetterau JR, Aggerbeck LP, Rall SC Jr, Weisgraber KH. Human apolipoprotein E3 in aqueous solution. I. Evidence for two structural domains. *J Biol Chem* 1988;263:6240–8.

43 Aggerbeck LP, Wetterau JR, Weisgraber KH, Wu C-S, Lindgren FT. Human apolipoprotein E3 in aqueous solution. II. Properties of the amino- and carboxyl-terminal domains. *J Biol Chem* 1988;263:6249–58.

44 Weisgraber KH. Apolipoprotein E distribution among human plasma lipoproteins: role of the cysteine–arginine interchange at residue 112. *J Lipid Res* 1990;31: 1503–11.

45 Small DM. *The Physical Chemistry of Lipids from Alkanes to Phospholipids. Handbook of Lipid Research Series*, Vol. 4 (ed. D Hanahan). New York: Plenum Press, 1986.

46 Janiak MJ, Small DM, Shipley GG. Temperature and compositional dependence of the structure of hydrated dimyristoyl lecithin. *J Biol Chem* 1980;255:9753–9.

47 Wald JH, Krul ES, Jonas A. Structure of apolipoprotein A-1 in three homogeneous, reconstituted high density lipoprotein particles. *J Biol Chem* 1990;265:20037–43.

48 Wald JH, Coormaghtigh, De Meutter J, Ruysschaert JM, Jonas A. Investigation of the lipid domains and apolipoprotein orientation in reconstituted high density lipoproteins by fluorescence and IR methods. *J Biol Chem* 1990;265:20044–50.

49 Yang C-Y, Kim TW, Weng S-A *et al.* Isolation and characterization of sulfhydryl and disulfide peptides of human apolipoprotein B-100. *Proc Natl Acad Sci USA* 1990;87:5523–7.

50 Yang CY, Gu Z-W, Weng S *et al.* Structure of apolipoprotein B-100 of human low density lipoproteins. *Arteriosclerosis* 1989;9:96–108.

51 Walsh MT, Atkinson D. Physical properties of apoprotein B in mixed micelles with sodium deoxycholate and in a vesicle with dimyristoylphosphatidylcholine. *J Lipid Res* 1986;27:316–25.

52 Walsh MT, Atkinson D. Calorimetric and spectroscopic investigation of the unfolding of human apolipoprotein B. *J Lipid Res* 1990;31:1051–62.

53 Ginsburg GS, Walsh MT, Small DM, Atkinson D. Reassembled plasma low density lipoproteins: Phospholipid–cholesterol ester–apoprotein B complexes. *J Biol Chem* 1984;259:6667–73.

54 Forte TM, Nordhausen RW. Electron microscopy of negatively stained lipoproteins. In *Plasma Lipoproteins, Part A. Preparation, Structure, and Molecular Biology. Methods in Enzymology*, Vol. 128 (eds JP Segrest, JJ Albers). Orlando: Academic Press, 1986: 442–57.

55 Phillips ML, Schumaker VN. Conformation of apolipoprotein B after lipid extraction of low density lipoproteins attached to an electron microscope grid. *J Lipid Res* 1989;30:415–22.

56 Atkinson D. Electron microscopy of unstained frozen hydrated low density lipoprotein (LDL). *Circulation* 1988;78:II287–1143a.

57 Aggerbeck LP, Gulik-Krzywicki T. Studies of lipoproteins by freeze-fracture and etching electron microscopy. In *Plasma Lipoproteins, Part A. Preparation, Structure, and Molecular Biology. Methods in Enzymology*, Vol. 128 (eds JP Segrest, JJ Albers). Orlando: Academic Press, 1986:457–72.

58 Chatterton J, Phillips ML, Curtiss LK *et al.* Mapping apolipoprotein B on the low density lipoprotein surface by immunoelectron microscopy. *J Biol Chem* 1991;266:5955–62.

59 Chapman MJ, Goldstein S, Mills GL. Limited tryptic digestion of human serum low-density lipoprotein isolation and characterization of the protein-deficient particle and of its apoprotein. *Eur J Biochem* 1978;87:475–88.

60 Chapman MJ, Millet A, Lagrange D *et al.* The surface-exposed trypsin-accessible

segments of apolipoprotein B in the low density lipoprotein of human serum. Fractionation and characterization of the liberated peptides. *Eur J Biochem* 1982;125:479−89.

61 Hahm K-S, Tikkanen MJ, Dargar R *et al.* Limited proteolysis selectively destroys epitopes on apolipoprotein B in low density lipoproteins. *J Lipid Res* 1983;24:877−85.

62 Forgez P, Gregory H, Young JA *et al.* Identification of surface-exposed segments of apolipoprotein B-100 epitopes. Comparisons of trypsin accessibility and immuno-reactivity and implications for apoB conformation. *Eur J Biochem* 1986;175:111−18.

63 Hirose N, Blankenship DT, Krivanek MA, Jackson RL, Cardin AD. Isolation and characterization of four heparin-binding cyanogen bromide peptides of human plasma apolipoprotein B. *Biochemistry* 1987;26:5505−12.

64 Cardin AD, Witt KR, Chao J *et al.* Degradation of apolipoprotein B-100 of human plasma low density lipoproteins by tissue and plasma kallikreins. *J Biol Chem* 1984; 259:8522−8.

65 Chen P-F, Marcel YL, Yang C-Y *et al.* Primary sequence mapping of human apolipoprotein B-100 epitopes. Comparisons of trypsin accessibility and immuno-reactivity and implications for apoB conformation. *Eur J Biochem* 1988;175:111−18.

66 Marcel YL, Hogue M, Theolis R Jr, Milne RW. Mapping antigenic determinants of human apolipoprotein B using monoclonal antibodies against low density lipoproteins. *J Biol Chem* 1982;257:13165−8.

67 Marcel YL, Innerarity TL, Spilman C *et al.* Mapping of human apolipoprotein B antigenic determinants. *Arteriosclerosis* 1987;7:166−75.

68 Milne RW, Blanchette L, Theolis R Jr *et al.* Monoclonal antibodies distinguish be-tween lipid-dependent and reversible conformational states of human apolipoprotein B. *Mol Immunol* 1987;24:435−47.

69 Innerarity TL, Mahley RW, Weisgraber KH *et al.* Familial defective apolipoprotein B100: A mutation of apolipoprotein B that causes hypercholesterolemia. *J Lipid Res* 1990;3:1337−49.

70 Young SG. Recent progress in understanding apolipoprotein B. *Circulation* 1990; 82:1574−94.

71 Deckelbaum RJ, Shipley GG, Small DM, Lees RS, George PK. Thermal transitions in human plasma low density lipoproteins. *Science* 1975;190:392−4.

72 Deckelbaum RJ, Shipley GG, Small DM. Structure and interactions of lipids in human plasma low density lipoproteins. *J Biol Chem* 1977;252:744−54.

73 Chen GC, Hardman DA, Hamilton RL *et al.* Distribution of lipid-binding regions in human apolipoprotein B-100. *Biochemistry* 1989;28:2477−84.

74 Herscovitz H, Hadzopoulou-Cladaras M, Walsh MT, Zannis VI, Small DM. The expression, secretion and lipid binding characterization of the N-terminal 17% of apolipoprotein B (apoB-17). *Proc Natl Acad Sci USA* 1991;88:7313−17.

75 Chen GC, Zhu S, Hardman DA *et al.* Structural domains of human apolipoprotein B-100. Differential accessibility to limited proteolysis of B-100 in low density and very low density lipoproteins. *J Biol Chem* 1989;264:14369−75.

76 Chen GC, Lau K, Hamilton RL, Kane JP. Differences in local conformation in human apolipoprotein B-100 of plasma low density and very low density lipoproteins as identified by cathepsin D. *J Biol Chem* 1992 (in press).

77 Kunitake ST, Young SG, Chen GC *et al.* Conformation of apolipoprotein B-100 in the low density lipoproteins of Tangier disease. Identification of localized conformational response to triglyceride content. *J Biol Chem* 1990;265:20739−46.

78 *Lipo-Proteins.* Discussions of the Faraday Society, No. 6. Aberdeen: Aberdeen University Press, 1949.

79 Dietschy JM, Gotto AM Jr, Ontko JA. *Disturbances in Lipid and Lipoprotein Metabolism.* Bethesda: American Physiological Society, 1978.

80 Lippel K. *Proceedings of the Workshop on Lipoprotein Heterogeneity.* NIH Pub. No. 87-2646, September 1987.

81 Tall A, Swenson T, Hesler C, Granot E. Mechanisms of facilitated lipid transfer mediated by plasma lipid transfer proteins. In *Plasma Lipoproteins. New Comprehensive Biochemistry*, Vol. 14 (ed. AM Gotto Jr). Amsterdam: Elsevier, 1987:277–98.

82 Borenstajn J. *Lipoprotein Lipase*. Chicago: Evener Publ., 1987.

83 Bensadoun A. Lipoprotein lipase. *Annu Rev Nutr* 1991;11:217–37.

84 Garfinkel AS, Schot MC. Lipoprotein lipase. In *Plasma Lipoproteins. New Comprehensive Biochemistry*, Vol. 14 (ed. AM Gotto Jr). Amsterdam: Elsevier, 1987:335–58.

85 Carey MC, Small DM, Bliss CM. Lipid digestion and absorption. *Annu Rev Physiol* 1983;45:651–77.

86 Small DM. The effects of glyceride structure on absorption and metabolism. *Annu Rev Nutr* 1991;11:413–34.

87 Kane JP, Havel RJ. Disorders of the biogenesis and secretion of lipoproteins containing the B apolipoproteins. In *Lipoprotein and Lipid Metabolism Disorders. The Metabolic Basis of Inherited Disease*, 6th edn, Vol. 1, Part 7 (eds CR Scriver, AL Beaudet, WS Sly, D Valle). New York: McGraw Hill, 1989:1139–64.

88 Hamilton JA, Small DM. Solubilization and localization of triolein in phosphatidylcholine bilayers: A ^{13}C NMR study. *Proc Natl Acad Sci USA* 1981; 78:6878–82.

89 Spooner PJR, Bennett Clark S, Gantz DL, Hamilton JA, Small DM. The ionization and distribution behavior of oleic acid in chylomicrons and chylomicron-like emulsion particles and the influence of serum albumin. *J Biol Chem* 1988;263:1444–53.

90 Spooner PJR, Gantz DL, Hamilton JA, Small DM. The distribution of oleic acid between chylomicron-like emulsions, phospholipid bilayers and serum albumin. A model for fatty acid distribution between lipoproteins, membranes, and albumin. *J Biol Chem* 1990;265:12650–5.

91 Ekman S, Derksen A, Small DM. The partitioning of fatty acid and cholesterol between core and surfaces of phosphatidylcholine-triolein emulsions at pH 7.4. *Biochim Biophys Acta* 1988;959:343–8.

92 Small DM. Physical properties of fatty acids and their extracellular and intracellular distribution. In *Nestle Nutrition Workshop Series* Vol. 28 (eds JJ Bisgro, RJ Deckelbaum). New York: Vevey/Raven Press, 1992:25–39.

93 Mahley RW, Hui DY, Innerarity TL, Weisgraber KH. Two independent lipoprotein receptors on hepatic membranes of dog, swine, and man. *J Clin Invest* 1981;68: 1197–206.

94 Kowal RC, Herz J, Weisgraber KH, Mahley RW, Brown MS. Opposing effects of apolipoproteins E and C on lipoprotein binding to low density lipoprotein receptor-related protein. *J Biol Chem* 1990;265:10771–9.

95 Weisgraber KH, Mahley RW, Kowal RC *et al.* Apolipoprotein C-I modulates the interaction of apolipoprotein E with β-migrating very low density lipoproteins (β-VLDL) and inhibits binding of β-VLDL to low density lipoprotein receptor-related protein. *J Biol Chem* 1990;265:22453–9.

96 Jones AL, Kradek GT, Hornick C *et al.* Uptake and processing of remnants of chylomicrons and very low density lipoproteins by rat liver. *J Lipid Res* 1984;25:1151–8.

97 Havel RJ, Hamilton RL. Hepatocytic lipoprotein receptors and intracellular lipoprotein catabolism. *Hepatology* 1988;8:1689–704.

98 Chao Y-S, Jones AL, Hradek GT, Windler EET, Havel RJ. Autoradiographic localization of the sites of uptake, cellular transport, and catabolism of low density lipoproteins in the liver of normal and estrogen-treated rats. *Proc Natl Acad Sci USA* 1981;78:597–601.

99 Hornick CVA, Jones CA, Renaud G, Hradek G, Havel RJ. Effect of chloroquine on low-density lipoprotein catabolic pathway in rat hepatocytes. *Am J Physiol* 1984;247:G187–G194.

100 Hornick CA, Hamilton RL, Spaziani E, Enders GH, Havel RJ. Isolation and

characterization of multivesicular bodies from rat hepatocytes: an organelle distinct from secretory vesicles of the Golgi apparatus. *J Cell Biol* 1985;199:1558–69.

101 Jost-Vu E, Hamilton RL, Hornick CA, Belcher JD, Havel RJ. Multivesicular bodies isolated from rat hepatocytes cytochemical evidence for transformation into secondary lysosomes by fusion with primary lysosomes. *Histochemistry* 1986;85: 457–66.

102 Goldstein JL, Brown MS. Familial hypercholesterolemia. In *Lipoprotein and Lipid Metabolism Disorders. The Metabolic Basis of Inherited Disease*, 6th edn, Vol. 1, Part 7 (eds CR Scriver, AL Beaudet, WS Sly, D Valle). New York: McGraw Hill, 1989;1215–50.

103 De Water R, Hessels EM, Bakkeren HF, Van Berkel TJ. Hepatic processing and biliary secretion of the cholesteryl esters from beta very low density lipoproteins in the rat. *Eur J Biochem* 1990;192:419–25.

104 Jones AL, Rudgerman NB, Herrera MG. Electron microscopic and biochemical study of lipoprotein synthesis in the isolated perfused rat liver. *J Lipid Res* 1967;8:429–46.

105 Hamilton RL, Regen DM, Grey ME, LeQuire VS. Lipid transport in liver. I. Electron microscopic identification of very low density lipoproteins in perfused rat liver. *Lab Invest* 1967;16:305–19.

106 Stein O, Stein Y. Lipid synthesis, intracellular transport, storage and secretion. Electron microscopic radioautographic studies of liver after injection of tritiated palmitate or glycerol in fasted and ethanol-treated rats. *J Cell Biol* 1967;33:319–39.

107 Alexander CA, Hamilton RL, Havel RJ. Subcellular localization of apoB apoprotein of plasma lipoproteins of rat liver. *J Cell Biol* 1976;69:214–63.

108 Davis RA, Prewett AB, Chan DC *et al.* Intrahepatic assembly of very low density lipoproteins: immunologic characterizations of apolipoprotein B in lipoproteins and hepatic membrane fractions and its intracellular distribution. *J Lipid Res* 1989; 30:1185–96.

109 Higgins JA, Hutson J. The roles of Golgi and endoplasmic reticulum in the synthesis and assembly of lipoprotein lipids in rat hepatocytes. *J Lipid Res* 1984;25:1295–305.

110 Boström K, Boren J, Wetstein M *et al.* Studies on the assembly of apoB-100-containing lipoproteins in Hep G2 cells. *J Biol Chem* 1988;263:4434–42.

111 Hamilton RL, Moorehouse A, Havel RJ. Isolation and properties of nascent lipoproteins from highly purified rat hepatocytic Golgi fractions. *J Lipid Res* 1991;32:529–43.

112 Imaizumi K, Fainaru M, Havel RJ. Composition of proteins of mesenteric lymph chylomicrons in the rat and alterations produced upon exposure of chylomicrons to blood serum and serum proteins. *J Lipid Res* 1978;19:712–22.

113 Malloy MJ, Kank JP, Hardman DA, Hamilton RL, Dalal KB. Normotriglyceridemic abetalipoproteinemia: Absence of the B-100 apolipoprotein. *J Clin Invest* 1981; 67:1441–50.

114 Hardman DA, Pullinger CR, Kane JP, Malloy MJ. Molecular defect in normotriglyceridemic abetalipoproteinemia. *Circulation* 1989;80(Suppl II):II-466.

115 McConathy WJ, Alaupovic P. Isolation and characterization of other apolipoproteins. In *Plasma Lipoproteins, Part A. Preparation, Structure, and Molecular Biology. Methods in Enzymology*, Vol. 128 (eds JP Segrest, JJ Albers). Orlando: Academic Press, 1986:297–310.

116 Nowicka G, Bruning T, Bottcher A, Kahl G, Schmitz G. Macrophage interaction of HDL subclasses separated by free flow isotachophoresis. *J Lipid Res* 1990;31:1947–63.

117 Castro GR, Fielding CJ. Early incorporation of cell-derived cholesterol into prebeta-migrating high density lipoprotein. *Biochemistry* 1988;27:25–9.

118 Hamilton RL, Williams MC, Fielding CJ, Havel RJ. Discoidal bilayer structure of nascent high density lipoproteins from perfused rat liver. *J Clin Invest* 1976;58: 667–80.

119 Marsh JB. Apoproteins of the lipoproteins in a nonrecirculating perfusate of rat liver. *J Lipid Res* 1976;17:85–90.

120 Green PHR, Tall AR, Glickman RM. Rat intestine secretes discoid high density lipoproteins. *J Clin Invest* 1978;61:528–34.

121 Green PHR, Glickman RM. Intestinal lipoprotein metabolism. *J Lipid Res* 1981;22:1153–73.

122 Driscoll DM, Getz GS. Extrahepatic synthesis of apolipoprotein E. *J Lipid Res* 1984;25:1368–79.

123 Sloop CH, Dory L, Roheim PS. Intestinal fluid lipoproteins. *J Lipid Res* 1987;28: 225–37.

124 Dory L, Boquet LM, Hamilton RL, Sloop CH, Roheim PS. Heterogeneity of dog interstitial fluid (peripheral lymph) high density lipoproteins: implications for a role in reverse cholesterol transport. *J Lipid Res* 1985;26:519–27.

125 Reichl D, Forte TM, Hong J-L, Rudra DN, Pflug J. Human lymphedema fluid lipoproteins: particle size, cholesterol and apolipoprotein distribution and electron microscopic structure. *J Lipid Res* 1985;26:1399–411.

126 Roheim PS, Sloop CH, Lefebre M. Interstitial fluid lipoprotein metabolism: implications for reverse cholesterol transport. In *High Density Lipoproteins and Atherosclerosis II* (ed. NE Miller). Amsterdam: Elsevier, 1989:269–76.

127 Roheim PS, Dory L, Lefevre M, Sloop CH. Lipoproteins in interstitial fluid of dogs: implications for a role in reverse cholesterol transport. *Eur Heart J* 1990;11(Suppl E):225–9.

128 Reichl D, Pflug JJ. The concentration of apolipoprotein A-I in human peripheral lymph. *Biochim Biophys Acta* 1982;710:456–63.

129 Reichl D. Lipoproteins of human peripheral lymph. *Eur Heart J* 1990;11(Suppl E):230–6.

130 Dory L, Boquet LM, Tate CR, Sloop CH. Peripheral synthesis and isoform distribution of dog apoprotein E. *J Biol Chem* 1986;261:811–16.

131 Francone OL, Fielding CJ. Initial steps in reverse cholesterol transport: the role of short-lived cholesterol acceptors. *Eur Heart J* 1990;II(Suppl E):218–24.

132 Francone O, Gurakar A, Fielding A. Distribution and functions of lecithin:cholesterol acyltransferase and cholesteryl ester transfer protein in plasma lipoproteins. *J Biol Chem* 1989;264:7066–71.

133 Glomset JA, Norum KR. The metabolic role of lecithin:cholesterol acyltransferase: Perspectives from pathology. *Adv Lipid Res* 1973;11:1–65.

134 Brouillette CG, Jones JL, Ng TC et al. Structural studies of apolipoprotein A-I/ phosphatidylcholine recombinants by high-field proton NMR, nondenaturing gradient gel electrophoresis and electron microscopy. *Biochemistry* 1984;23:359–67.

135 Tall AR, Blum CB, Forester GP, Nelson CA. Changes in the distribution and composition of plasma high density lipoproteins after ingestion of fat. *J Biol Chem* 1982;257:198–207.

136 Mahley RW, Innerarity TL, Weisgraber KH. Alterations in metabolic activity of plasma lipoproteins following selective chemical modification of the apoproteins. *Ann NY Acad Sci* 1980;348:265–77.

137 Yamashita S, Sprecher DL, Sakai N et al. Accumulation of apolipoprotein E-rich high density lipoproteins in hyperalphalipoproteinemic human subjects with plasma cholesteryl ester transfer protein deficiency. *J Clin Invest* 1990;86:688–95.

138 Van Tol A, Scheek LM, Groener JE. Net mass transfer of cholesteryl esters from low density lipoproteins to high density lipoproteins in plasma from normolipidemic subjects. *Arterioscler Thromb* 1991;11:55–63.

139 Azema C, Marques-Vidal P, Lespine A et al. Kinetic evidence for phos- phatidylethanolamine and triacylglycerol as preferential substrates for hepatic lipase in HDL subfractions: modulation by changes in the particle surface, or in the lipid core. *Biochim Biophys Acta* 1990;1046:73–80.

140 Goldberg DI, Beltz WF, Pittman RC. Evaluation of pathways for the cellular uptake of high density lipoprotein cholesterol esters in rabbits. *J Clin Invest* 1991;87:331–46.

141 Sparrow CP, Pittman RC. Cholesterol esters selectively taken up from high-density lipoproteins are hydrolyzed extralysosomally. *Biochim Biophys Acta* 1990;1043: 203–10.

Chapter 4
Role of Low-density Lipoproteins in Development of Coronary Artery Atherosclerosis

SCOTT M. GRUNDY

High serum cholesterol is a major risk factor for coronary heart disease (CHD). The major cholesterol-carrying lipoprotein in the serum is low-density lipoprotein (LDL), and LDL has been recognized by the National Cholesterol Education Program (NCEP) as the major atherogenic lipoprotein [1]. In accord, the NCEP [1] identified LDL, specifically LDL cholesterol, as the primary target of cholesterol intervention. The purpose of this chapter is to examine evidence linking LDL to atherogenesis and CHD. In recent years, the mechanisms whereby LDL directly promotes atherogenesis have become much better understood. Further, there is growing evidence that LDL is heterogeneous in both physical properties and chemical composition, and different forms of LDL may have different tendencies to induce atherosclerosis. This chapter will first summarize current concepts of the structure and metabolism of LDL before turning to the possible links between LDL and atherosclerosis.

Structure of LDL

Particle size and molecular weight

LDL consists of spherical lipoprotein particles, and most particles have a diameter ranging from 21.0 to 25.0 nm. All LDL particles are not identical in diameter but have a spectrum of sizes. Likewise, molecular weights range from 2.43×10^6 to 2.98×10^6 [2,3]. The size of LDL probably has significance for atherogenesis because it allows LDL particles to be filtered into the arterial wall where it can initiate the atherosclerotic process. In this respect it differs from still lower density lipoproteins, i.e., very low-density lipoproteins (VLDL) and chylomicrons, which are filtered more slowly into the arterial wall [4].

Apolipoprotein B_{100} (apo B_{100})

When LDL is isolated by preparative ultracentrifugation, apo B_{100} generally is the sole apolipoprotein present on LDL particles. Current evidence indicates that every LDL particle has one, and only one, molecule of apo B_{100}. Apo B_{100} is synthesized primarily in the liver. The apo B gene resides on the short arm of chromosome 2. The protein contains 4563 amino acids, and it is covalently linked to small amounts of carbohydrate. In newly secreted lipoproteins, apo B_{100} has $8-10\%$ carbohydrate. Seemingly, the apo B_{100} molecule is synthesized on the inner leaflet of the endoplasmic reticulum, whereas the lipids that bind to the protein are produced on the outer leaflet. The amount of apo B_{100} actually used for formation of lipoproteins depends on at least two factors: the rates of formation and the rate of breakdown of apo B_{100} before combining with lipids. The regulation of these two processes is not well understood, but both processes could be important for regulating lipoprotein levels.

Metabolic origins and fates of LDL

According to current concepts, LDL is derived from the catabolism of VLDL, and VLDL is secreted by the liver. VLDL is a triglyceride-rich lipoprotein that contains apo B_{100}; it also contains other apolipoproteins—apo Cs and apo Es. One form of apo C, i.e., apo C-II, activates lipoprotein lipase (LPL), an enzyme located on the surface of capillary endothelial cells; this enzyme hydrolyzes most of the triglycerides of VLDL. VLDL remnants are the result, and these particles can be converted into LDL. The precise mechanisms whereby VLDL remnants are converted to LDL are not well understood. Whether the liver is required for this conversion is not known, although some workers speculate that hepatic triglyceride lipase (HTGL) is required to hydrolyze the remaining triglycerides of VLDL remnants to form LDL.

VLDL particles also contain apo E that likewise affects VLDL metabolism. The liver expresses lipoprotein receptors, called LDL receptors, that recognize apo E as well as apo B_{100}, and LDL receptors normally remove a portion of VLDL and VLDL remnants before they are converted into LDL. Available evidence suggests that at least half, and perhaps more, of VLDL and VLDL remnants are removed directly by the liver and thus are not degraded to LDL. An important question about apo E, which is of great interest but not resolved, is whether a unique apo E receptor exists independently of the LDL receptor. If so, this second receptor could enhance the removal of triglyceride-rich precursors of LDL, further reducing the conversion of VLDL to LDL; such an effect should lower serum LDL levels. Intense research currently is underway to identify a separate apo E receptor.

Another parameter that affects LDL levels is the rate of hepatic secretion of VLDL particles. For example, if synthesis of apo B_{100} were to be increased, more VLDL might be secreted, with more conversion to LDL. For many years, variability in hepatic synthesis of apo B_{100} was thought to be an important determinant of LDL levels. More recently, however, the question has been raised whether synthesis of apo B_{100} is truly variable, or instead is relatively constant. Studies in laboratory animals have suggested that various dietary perturbations may markedly alter metabolism of lipids, but synthesis of apo B_{100} remains essentially constant. Therefore, the extent to which variability in synthesis rate for apo B_{100} affects serum LDL levels remains an open question.

Several investigators have postulated that a portion of serum LDL enters the circulation directly, independent of the VLDL pathway. But how could this occur? Does the liver actually synthesize apo B-containing lipoproteins that are very poor in triglycerides and rich in cholesterol esters? In some cholesterol-fed animals this process may occur, but in humans it seems unlikely; although isotope kinetic studies have suggested that some LDL may arise "directly" from the liver, other explanations of the data cast doubt on this mechanism [5].

Let us next ask how LDL is removed from the circulation. Key questions are: (i) What is the distribution of removal of LDL between the liver and other tissues? (ii) How is LDL uptake distributed between LDL receptor and nonreceptor pathways? Although early studies in animals suggested that LDL might be largely cleared by extrahepatic tissues, more recent investigations indicate that the liver is the major site of LDL uptake. In accord, transplantation of a normal liver in a patient who was genetically devoid of LDL receptors caused a marked reduction in LDL level [6], indicating that the liver has a great capacity to remove LDL via LDL receptors. But does the liver remove *all* circulating LDL? In the patient mentioned, LDL levels did not completely normalize after liver transplantation, suggesting that peripheral tissues normally remove a portion, perhaps 25%, of circulating LDL [6].

It appears that most LDL particles are cleared via the LDL receptor, but LDL also can exit via other pathways. In general, nonreceptor pathways seem to be nonspecific and probably represent bulk-phase phagocytosis. About 10% of the circulating pool of LDL is removed each day by nonreceptor pathways. This percentage is independent of the plasma pool size of LDL, supporting the concept of bulk-phase phagocytosis. This 10% per day is similar to that for serum albumin, which apparently is removed entirely by nonreceptor pathways.

Evidence for atherogenicity of LDL

Animal studies

The feeding of high-cholesterol diets to many animal species (e.g., rabbits, nonhuman primates) induces hypercholesterolemia and atherosclerosis [7–10]. We therefore must ask whether the hypercholesterolemia– atherosclerosis link in various species can be explained entirely by an increase in LDL. In rabbits, high cholesterol intake results in a marked increase in plasma β-VLDL, with a lesser increase in LDL. β-VLDL are large, cholesterol-rich VLDL, and they differ from normal LDL in several ways: (i) they have more cholesterol ester molecules per lipoprotein particle; (ii) they are larger particles; (iii) they contain more triglycerides than LDL; and (iv) they contain apo Es and apo Cs, which LDL do not [11]. Almost certainly, β-VLDL are atherogenic in cholesterol-fed rabbits, and since LDL are not uniquely raised in these animals, we cannot be certain that LDL *per se* contribute to atherosclerosis in rabbits. In the Watanabe rabbit, which has a genetic deficiency of LDL receptors, LDL-like particles are however increased, and atherosclerosis develops without cholesterol feeding. The LDL of Watanabe rabbits are triglyceride rich and are not identical to human LDL; nonetheless, they provide better evidence for the atherogenic potential of LDL than do the β-VLDL of cholesterol-fed rabbits.

In some cholesterol-fed primates, the increase in serum cholesterol occurs mainly in the LDL fraction, and in these the elevated LDL almost certainly are atherogenic. However, the LDL particles in cholesterol-fed primates are increased in size and cholesterol ester content [12]. Since the oversized LDL particles in cholesterol-fed animals are not entirely the same as human LDL, their atherogenicity in primates does not necessarily prove that human LDL are atherogenic.

Epidemiologic evidence

Worldwide epidemiologic studies provide strong evidence that high plasma total cholesterol levels increase risk for CHD. These include investigations both between populations [13] and within populations [14]. We must ask whether these studies support the concept that LDL *per se* is a risk factor for CHD. Certainly elevated total cholesterol concentrations in populations generally reflect an increase in LDL cholesterol levels, which suggests that high LDL levels are atherogenic. Further, in epidemiologic surveys [15], in which lipoprotein levels have been determined, LDL concentrations were "independently" correlated with CHD risk. This statistical correlation between LDL and CHD events implies a causative connection between LDL and atherogenesis, although conclusions from epidemiologic investigations always can be marred by confounding variables.

Genetic hypercholesterolemia

Perhaps the strongest evidence that LDL is atherogenic comes from the genetic disorder called familial hypercholesterolemia (FH) [16]. In this disorder, the gene encoding the LDL receptor is defective or absent. The result is a major increase in LDL levels. In patients with heterozygous FH, one allele for the LDL receptor is defective, and as a result LDL levels are twice normal; in homozygous FH, in which both alleles are defective, serum LDL levels are fourfold increased. For both forms of FH, atherogenesis is greatly accelerated, more so in the homozygous form than in the heterozygous form. Enhanced atherogenesis in these patients almost certainly can be explained by an excess of circulating LDL. In these patients there are small increases in VLDL remnants, also secondary to a deficiency of LDL receptors; some workers have speculated that VLDL remnants contribute to (or even explain) the accelerated atherogenesis in FH patients, but the general consensus is that LDL is the most important atherogenic factor in these patients.

Clinical trials

Another argument for the atherogenic potential of LDL comes from clinical trials in which LDL lowering by diet or drugs prevents the development of CHD. The best example of such a trial is the Lipid Research Clinics (LRC) Coronary Primary Prevention Trial (CPPT) [17,18]. In this trial, lowering of LDL cholesterol levels in hypercholesterolemic patients by cholestyramine therapy reduced the risk for CHD, compared to placebo. Although patients treated with cholestyramine respond with a modest rise in HDL levels, the major lipoprotein change is a fall in LDL levels. Other cholesterol-lowering trials [19–24] also indicate that therapeutic modification of lipoproteins will retard coronary atherogenesis and/or prevent CHD, although a fall in LDL levels in these trials was only one of other lipoprotein changes, e.g., a fall in VLDL and a rise in HDL were observed. Therefore, the best clinical-trial evidence that LDL is atherogenic comes from the LRC-CPPT, in which cholestyramine was used as the LDL-lowering agent.

Pathologic investigations

Chemical analysis of atherosclerotic plaques strongly suggests that the cholesterol accumulated in plaques is derived from the serum cholesterol

[25]. The striking correspondence of the fatty acids of cholesterol esters of serum cholesterol and cholesterol in advanced atheroma is suggestive of plasma origin. The demonstration of the presence of apo B_{100} in atherosclerotic lesions gives further evidence for the lipoprotein origin of serum cholesterol [26]. Since LDL is the major apo B-containing lipoprotein, it is reasonable that LDL itself contributes to atheroma cholesterol. Finally, LDL has been shown to be present in atherosclerotic lesions [27]. These several observations are consistent with an etiologic role for LDL in the pathogenesis of atherosclerosis.

Summary

There are several lines of circumstantial evidence that LDL is atherogenic. Many epidemiologic investigations reveal a positive correlation between serum LDL concentrations and CHD. Animal studies reveal without doubt that at least some forms of cholesterol-rich lipoproteins, including those in the LDL density range, can promote deposition of cholesterol within the arterial wall. Clinical trials have demonstrated that LDL lowering in hypercholesterolemic patients will retard atherogenesis and prevent CHD, and pathologic studies of the arterial wall are consistent with an atherogenic role for LDL. Each of these approaches have limitations in defining an etiologic role of specific lipoproteins, but taken together they strongly suggest that LDL is an atherogenic lipoprotein. Finally, the premature atherosclerosis occurring in patients with the genetic disorder FH provide very strong evidence that high concentrations of LDL alone can cause atherosclerosis without the need for concomitant risk factors.

Mechanisms of atherogenicity of LDL

Filtration of LDL into the arterial wall

One requirement for a lipoprotein to be atherogenic is that it must be able to be filtered into the arterial wall. Very large lipoproteins, such as chylomicrons and large VLDL, seemingly cannot penetrate through endothelial cells and thus do not contribute their cholesterol to plaque formation. LDL particles in contrast are small enough to penetrate between (or through) endothelial cells, and they therefore can accumulate within the intima. Apparently, the rate of filtration of LDL into the arterial wall is a function of the LDL plasma concentration [4]. Thus, the "pores" through which LDL particles pass are not saturated at lower plasma concentrations of LDL, since higher concentrations result in more particles being filtered. The possibility has been raised that LDL receptors on endothelial cells may be required for LDL particles to pass through them, analogous to the mechanism for insulin transport, but this mechanism seems unlikely since severe atherosclerosis develops in hypercholesterolemic patients who are completely devoid of LDL receptors [16].

Role of apo B_{100}

The apo B_{100} on LDL particles appears to play a key role in atherogenesis. There is no evidence that lipoproteins containing no apo B are atherogenic. For example, people with high cholesterol levels on the basis of elevated high-density lipoprotein (HDL) cholesterol are not at increased risk for CHD. If anything, they are protected against CHD. Thus, only lipoproteins containing apo B are atherogenic. Undoubtedly, this fact must be related to the unique characteristics of the apo B species, especially apo B_{100}. This protein is extremely large, and highly insoluble in aqueous solutions. Thus, it is prone to precipitation and probably is difficult to remove from the arterial wall. In the discussion to follow, these factors will be examined as they pertain to the role of apo B_{100} in atherogenesis.

Interaction of LDL with proteoglycans and elastin

One way in which LDL apo B_{100} might promote atherosclerosis is by its interaction with proteoglycans in the arterial wall. Apo B_{100} appears to have a high affinity for proteoglycans, and this interaction could interfere with removal of LDL components from the arterial wall [28–30]. A similar binding of LDL to arterial wall elastin may occur [31–35]. It should be extremely difficult to remove cholesterol ester from LDL particles that have been bound to the connective tissue elements. Certainly, HDL is not a good acceptor for precipitated cholesterol ester. Cellular engulfment of cholesterol ester is a possible mechanism for removal of extracellular HDL, but this would only lead to foam-cell formation, which would further increase plaque size. Thus, the interaction of LDL with proteoglycans and elastin may be a key first step in the pathogenesis of atherosclerosis.

Modification of LDL

SELF-AGGREGATION OF LDL

Apo B_{100} is a highly insoluble apolipoprotein, and it is prone to aggregation. Even moderate shaking of a solution of LDL will cause the particles to self-aggregate [36]. A similar process could occur in the arterial wall where migration of LDL is sluggish and precipitating factors may be present. Once LDL has self-aggregated, removal of its components should be delayed, promoting atherogenesis. The extent of LDL self-aggregation in the arterial wall is unknown, but this is a potential mechanism for atherogenesis. Once LDL has precipitated it may be engulfed by macrophages to promote foam-cell formation. [36].

DERIVATIZATION

Goldstein *et al.* [37] observed earlier that pure LDL *cannot* transform macrophages into cholesterol ester-laden foam cells, even though LDL receptors are present on these cells. Apparently, uptake of LDL cholesterol via LDL receptors suppresses receptor synthesis; uptake of LDL then declines and cholesterol esters do not accumulate. On the other hand, if LDL is acetylated, uptake by macrophages proceeds without inhibition, and foam cells result [37]. Uptake of acetylated LDL occurs via a separate receptor, the acetyl-LDL receptor [38]. Other derivatives of LDL, e.g., malonaldehyde LDL, also produce foam cells [39,40]. Although the derivatization of LDL as a potentially atherogenic mechanism is attractive, appreciable amounts of derivative LDL have not been demonstrated in the arterial wall; thus it is uncertain the extent to which this mechanism occurs.

"OXIDATION" OF LDL

One of the most interesting potential modifications of LDL is its oxidation by various species of "active" oxygen that are released by macrophages and other cells in the arterial wall [41,42]. Various oxygen radicals can attack both protein and lipid components of LDL. When LDL lipids are enriched with polyunsaturated fatty acids, LDL particles are particularly susceptible to oxidation [43,44]. When LDL has been partially oxidized, its properties are changed in a way that may enhance its atherogenicity. For example, oxidized LDL may be recognized by the scavenger receptor of macrophages [41,42]; its uptake by these receptors may promote formation of foam cells and thus enhance cholesterol accumulation in the arterial wall. In addition, oxidized LDL may have other adverse effects within the arterial wall. It may activate inflammatory and immune responses, promote coagulation, and regulate vascular tone [45–48]. Recently, Berliner *et al.* [49] and Liao *et al.* [50] reported that even minimally oxidized LDL induces the binding of monocytes to cultured endothelial cells, stimulates endothelial cell production of colony stimulating factors, and triggers early inflammatory reactions, all of which may contribute to the early stages of atherosclerosis.

Relation of LDL to other risk factors

There appears to be an interplay between LDL and other risk factors in atherogenesis. Even so, a strong argument can be made that LDL is the "primary" risk factor because in populations in which LDL levels are low, rates of CHD also are low, even when other risk factors—smoking, hypertension, low HDL, or diabetes mellitus—are common. In contrast, when LDL levels are relatively high, other risk factors assume enhanced importance as causes of CHD. The ways in which these risk factors interact with LDL to promote atherogenesis are not fully understood. In some cases, they may modify LDL in a way to make it more atherogenic, as will be considered in the following section. Alternately, they may enhance atherogenesis independently of LDL but in conjunction with it. This latter possibility will be considered briefly in this section.

SMOKING

Cigarette smoking is a powerful risk factor for CHD. Its effect may be due to two processes. First, smoking may accelerate the development of coronary atherosclerosis in the presence of higher levels of LDL. Epidemiologic autopsy studies [51,52] provide strong evidence that smoking promotes development of aortic and peripheral vascular atherosclerosis. In contrast, the evidence that cigarette smoking enhances coronary atherogenesis is less strong, even though it is definitely a risk factor for clinical CHD [53–55]. Some investigators thus believe that cigarette smoking predisposes to myocardial infarction only when there is underlying coronary atherosclerosis from other causes [53–56]. This latter effect might be the result of either modification of the clotting system or promotion of plaque fissure, the terminal event precipitating coronary thrombosis. Although it is likely that smoking predisposes to coronary thrombosis, that it also promotes coronary atherosclerosis has by no means been ruled out [51].

In recent years, the cellular events underlying atherogenesis have come under increasing scrutiny. Several cells—macrophages, endothelial cells, and smooth-muscle cells—participate in the process. A variety of growth factors, chemotoxic factors, proteolytic enzymes, and lipoxygenases are released by these cells and may modulate various atherogenic steps. Products entering the circulation from tobacco smoke theoretically could modify these listed factors. Even if LDL is the primary factor initiating atherosclerosis, cigarette smoking could play an aggravating role. The concept that smoking acts as an accelerating factor rather than an initiating factor is supported by the observation that smoking apparently does not predispose to premature CHD in populations having low levels of LDL [57,58].

HYPERTENSION

Like cigarette smoking, hypertension is a major risk factor for CHD [59–61]; but again this is true only in populations in which average LDL levels are relatively high [62,63]. Hypertension could accelerate coronary atherosclerosis in several ways. For example, it may enhance the filtration of LDL into the arterial wall. In the presence of hypertension, increased lateral pressure within the arterial lumen should raise the concentration of LDL adjacent to the arterial wall; if so, the effective concentration of serum LDL for filtration of LDL into the arterial wall should be increased. Moreover, increased lateral pressure itself should cause "hyperfiltration" of LDL into the arterial intima. And finally, hypertension may mechanically injure the arterial wall in a way to allow more influx of LDL. The precise nature of this injurious process has not been determined.

DIABETES MELLITUS

Persistent hyperglycemia may act at several levels in the causation of CHD. For example, it may promote development of atherosclerosis, increase risk for coronary thrombosis, and impair myocardial response to coronary artery disease. Once again, all the manifestations of CHD in diabetic patients occur less frequently in populations having low LDL levels [64–66]; thus diabetes appears to be more of an accelerator than an initiator of coronary atherosclerosis. As with the other risk factors, the precise mechanisms whereby diabetes promotes atherogenesis are not known. Several processes, however, have been implicated: (i) glycosylation of arterial wall proteins; (ii) microvascular disease of the vasa vasorum of the coronary arteries; (iii) enhanced "aging" of the cells of the arterial walls; and (iv) altered cell responses, both in the release and response to various factors produced by endothelial cells, macrophages, and endothelial cells. Intense investigations are being carried out to better understand the pathogenesis of atherosclerosis, and these studies may reveal new mechanisms whereby diabetes promotes atherosclerosis in patients having relatively high levels of LDL.

Finally, low HDL cholesterol concentrations are a risk factor for CHD; but again, this is true only when LDL levels are relatively high [67–69]. The inverse relation between HDL concentrations and CHD rates may have several explanations. First, a low HDL level commonly occurs in the presence of other CHD risk factors, i.e., smoking, obesity, and diabetes mellitus; in such cases, the low HDL concentration may be secondary to the other risk factor, and if so, the low HDL is not necessarily an etiologic factor for atherosclerosis and CHD. Second, a low HDL cholesterol can be secondary to various dyslipidemias, i.e., high triglycerides, increased remnant lipoproteins, and even high LDL; these latter abnormalities (and not necessarily the low HDL) may be the true atherogenic factors. And third, a low HDL level may directly prevent the development of atherosclerosis by promoting mobilization of cholesterol from the arterial wall (reverse cholesterol transport). Thus, the strong, inverse relationship between low HDL and CHD in part may be the result of confounding factors and partly from a true etiologic relationship. Finally, recent reports suggest that there may be a direct interaction between HDL and LDL that can occur in a way to reduce the atherogenicity of LDL. One study has shown that apo A-I, the major apolipoprotein of HDL, prevents oxidation of LDL [70]. Since HDL filters more readily into the arterial wall than LDL, it should be present in much greater concentrations than LDL within the arterial wall, and thus it should be readily available to interfere with LDL oxidation. Another report [71] indicates that HDL can interfere with the self-aggregation of LDL, the latter being a potential modification of LDL that promotes atherogenesis. These latter two reports [70,71] thus raise the possibility that HDL may directly interfere with the atherogenicity of LDL. This putative mechanism is supported by epidemiologic data indicating that the LDL/HDL ratio is the single strongest lipoprotein parameter predicting the occurrence of CHD [72]. Indeed, this ratio might have a direct pathogenetic role rather than being an artifact of two independent risk factors.

Atherogenicity of different forms of LDL

In recent years growing evidence shows that LDL is not a homogeneous group of molecular complexes, but rather is heterogeneous in a number of respects—molecular size, chemical composition, immunologic reactivity, and affinity for receptors. The recognition of this heterogeneity raises the possibility that all forms of LDL do not have the same atherogenic potential. Since there are several steps whereby LDL promotes athero-sclerosis (e.g., filtration into the arterial wall, interaction with extra-cellular matrix, modification, and uptake by cells), different subfractions of LDL might react differently at these various steps and hence modify the rate of atherogenesis. For this reason, we can consider the different forms of LDL and speculate on how each might uniquely promote atherogenesis.

Cholesterol-enriched LDL

When some primates are fed cholesterol, they respond with an increase in LDL cholesterol concentrations. This increase is due to two factors: (i) an increase in the number of LDL particles in circulation; and (ii) enrichment of LDL particles with cholesterol. Rudel *et al.* [12] noted that the molecular weight of LDL particles increases substantially in cholesterol-fed primates, and these workers speculated that cholesterol-enriched LDL have an increased atherogenic potential. Certainly each cholesterol-enriched LDL particle will deliver more cholesterol into the arterial wall than will a normal LDL particle. Whether an excess cholesterol carried in LDL is offset by a reduced rate of filtration of somewhat larger particles is unknown; nonetheless, without question atherosclerosis can be induced by cholesterol-enriched LDL produced in cholesterol-fed primates.

Studies from our laboratory [73] have shown that one cause of moderate hypercholesterolemia is an enrichment of LDL particles with cholesterol. Patients with this condition do not have an increased number of circulating LDL particles, as indicated by their normal levels of LDL apo B_{100}, but instead they have abnormally high LDL cholesterol levels due entirely to an increase in the amount of cholesterol in each particle. An important question is whether humans having cholesterol-enriched LDL are at a greater risk for CHD than are people with normal LDL particles, at the same concentration of total particles. Certainly the former people have a higher LDL cholesterol level. At present no data suggest that hypercholesterolemia on the basis of cholesterol-enriched LDL is more "benign" than the same degree of hypercholesterolemia due to an increased number of LDL particles having a normal cholesterol ester content. If the level of LDL cholesterol and not the number of LDL particles is the critical risk factor, this would mean that cholesterol-enriched LDL particles are more atherogenic than LDL particles having a normal cholesterol content. This important issue requires further investigation.

Small, dense LDL

Another category of LDL includes particles that are smaller than normal. Recently, Austin et al. [74] have defined two types of LDL that differ mainly in particle size. By their criteria, Type 4 LDL have a mean particle diameter greater than 25.5 nm, whereas Type B LDL have diameters below this value. These workers suggest that the two forms of LDL are genetically determined, although the reasons for these size differences have not been elucidated. Austin et al. [75] further propose that Type B LDL are more atherogenic than Type A LDL. This latter hypothesis is difficult to prove because the smaller, dense LDL (Type B LDL) usually are accompanied with relatively low HDL cholesterol and high−normal triglyceride levels; these latter abnormalities could be confounding variables to explain increased CHD rates. Nonetheless, it is still possible that Type B LDL are more atherogenic than Type A LDL. If so, one reason may be that the smaller LDL filter more readily into the arterial wall than larger LDL. Another possibility is that Type B LDL are more susceptible to modification (e.g., oxidation or self-aggregation).

"Hypertriglyceridemic" LDL

LDL particles of hypertriglyceridemic patients are unusually hetero-geneous in both size and chemical composition [76,77]. Some particles are relatively large and of lower density, whereas others are unusually small and dense. Both kinds of LDL have a relatively low cholesterol content; the less dense particles are enriched in triglycerides, but the more dense particles are poor in core lipids, i.e., both cholesterol ester and triglycerides. The latter particles generally are smaller and denser than Type B LDL found in normotriglyceridemic subjects [77]. Various investigators have speculated that the abnormal LDL observed in hyper-triglyceridemic patients are more atherogenic than normal LDL. The triglyceride-enriched LDL may have a greater propensity for oxidation because of the susceptibility of excess triglycerides for free radical attack, or they may have a greater affinity for "scavenger" receptors of macrophages [78,79]. The very small and dense LDL in hyper-triglyceridemic patients may filter more readily into the arterial wall or be unusually susceptible to modification, because of increased exposure of apo B on the surface of LDL particles. These various potentially atherogenic mechanisms of course lie in the realm of speculation since they have not been tested directly.

"Diabetic" LDL

The LDL particles in patients with diabetes mellitus frequently resemble those found in hypertriglyceridemic subjects. They tend to be heterogeneous, or polydisperse [80]; some particles are triglyceride rich, and others are small and very dense. These changes may be related in part to the tendency of diabetic patients to be hypertriglyceridemic, but triglyceride enrichment could also be a function of the diabetic condition. Again, these various changes could enhance the atherogenicity of "diabetic" LDL possibly by increasing susceptibility of LDL to oxidation [81−83]. Furthermore, some of the apo B of LDL may be glycosylated in diabetic patients which could promote their susceptibility to uptake by "scavenger" receptors of macrophages.

Smokers' LDL

One mechanism whereby cigarette smoking could promote atherogenesis is by rendering LDL more susceptible to modification within the arterial wall. Several studies suggest that smoking predisposes LDL to oxidation [84−86]. For oxidation of LDL to occur, it is necessary to have a minor oxidation product that can prime the particle for propagation of free-radical oxidation. Smoking thus could act as an initiator for LDL oxidation. A recent study [86] indicates that administration of antioxidants to smokers may eliminate the tendency of LDL to undergo oxidation. Therefore, if the process of LDL oxidation proves to be a critical step in the chain of atherogenesis, cigarette smoking could promote atherosclerosis by conditioning LDL particles for oxidation.

Classification of hypercholesterolemia

The epidemiologic database relating total cholesterol (and LDL cholesterol) levels to risk for CHD provides a basis upon which to classify elevated cholesterol concentrations. In this review, the term "hypercholesterolemia" will be used synonymously with high LDL cholesterol levels; for whole populations, a high correlation exists between total cholesterol and LDL cholesterol concentrations. The nomenclature used in this review is similar to that employed by the NCEP [1].

Desirable serum cholesterol

The NCEP defined a desirable serum cholesterol as a total cholesterol of less than 200 mg/dl (LDL cholesterol of less than 130 mg/dl). In populations around the world in which the average total cholesterol is below 200 mg/dl, the risk for CHD is relatively low [13]; the lower the cholesterol level, the lower is the risk for CHD. Within the USA the curve relating cholesterol levels to CHD is not linear, but is curvilinear [87]; in other words, raising the total cholesterol levels from 150 to 200 mg/dl increases the CHD risk by only 30%, but above 200 mg/dl, an increment of 50 mg/dl increases the risk by approximately 50%, or even more at very high cholesterol levels.

The argument has been made that lowering the total cholesterol to 200 mg/dl is not enough for primary prevention, because many people who manifest CHD have total cholesterol concentrations in the range 150–200 mg/dl. However, a review of the epidemiologic data indicates that when CHD occurs in people having a total cholesterol in the range 150–200 mg/dl (LDL cholesterol 100–130 mg/dl) other CHD risk factors (e.g., smoking, hypertension, or low HDL) usually are present. In the absence of these additional risk factors, rates of CHD are quite low when cholesterol levels are below 200 mg/dl [87]; certainly, total cholesterol levels between 150 and 200 mg/dl are high enough to allow for the development of significant atherosclerosis when other CHD risk factors are present. Thus, the term "desirable" when applied to cholesterol levels is relative, and not absolute. At still lower total cholesterol levels (i.e., below 150 mg/dl), atherogenesis rates seldom lead to clinical events even in the presence of other risk factors.

The term "desirable" applied to cholesterol levels may be relative in another sense. Even at low serum concentrations of LDL there is continuous influx of LDL into the arterial wall and hence atherogenesis still progresses, albeit at a low rate [88]. Nonetheless, the continuous progression of atherosclerosis may eventually lead to a critical degree of arterial narrowing at an advanced age [89]. The term "desirable" thus applies primarily to prevention of premature CHD, and desirable levels will not necessarily prevent CHD in the 70s or 80s. This is especially so if these levels are accompanied by mild hypertension, which is especially common late in life. There is growing evidence that LDL levels are related to CHD risk even into old age [90].

Borderline-high cholesterol (borderline hypercholesterolemia)

Approximately 40% of the general population has a borderline-high serum cholesterol, and about 40% of all CHD in people occurs with cholesterol levels in this category [87]. The risk ratio for CHD (compared to a ratio of 1.0 for desirable cholesterol levels) increases progressively from 1.0 to 2.0 as total cholesterol levels increase from 200:240 mg/dl.

Certainly, the risk of borderline-high cholesterol is enhanced greatly by the presence of other risk factors, such as hypertension, smoking, diabetes mellitus, and low HDL cholesterol levels.

Without any question atherogenesis is enhanced when LDL cholesterol levels are borderline high (130–159 mg/dl) as compared to levels below 130 mg/dl. As indicated before, even when concentrations are in this range, premature CHD may not be frequent when other CHD risk factors are absent, but development of CHD is relatively common later in life. Thus, if the focus of CHD prevention should turn more toward prevention of CHD in the elderly, then more consideration will have to be given to reduction of borderline-high LDL levels. Prevention of clinically significant coronary atherosclerosis in the elderly may require that borderline-high LDL levels be reduced to the low desirable range starting relatively early in life. Unfortunately, it may not be possible to achieve this aim by dietary modification alone for many people; instead, prevention of CHD in the elderly may require either pharmacologic therapy of borderline-high LDL levels for many years, or discovery of new methods to prevent coronary atherosclerosis (e.g., increased intake of dietary antioxidants to block oxidation of LDL within the arterial wall).

High serum cholesterol (definite hypercholesterolemia)

PRIMARY MODERATE HYPERCHOLESTEROLEMIA

This condition is defined as a total cholesterol in the range 240–300 mg/dl (LDL cholesterol 160–210 mg/dl). Approximately 20% of the total adult population in the USA has cholesterol levels in this range [1], and this accounts for about 30% of all myocardial infarctions in middle-aged men [87]. Risk for CHD is increased by two- to fourfold, as compared to cholesterol levels in the desirable range. This increase in risk seemingly can be accounted for almost entirely by an increase in LDL cholesterol concentrations. When primary moderate hypercholesterolemia is present, men in particular are at significant risk for premature CHD even in the absence of other risk factors, although risk is raised even more when other risk factors are present. In view of the large fraction of the general population having primary moderate hypercholesterolemia, this condition represents one of the most important causes of CHD in our society.

PRIMARY SEVERE HYPERCHOLESTEROLEMIA

When the total cholesterol (or LDL cholesterol) exceeds the 95th percentile for the adult population of the USA, this condition can be called *severe hypercholesterolemia*. CHD risk is over fourfold elevated, and approximately 10% of patients with *premature* CHD have levels in this range. Thus, severely elevated LDL concentrations are highly atherogenic, and commonly lead to premature CHD. Patients who have heterozygous FH have sustained lifelong elevations of LDL cholesterol levels, and they are especially prone to CHD [16]. For men with heterozygous FH, clinically manifested CHD commonly occurs in the 30s and 40s, whereas in women with this condition, onset of CHD usually is in the 50s or 60s. Since many patients with heterozygous FH have no other CHD risk factors, the common occurrence of CHD with this genetic disease provides a strong argument for the atherogenicity of LDL.

Causes of hypercholesterolemia: relation to CHD

A final question to be raised is whether the atherogenicity of LDL in hypercholesterolemic patients might be related to the particular causes of elevated serum cholesterol. Above we have considered whether associated conditions (e.g., hypertriglyceridemia and diabetes mellitus) might enhance the potential of LDL to promote atherosclerosis; but even under the general heading of "primary hypercholesterolemia" there are multiple causes of elevated LDL, and each of these etiologies could impart a different risk for CHD, even at the same LDL cholesterol concentration. For this reason, we can explore the various mechanisms for elevated LDL concentrations, and review available data on their propensity to induce atherosclerosis and CHD.

Borderline-high cholesterol

Several different causes for borderline-high levels of total cholesterol and LDL cholesterol have been identified. These are responsible for raising the cholesterol level by about 80–100 mg/dl above the cholesterol levels that occur normally in nonobese, mature teenagers consuming a desirable diet (7% saturates and less than 200 mg/dl cholesterol). In such teenagers, the total cholesterol level averages about 140 mg/dl. In middle-aged American men, in contrast, the average total cholesterol concentration is 220 mg/dl, and in postmenopausal women it averages 240 mg/dl. Factors that contribute to these high cholesterol levels in middle-aged Americans appear to be the following: high intakes of saturated fatty acids and cholesterol, increasing obesity with age, an unexplained rise of cholesterol levels with aging, and in women, loss of estrogen after the menopause. The relation of each of these factors to CHD can be considered.

SATURATED FATTY ACIDS AND CHOLESTEROL

High-risk populations such as the American public have relatively high intakes of both saturated fatty acids and cholesterol. Dietary cholesterol raises the plasma LDL level in large part by inhibition of LDL receptor synthesis [91]. The former, saturated fatty acids, probably act through a similar mechanism [92–94]. It can be estimated from metabolic ward studies that the relatively high intakes of these two cholesterol-raising nutrients increase the plasma cholesterol level by about 25 mg/dl, compared to the level on the desirable diet [95,96]. Since a high intake of these nutrients is maintained throughout life, the higher serum cholesterol level persists throughout life. The atherogenic effect of a high intake of saturated fatty acids and cholesterol therefore is lifelong, which should make it a greater atherogenic factor over the whole of the lifespan than other factors that raise cholesterol levels only in later life. For example, it has been shown that high LDL levels, presumably induced by diet, promote coronary atherosclerosis even in the teens and 20s [97]. A lifelong habit of high intakes of saturates and cholesterol therefore must be considered to be relatively high on the list of atherogenic factors causing borderline-high cholesterol levels.

OBESITY

There is a progressive increase in body fat with increasing age in most American adults. Approximately 30% of middle-aged Americans can be classified as obese, but an even greater percentage have a higher percent body fat than was present at age 20. Certainly, most of the increase in body weight with age after age 20 is due to accumulation of fat. Growing evidence indicates that increasing weight contributes importantly to the rise of total cholesterol (and LDL cholesterol) levels with age [98–100]. The mechanism for obesity-induced increase in LDL levels probably is multifactorial, i.e., overproduction of apo B-containing lipoproteins by the liver (due to hepatic substrate overload) [101–103], and reduced activity of LDL receptors (due to high cholesterol synthesis and increased intakes of saturated fatty acids and cholesterol). The rise of serum total cholesterol resulting from increasing body weight apparently averages 25–30 mg/dl [98–100]. On the one hand, the delay in rise of cholesterol levels due to obesity until near middle age might be considered to be less atherogenic than that due to saturated fatty acids and cholesterol, since the latter effect is lifelong. It must be noted however that obesity also raises VLDL and reduces HDL levels [104], both of which appear to promote atherosclerosis; thus, the multiple adverse effects of obesity on lipoprotein metabolism may offset the delayed rise in LDL cholesterol levels.

UNEXPLAINED RISE OF CHOLESTEROL LEVELS WITH AGE

Dietary factors (saturated fatty acids, cholesterol, and obesity) cannot explain all of the rise in cholesterol levels with age. There is an additional increment in LDL cholesterol levels that occurs between ages 20 and 50 years, both in men and women. The mechanism for this rise is unknown, but it probably is due to a gradual decline in activity of LDL receptors [105–107]. Whether this decline is the result of cellular aging or a change in hormonal status remains to be determined. Since this rise does not begin until after age 20, it probably is not as atherogenic as the increase in LDL levels due to dietary saturated fatty acids and cholesterol which persists lifelong. Nonetheless, if it were not for this approximately 30 mg/dl rise of serum cholesterol with age, most people with borderline-high cholesterol levels would maintain cholesterol levels in the desirable range, and risk for CHD would be much lower. Thus, the unexplained rise in cholesterol levels with aging probably contributes substantially to the increased risk for CHD in high-risk populations.

LOSS OF ESTROGENS

The serum cholesterol concentration in postmenopausal women is approximately 20–25 mg/dl higher than in men of the same age. This higher cholesterol level in women almost certainly can be explained by the loss of estrogen-stimulated LDL receptor activity after the menopause [108,109]. Before the menopause, women are protected against CHD; although the reason for this protection is not entirely understood, lower levels of LDL cholesterol may be a factor. After the menopause, the risk for CHD increases sharply, and ultimately just as many women develop CHD as men [110]. This rise in LDL levels after the menopause probably explains why CHD rates in women eventually "catch up" to those in men. The postmenopausal rise in CHD risk occurring in parallel with an increase in LDL concentrations provides additional support for the concept that LDL is an important atherogenic agent. It might be thought that HDL cholesterol levels would decline after the menopause, because estrogens supposedly raise HDL levels, but in fact HDL cholesterol levels on the average do not decrease post-menopausally. The only significant change in the lipoprotein pattern after the menopause is an increase in LDL cholesterol levels.

Primary moderate hypercholesterolemia

In the USA, patients with primary moderate hypercholesterolemia have the usual causes of borderline-high cholesterol listed above *plus* additional factors. The latter in general are not well understood, but probably are both genetic and acquired in origin. Studies carried out recently in our laboratory have defined several general categories of primary moderate hypercholesterolemia based on general categories of defects in LDL metabolism [73]. Available evidence indicates that each of these categories can have several different causes, some of which almost certainly are genetic in origin. These general categories can be reviewed, and we might speculate on the relation of each to atherogenesis.

DEFECTIVE LDL RECEPTOR GENE (FH)

The most commonly recognized clinical presentation of heterozygous FH is severe hypercholesterolemia, which will be considered in the next section. Several recent reports however indicate that heterozygous FH can manifest as moderate hypercholesterolemia [111–114]. Mitigating factors apparently can lessen the severity of LDL elevation. One family of this type, which carries the FH gene, has been investigated by Hobbs *et al.* [113]. This family apparently carries an LDL-lowering "gene" that partially offsets hypercholesterolemia even in patients with proven heterozygous FH. The precise nature of this LDL-lowering factor has not been determined, but Vega *et al.* [114] recently reported that several members of this same family have an unusually low input of LDL, suggesting a modification in metabolism of LDL precursors (e.g., VLDL). The most likely change in VLDL metabolism in these patients is an enhanced direct clearance of VLDL by the liver so that less VLDL is converted to LDL. This family does not appear to be afflicted with premature CHD, and thus mitigating factors seemingly reduce the atherogenic potential of FH in this family. The proportion of people in the general population with moderate hypercholesterolemia who in fact have a mild form of FH has not been determined. It would seem important to be able to detect such patients since they presumably have had elevated LDL levels lifelong and thus deserve more aggressive lowering of their LDL levels than people who develop hypercholesterolemia later in life.

DOWNREGULATION OF LDL RECEPTOR ACTIVITY

The number of LDL receptors expressed on the surface of liver cells is determined not only by the structure of the LDL receptor gene but also by the activity of this gene. In fact, LDL receptor activity is highly regulated, the purpose of which is to provide optimal amounts of cholesterol for liver cells. When the concentration of cholesterol in the liver cells falls, LDL receptors are upregulated. A small amount of hepatic cholesterol apparently is converted into an oxysterol derivative, which interacts with nuclear regulatory proteins that act on the promoter region of the LDL receptor to control gene transcription. Through this sequence of steps, any factor that raises the hepatic cholesterol content downregulates LDL receptor synthesis and raises LDL cholesterol levels. It is likely that abnormalities in any one of several factors regulating hepatic cholesterol concentrations could be responsible for moderate hypercholesterolemia.

The major endogenous factors that determine levels of hepatic cholesterol are: (i) the capacity of the intestine to absorb cholesterol; (ii) the body's synthesis of cholesterol; (iii) the liver's ability to secrete cholesterol into bile; (iv) the rate of conversion of cholesterol into bile acids; and (v) the equilibrium between esterified and unesterified cholesterol in the hepatocyte. Regarding the latter, it apparently is the hepatic content of unesterified cholesterol (not total hepatic cholesterol) that influences LDL receptor synthesis. Indeed, within the total intracellular pool of unesterified cholesterol, only a small portion, a metabolically active pool, may be the true regulator of the receptor gene. Abnormalities in any pathways listed above could lead to higher concentrations of cholesterol in the metabolically active pool, and hence to downregulation of LDL receptor activity. In addition, abnormalities in LDL receptor function—defects in the promoter region of the LDL receptor, in the transport of newly synthesized receptors to the cell surface and to their active site in coated pits, and in their rate of binding the ligand, internalization uncoupling from the ligand, and returning to the cell surface—may affect LDL receptor "activity." Finally, there are scattered reports that some patients with primary hypercholesterolemia have abnormalities in cholesterol metabolism, but the genetic defects responsible for these abnormalities have not been clearly elucidated. Nonetheless, genetic abnormalities in the metabolism of cholesterol could be an important cause of primary hypercholesterolemia, and hence atherogenesis.

One category of patients with defective regulation of LDL receptor activity may be those who are "diet sensitive," i.e., those who respond to usual intakes of saturated fatty acids and cholesterol with an excessive rise in LDL cholesterol levels [115]. Certainly, everyone does not respond equally to the cholesterol-raising actions of saturated fatty acids and cholesterol, and some people may develop definite hypercholesterolemia when these nutrients are consumed in excess, whereas the majority of people on the same diet will manifest only borderline-high cholesterol levels. The former individuals likely have an abnormality in regulation of cholesterol metabolism, as described above, but their defect becomes apparent only when they consume a diet high in saturated fatty acids and cholesterol.

FAMILIAL DEFECTIVE APO B_{100}

Another possible cause of hypercholesterolemia is a defect in LDL apo B_{100}, in which the apo B_{100} does not interact normally with LDL receptors. Studies carried out in our laboratory first identified patients in whom LDL particles failed to bind normally to LDL receptors *in vivo* [116]. Follow-up collaborative studies on these patients with investigators in San Francisco [117–120] revealed that one of the patients definitely had an abnormality in apo B_{100}, which was shown to be a glutamine for arginine transformation at position 3500 in the apo B_{100} molecule. This condition was named familial defective apo B_{100} (FDB), and this patient's specific defect can be called FDB (3500). Thus far, several different families have been identified that carry FDB (3500); their abnormality is usually expressed in the heterozygous form. Typically, affected patients have moderate hypercholesterolemia, although recently some have been found to have severe elevations of LDL cholesterol and even tendon xanthomas [121,122]. Since patients with FDB have elevations only in LDL, and not in LDL precursors, the finding of premature atherosclerosis in FDB (3500) would strongly support the concept that LDL is atherogenic, independent of LDL precursors. Indeed, several patients with FDB (3500) have now been shown to have premature CHD. Although several other patients in our series of turnover studies appeared to have FDB [116], they were not found to have the 3500 defect. It is therefore likely that other mutations in the apo B_{100} molecule also exist and produce hypercholesterolemia.

APOLIPOPROTEIN E-IV (APO E-IV)

Among the three isoforms of apo E (E-II, E-III, and E-IV), apo E-IV imparts the highest average levels of LDL cholesterol [123–125]. The mechanism for this "hypercholesterolemic" action of apo E-IV is not understood, but it may be related to the ability of LDL precursors having apo E-IV to bind to LDL receptors more avidly than those with other forms of apo E. The uptake of VLDL particles by LDL receptors may enhance hepatic concentrations of cholesterol and thus downregulate LDL receptors. Presumably patients with apo E-IV have higher LDL cholesterol levels throughout life, and thus coronary atherosclerosis should be promoted for a long time. Because of lifelong higher levels of LDL, apo E-IV may be more atherogenic than would be predicted from the somewhat higher LDL levels noted in patients with this apo E isoform.

HYPERSECRETION OF APO B-CONTAINING LIPOPROTEINS

Another possible mechanism for hypercholesterolemia is an excessive secretion of apo B-containing lipoproteins. Presumably, everyone does not secrete the same number of VLDL particles, and those at the top end of the spectrum might be expected to have higher LDL levels than those at the lower end. It has been postulated that patients with the condition called *familial combined hyperlipidemia* have hypersecretion of apo B-containing lipoproteins [126–129]. Unfortunately, with currently available technology, hepatic secretion rates of VLDL cannot be determined with precision, and thus in any given individual we cannot be certain whether hypersecretion of lipoproteins actually exists. Recent studies in laboratory animals suggest that hepatic synthesis rates of apo B are relatively constant regardless of the nutritional state of the animal. On the other hand, hepatic apo B_{100} may have two fates: (i) it can be incorporated into lipoproteins and secreted into the circulation; or (ii) it can be degraded in the liver cell and never used. The distribution between these two fates in turn may depend on the nutritional state of the individual. For example, several lines of evidence suggest that obese people oversecrete apo B-containing lipoproteins, suggesting that they recruit more apo B_{100} for incorporation into lipoproteins. A study from our laboratory is consistent with the concept that some patients are "hypersensitive" to obesity and respond in hepatic secretion of VLDL excessively [73]. This oversecretion of apo B-containing lipoproteins may be one cause of moderate hypercholesterolemia.

DEFECTIVE DIRECT REMOVAL OF LDL PRECURSORS

If VLDL and VLDL remnants were to be removed sluggishly from the circulation, they should be converted to LDL in higher amounts. This mechanism likewise should lead to "overproduction" of LDL and high LDL concentrations. Since VLDL apparently is a relatively poor ligand in these patients, fewer LDL receptors are occupied by LDL precursor lipoproteins; consequently, the number of receptors available for LDL clearance are relatively high, and the fractional clearance of LDL is high. This pattern of high input and high clearance of LDL, which can be called "high LDL flux," is a relatively common pattern of LDL metabolism noted in patients with moderate hypercholesterolemia [73]. These patients have hypercholesterolemia in spite of a relatively high clearance rate for LDL because the input rate for LDL likewise is high; since normal LDL is a relatively poor ligand for LDL receptors, compared to LDL precursors containing apo E, the high input of LDL should raise its concentration. An important question is whether the pattern of high LDL flux is atherogenic, independent of LDL cholesterol concentrations. Circumstantial data suggest that patients with high LDL flux are predisposed to CHD [130,131], although too few patients of this type have been investigated to be certain. If such holds, either the LDL particles present in patients with high LDL flux are unusually atherogenic or the abnormality in metabolism of LDL precursors is somehow atherogenic beyond that reflected by LDL cholesterol concentrations.

CHOLESTEROL-ENRICHED LDL

Finally, some patients with moderate hypercholesterolemia have a normal metabolism of apo B_{100} but demonstrate elevated LDL cholesterol concentrations because their LDL particles are overloaded with cholesterol ester. These abnormal LDL particles typically are larger than normal LDL particles [73]. Whether they are excessively atherogenic remains to be determined. However, since cholesterol-enriched LDL of cholesterol-fed primates appear to have an unusually high atherogenic potential [12], it is possible that cholesterol-enriched LDL in humans likewise carries increased risk for CHD. The mechanisms underlying cholesterol enrichment of LDL have not been determined.

Primary severe hypercholesterolemia

The most dramatic cause of severe hypercholesterolemia is heterozygous FH [16]. The LDL cholesterol levels in this condition are at least twice normal due to a defective allele in the gene regulating LDL receptor synthesis. Hypercholesterolemia is present throughout life, and as a result enhanced atherogenesis begins early in life. The consequence is premature CHD. In men, CHD often develops in the 30s or 40s, whereas in women CHD frequently occurs in the 50s or 60s. The occurrence of premature CHD in FH heterozygotes in the absence of other risk factors is strong evidence for the unique atherogenicity of LDL.

Severe hypercholesterolemia occurs in approximately 5% of the adult American population, but only one in 500 people have heterozygous FH; seemingly the remainder do not have severe elevations of LDL on the basis of defects in the gene-encoding LDL receptors. Indeed, our studies [73] have shown that a variety of defects in LDL metabolism appear to exist in patients with severe hypercholesterolemia of the non-FH variety. In most of these patients, in fact, there appears to be more than one defect present. Usually two of the defects causing moderate hypercholesterolemia coexist to yield severe hypercholesterolemia. In almost all cases, the patients had overloading of LDL with cholesterol, besides having a defect in the metabolism of LDL apo B. On the basis of previous investigations, severe hypercholesterolemia of this type has not been present lifelong, and whereas CHD may be "premature," it usually surfaces much later than occurs in heterozygous FH patients. Again, the duration of elevation of LDL cholesterol apparently is an important determinant of the time of onset of CHD.

Conclusions

The evidence reviewed in this chapter provides strong support for the concept that LDL is atherogenic. Indeed, LDL can be considered the primary cause of human atherosclerosis, because in the absence of at least modest elevations in LDL cholesterol levels CHD is relatively rare. In other words, unless LDL is present in sufficient amounts to interact with the arterial wall, very little atherosclerosis develops. On the other hand, when LDL is present at relatively high concentrations, other risk factors contribute significantly to acceleration of the atherosclerotic process. Besides the standard risk factors—smoking, hypertension, diabetes, and low HDL—several other factors modify the atherogenic potential of LDL. These include duration of hypercholesterolemia and physical–chemical properties of LDL, i.e., particle size and composition. In summary, the evidence underlying the concept that LDL is an atherogenic lipoprotein provides strong support for a major effort at both a public health and clinical level to favorably modify the concentration and composition of LDL for the prevention of CHD.

References

1 The Expert Panel. Report of the National Cholesterol Education Program Expert Panel on detection, evaluation, and treatment of high blood cholesterol in adults. *Arch Intern Med* 1988;148:36–69.
2 Adams GH, Schumaker VN. Polydispersity of human low density lipoproteins. *Ann N Y Acad Sci* 1969;164:130–46.

3 Fisher WR, Granade ME, Mauldin JL. Hydrodynamic studies of human low density lipoproteins. Evaluation of the diffusion coefficient and the preferential hydration. *Biochemistry* 1971;10:1622–9.

4 Stender S, Zilversmit DB. Transfer of plasma lipoprotein components and of plasma proteins into aortas of cholesterol-fed rabbits: molecular size as a determinant of plasma lipoprotein influx. *Arteriosclerosis* 1981;1:28–49.

5 Beltz WF, Kesaniemi YA, Howard BV, Grundy SM. Development of an integrated model for analysis of the kinetics of apolipoprotein B in plasma lipoproteins VLDL, IDL, and LDL. *J Clin Invest* 1985;76:575–85.

6 Bilheimer DW, Goldstein JL, Grundy SM, Starzl TE, Brown MS. Liver transplantation to provide low-density-lipoprotein receptors and lower plasma cholesterol in a child with homozygous familial hypercholesterolemia. *N Engl J Med* 1984;311:1658–64.

7 Katz LN, Stamler J. Experimental atherosclerosis. In *Bannerstone Division of American Lectures in Metabolism*. Publication No. 124, American lecture series. Springfield, Illinois: Charles C. Thomas, 1953.

8 Strong JP, McGill HC Jr. Diet and experimental atherosclerosis in baboons. *Am J Pathol* 1967;50:669–90.

9 Taylor CB, Patton DE, Cox GE. Atherosclerosis in Rhesus monkeys. VI. Fatal myocardial infarction in a monkey fed fat and cholesterol. *Arch Pathol* 1963;76:404–23.

10 McGill HC Jr, McMahan CA, Kruski AW, Mott GE. Relationship of lipoprotein cholesterol concentrations to experimental atherosclerosis in baboons. *Arteriosclerosis* 1981;1:3–12.

11 Mahley RW. Atherogenic hyperlipoproteinemia: the cellular and molecular biology of plasma lipoproteins altered by dietary fat and cholesterol. *Med Clin North Am* 1982;66:375–402.

12 Rudel LL, Parks JS, Bond MG. LDL heterogeneity and atherosclerosis in nonhuman primates. *Ann N Y Acad Sci* 1985;454:248–53.

13 Keys A. Coronary heart disease in seven countries. *Circulation* 1970;40:I-1–I-211.

14 Kannel WB, Castelli WP, Gordon T, McNamara PM. Serum cholesterol, lipoproteins, and risk of coronary heart disease. *Ann Intern Med* 1971;74:1–12.

15 Kannel WB, Castelli WP, Gordon T. Cholesterol in the prediction of atherosclerotic disease: new perspectives based on the Framingham Study. *Ann Intern Med* 1979;90:85–91.

16 Goldstein JL, Brown MS. Familial hypercholesterolemia. In *The Metabolic Basis of Inherited Disease*, 5th edn (eds JB Stanbury, JB Wyngaarden, DS Fredrickson, JL Goldstein, MS Brown). New York: McGraw-Hill, 1973:672–713.

17 Lipid Research Clinics Program. The lipid research clinics coronary primary prevention trial results. I. Reduction in the incidence of coronary heart disease. *JAMA* 1984;251:351–64.

18 Lipid Research Clinics Program. The Lipid Research Clinics Coronary Primary Prevention Trial Results. II. The relationship of reduction in incidence of coronary heart disease to cholesterol lowering. *JAMA* 1984;251:365–74.

19 Oliver M. A co-operative trial in the primary prevention of ischaemic heart disease using clofibrate. Report from the Committee of Principal Investigators. *Br Heart J* 1978;40:1069–118.

20 Canner PL, Berge KG, Wenger NK *et al.* Coronary drug project research group. Fifteen year mortality in coronary drug project patients: Long-term benefit with niacin. *J Am Coll Cardiol* 1986;8:1245–55.

21 Frick MH, Elo MO, Haapa K *et al.* Helsinki Heart Study: Primary prevention trial with gemfibrozil in middle-aged men with dyslipidemia. *N Engl J Med* 1987;317:1237–45.

22 Carlson LA, Rosenhamer G. Reduction of mortality in the Stockholm Ischaemic Heart Disease Secondary Prevention Study by combined treatment with clofibrate and

nicotinic acid. *Acta Med Scand* 1988;223:405−18.

23 Blankenhorn DM, Nessim SA, Johnson RL *et al*. Beneficial effects of combined colestipol−niacin therapy on coronary atherosclerosis and coronary venous bypass grafts. *JAMA* 1987;257:3233−40.

24 Brown G, Albers JJ, Fisher LD *et al*. Regression of coronary artery disease as a result of intensive lipid-lowering therapy in men with high levels of apolipoprotein B. *N Engl J Med* 1990;323:1289−98.

25 Small DM. Progression and regression of atherosclerotic lesions; insights from lipid physical biochemistry. *Arteriosclerosis* 1988;8:103−29.

26 Hoff HF, Karagas M, Heideman, CL, Gaubatz, JW, Gotto AM Jr. Correlation in human aorta of apo B fractions with tissue, cholesterol, and collagen content. *Atherosclerosis* 1979;32:259−68.

27 Hoff HF, Bradley WA, Heideman CL *et al*. Characterization of low density lipoprotein-like particles in human aorta from grossly normal and atherosclerotic regions. *Biochim Biophys Acta* 1979;573:361−74.

28 Srinivasan SR, Radhakrishnamurthy B, Pargainkar PS, Berenson GS, Dolan P. Lipoprotein-acid mucopolysaccharide complexes of human atherosclerotic lesions. *Biochim Biophys Acta* 1975;388:58−70.

29 Hollander W. Unified concept on the role of acid mucopolysaccharides and connective tissue proteins in the accumulation of lipids, lipoproteins, and calcium in the atherosclerotic plaque. *Exp Mol Pathol* 1976;25:106−20.

30 Sambandam T, Baker JR, Christner JE, Ekborg SL. Specificity of low density lipoprotein−glycosaminoglycan interaction. *Arterioscler Thromb* 1991; 11:561−8.

31 Kramsch DM, Franzblau C, Hollander W. Components of the protein−lipid complex of arterial elastin: their role in the retention of lipid in atherosclerotic lesions. *Adv Exp Med Biol* 1973;43:193−210.

32 Guyton JR, Bocan TMA, Schifani TA. Quantitative ultrastructural analysis of perifibrous lipid and its association with elastin in nonatherosclerotic human aorta. *Arteriosclerosis* 1985;5:644−52.

33 Winlove CP, Parker KH, Ewins AR. Reversible and irreversible interactions between elastin and plasma lipoproteins. *Biochim Biophys Acta* 1985;838:374−80.

34 Bocan TMA, Guyton JR. Human aortic fibrolipid lesions: progenitor lesions for fibrous plaques, exhibiting early formation of the cholesterol-rich core. *Am J Pathol* 1985;120:193−206.

35 Podet EJ, Shaffer DR, Gianturco SH *et al*. Interaction of low density lipoproteins with human aortic elastin. *Arterioscler Thromb* 1986;6:116−22.

36 Khoo JC, Miller E, McLaughlin P, Steinberg D. Enhanced macrophage uptake of low density lipoproteins after self-aggregation. *Arteriosclerosis* 1988;8:348−58.

37 Goldstein JL, Ho YK, Basu SK, Brown MS. Binding site on macrophages that mediates uptake and degradation of acetylated low density lipoprotein, producing massive cholesterol deposition. *Proc Natl Acad Sci USA* 1979;76:333−77.

38 Brown MS, Goldstein JL. Lipoprotein metabolism in the macrophage: implications for cholesterol deposition in atherosclerosis. *Annu Rev Biochem* 1983;52:223−61.

39 Fogelman AM, Schechter JS, Hokom M, Child JS, Edwards PA. Malondialdehyde alteration of low density lipoprotein leads to cholesterol accumulation in human monocyte-macrophages. *Proc Natl Acad Sci USA* 1980;77:2214−18.

40 Schecter I, Fogelman AM, Haberland ME *et al*. The metabolism of nature and malondialdehyde-altered low density lipoproteins by human monocyte-macrophages. *J Lipid Res* 1980;22:63−71.

41 Henriksen T, Mahoney EM, Steinberg D. Enhanced macrophage degradation of low density lipoprotein previously incubated with cultured endothelial cells: recognition by the receptor for acetylated low density lipoproteins. *Proc Natl Acad Sci USA* 1981;78:6499−503.

42 Steinberg D, Parthasarathy S, Carew TE, Khoo JC, Witztum JL. Beyond cholesterol:

Modifications of low-density lipoproteins that increase its atherogenicity. *N Engl J Med* 1989;320:915–23.

43 Parthasarathy S, Khoo JC, Miller E *et al.* Low density lipoprotein high in oleic acid is protected against oxidative modification: implications for dietary prevention of atherosclerosis. *Proc Natl Acad Sci USA* 1990;87:3894–8.

44 Berry EM, Eisenberg S, Haratz D *et al.* Effects of diets rich in monounsaturated fatty acids on plasma lipoproteins—the Jerusalem Nutrition Study: high MUFAs vs high PUFAS. *Am J Clin Nutr* 1991;53:899–907.

45 Tanner FC, Noll G, Boulanger CM, Luscher TF. Oxidized low density lipoproteins inhibit relaxations of porcine coronary arteries: role of scavenger receptor and endothelium-derived nitric acid. *Circulation* 1991;83:2012–20.

46 Rosenfeld ME. Oxidized LDL affects multiple atherogenic cellular responses. *Circulation* 1991;83:2137–9.

47 Cathcart MK, Morel DW, Chisolm GM. III. Monocytes and neutrophils oxidize low density lipoproteins making it cytotoxic. *J Leuk Biol* 1985;38:341–50.

48 Chisolm GM, Morel DW. Lipoprotein oxidation and cytotoxicity: effect of probucol on sterptozotocin-treated rats. *Am J Cardiol* 1988;62:20B–26B.

49 Berliner JA, Territo MC, Sevanian A *et al.* Minimally modified low density lipoprotein stimulates monocyte endothelial interactions. *J Clin Invest* 1990;85:1260–6.

50 Liao F, Berliner JA, Mehrabian M *et al.* Minimally modified low density lipoprotein is biologically active *in vivo* in mice. *J Clin Invest* 1991;87:2253–7.

51 Strong JP, Richards ML. Cigarette smoking and atherosclerosis in autopsied men. *Atherosclerosis* 1976;23:451–76.

52 Solberg LA, Strong JP. Risk factors and atherosclerotic lesions: a review of autopsy studies. *Arteriosclerosis* 1983;3:187–98.

53 Kannel WB, McGee DL, Castelli WP. Latest perspective on cigarette smoking and cardiovascular disease: The Framingham Study. *J Cardiac Rehab* 1989;4:267–77.

54 Wilhelmsen L. Coronary heart disease: Epidemiology of smoking and intervention studies of smoking. *Am Heart J* 1988;115:242–9.

55 Hagman M, Wilhelmsen L, Wedel H, Pennert K. Risk factors for angina pectoris in a population study of Swedish men. *J Chron Dis* 1987;40:265–75.

56 Friedman GD, Siegelaub AB, Dales LG. Cigarette smoking and chest pain. *Ann Intern Med* 1975;83:1–7.

57 Todd GF. Cigarette consumption per adult of each sex in various countries. *J Epidemiol Community Health* 1986;32:289–93.

58 Balaguer-Vintro I, Sans S. Coronary heart disease mortality trends and related factors in Spain. *Cardiology* 1985;72:97–104.

59 Pooling project research group. Relationship of blood pressure, serum cholesterol, smoking habit, relative weight, and ECG abnormalities to incidence of major coronary events: final report of the pooling project. *J Chron Dis* 1978;31:201–306.

60 Kannel WB, Castelli WP, Gordon T. Cholesterol in the prediction of atherosclerotic disease: New perspectives in the Framingham Study. *Ann Intern Med* 1979;90:85–91.

61 Salonen JT, Puska P, Kottke TE. Smoking, blood pressure and serum cholesterol as risk factors of acute myocardial infarction and death among men in eastern Finland. *Eur Heart J* 1981;2:365–73.

62 Matova EE, Vihart AM. Atherosclerosis and hypertension. *Bull WHO* 1976;53:539–46.

63 Robertson WB, Strong JP. Atherosclerosis in persons with hypertension and diabetes mellitus. *Lab Invest* 1968;78:538–51.

64 Ingelfinger JA, Bennett PH, Liebow IM, Miller M. Coronary heart disease in Pima Indians: Electrocardiographic findings and postmortem evidence of myocardial infarction in a population with high prevalence of diabetes mellitus. *Diabetes* 1976;25:561–5.

65 Consensus Development Conference. Treatment of hypertriglyceridemia. *JAMA*

1984;251:1196—200.
66 Pan X-R, Walden CE, Warnick GR *et al*. Comparison of plasma lipoproteins and apoproteins in Chinese and American non-insulin-dependent diabetic subjects and controls. *Diabetes Care* 1986;9:395—400.
67 Miller GJ, Miller NE. Plasma high density lipoprotein concentration and development of ischaemic heart disease. *Lancet* 1975;i:16—19.
68 Castelli WP, Doyle JR, Gordon T *et al*. HDL cholesterol and other lipids in coronary heart disease. The cooperative lipoprotein phenotyping study. *Circulation* 1977; 55:767—72.
69 Goldbourt V, Holtzman E, Neufeld HN. Total and high density lipoprotein cholesterol in the serum and risk of mortality: evidence of a threshold effect. *Br Med J* 1985;290:1239—43.
70 Parthasarathy S, Barnett J, Fong LG. High density lipoprotein inhibits the oxidative modification of low density lipoprotein. *Biochim Biophys Acta* 1990;1044:275—83.
71 Khoo JC, Miller EA, McLoughlin P, Steinberg D. Prevention of low density lipoprotein aggregation by high density lipoprotein or apolipoprotein A-I. *J Lipid Res* 1990;31:645—52.
72 Castelli WP, Abbott RD, McNamara PM. Summary estimates of cholesterol used to predict coronary heart disease. *Circulation* 1983;67:730—4.
73 Vega GL, Denke MA, Grundy SM. Metabolic basis of hypercholesterolemia. *Circulation* 1991;84:118—28
74 Austin MA, King MC, Vranizan KM, Newman B, Krauss RM. Inheritance of low density lipoprotein subclass patterns: Results of complex segregation analysis. *Am J Hum Genet* 1988;43:838—46.
75 Austin MA, Breslow J, Hennekens CH *et al*. Low-density lipoprotein subclass patterns and risk of myocardial infarction. *JAMA* 1988;260:1917—21.
76 Kleinman Y, Eisenberg S, Oschry Y *et al*. Defective metabolism of hypertriglyceridemic lipoprotein in cultured human skin fibroblasts. Normalization with bezafibrate. *J Clin Invest* 1985;75:1786—803.
77 Vega GL, Grundy SM. Kinetic heterogeneity of low density lipoproteins in primary hypertriglyceridemia. *Arteriosclerosis* 1986;6:395—406
78 Naruszewicz M, Mirkiewicz E, Klosiewicz-Latoszek L. Modification of low density lipoproteins from hypertriglyceridemic patients by macrophages *in vitro* and the effect of bezafibrate treatment. *Atherosclerosis* 1989;79:261—5.
79 de Graaf J, Hak-Lemmers HLM, Hectors MPC *et al*. Enhanced susceptibility to *in vitro* oxidation of the dense low density lipoprotein subfraction in healthy subjects. *Arterioscler Thromb* 1991;11:298—306.
80 Fielding CJ. The origin and properties of free cholesterol potential gradients in plasma, and their relation of atherogenesis. *J Lipid Res* 1984;25:1624—8.
81 Lorenzi M, Cagliero E, Markey B *et al*. Interaction of human endothelial cells with elevated glucose concentrations and native and glycosylated low density lipoproteins. *Diabetologia* 1984;26:218—22.
82 Hunt JV, Smith CCT, Wolff SP. Autoxidative glycosylation and possible involvement of peroxides and free radicals in LDL modification by glucose. *Diabetes* 1990;39: 420—4.
83 Sakurai T, Kimura S, Nakano M, Kimura H. Oxidative modification of glycated low density lipoprotein in the presence of iron. *Biochem Biophys Res Commun* 1991;177:433—9.
84 Yokode M, Kita T, Arai H, Kawai C, Narumiya S. Cholesteryl ester accumulation in macrophages incubated with low density lipoprotein pretreated with cigarette smoke extract. *Proc Natl Acad Sci USA* 1988;85:2344—8.
85 Harats D, Ben-Naim M, Dabach Y *et al*. Cigarette smoking renders LDL susceptible to peroxidative modification and enhanced metabolism by macrophages. *Atherosclerosis* 1989;79:245—52.

86 Harats D, Ben-Naim M, Dabach Y *et al.* Effect of vitamin C and E supplementation on susceptibility of plasma lipoproteins to peroxidation induced by acute smoking. *Atherosclerosis* 1990;85:47−54.

87 Stamler J, Wentworth D, Neaton JD. Is the relationship between serum cholesterol and risk of premature death from coronary heart disease continuous or graded? Findings in 356 222 primary screenees of the Multiple Risk Factor Intervention Trial (MRFIT). *JAMA* 1986;256:2823−8.

88 McGill HC (ed.). *The Geographic Pathology of Atherosclerosis*. Baltimore: Williams and Wilkins, 1968.

89 Grundy SM. Cholesterol and coronary heart disease. A new era. *JAMA* 1986;256:2849−58.

90 Castelli WP, Garrison RJ, Wilson PWF *et al.* Incidence of coronary heart disease and lipoprotein cholesterol levels: the Framingham Study. *JAMA* 1986;256:2835−8.

91 Sorci-Thomas M, Wilson MD, Johnson FL, Williams DL, Rudel LL. Studies on the expression of genes encoding apolipoproteins B100 and B48 and the low density lipoprotein receptor in nonhuman primates. *J Biol Chem* 1989;264:9039−45.

92 Spady DK, Dietschy JM. Dietary saturated triglycerides suppress hepatic low density lipoprotein receptors in the hamster. *Proc Natl Acad Sci USA* 1985;82:4526−30.

93 Fox JC, McGill HC Jr, Carey KD, Getz GS. *In vivo* regulation of hepatic LDL receptor mRNA in the baboon: Differential effects of saturated and unsaturated fat. *J Biol Chem* 1987;262:7014−20.

94 Nicolosi RJ, Stucchi AF, Kowala MC *et al.* Effect of dietary fat saturation and cholesterol on LDL composition and metabolism. *Arteriosclerosis* 1990;10:119−28.

95 Keys A, Anderson JT, Grande F. Serum cholesterol response to changes in the diet. IV. Particular saturated fatty acids in the diet. *Metabolism* 1965;14:776−87.

96 Hegsted DM, McGandy RB, Myers ML, Stare FJ. Quantitative effects of dietary fat on serum cholesterol in man. *Am J Clin Nutr* 1987;17:281−95.

97 Pathological Determinants of Atherosclerosis in Youth (PDAY) Research Group. Relationship of atherosclerosis in young men to serum lipoprotein cholesterol concentrations and smoking. *JAMA* 1990;264:3018−24.

98 Keys A. *Seven Countries: A Multivariate Analysis on Death and Coronary Heart Disease.* Cambridge, MA: University Press, 1980.

99 Ashley FW Jr, Kannel WB. Relation of weight change to changes in atherogenic traits: The Framingham Study. *J Chron Dis* 1974;27:103−14.

100 Kannel WB, Gordon T, Castelli WP. Obesity, lipids, and glucose intolerance: The Framingham Study. *Am J Clin Nutr* 1979;32:1238−45.

101 Kesaniemi YA, Beltz WF, Grundy SM. Comparisons of metabolism of apolipoprotein B in normal subjects, obese patients, and patients with coronary heart disease. *J Clin Invest* 1985;76:586−95.

102 Egusa G, Beltz WF, Grundy SM, Howard BV. Influence of obesity on the metabolism of apolipoprotein B in man. *J Clin Invest* 1985;76:596−603.

103 Kesaniemi YA, Grundy SM. Increased low density lipoprotein production associated with obesity. *Arteriosclerosis* 1983;3:170−7.

104 Wolf R, Grundy SM. Influence of weight reduction on plasma lipoproteins in obese patients. *Arteriosclerosis* 1983;3:160−9.

105 Miller NE. Why does plasma low density lipoprotein concentration in adults increase with age? *Lancet* 1984;i:263−6.

106 Grundy SM, Vega GL, Bilheimer DW. Kinetic mechanisms determining variability in low density lipoprotein levels and rise with age. *Arteriosclerosis* 1985;5:623−30.

107 Ericsson S, Eriksson M, Vitols S *et al.* Influence of age on the metabolism of plasma low density lipoproteins in healthy males. *J Clin Invest* 1991;87:591−6.

108 Ma PT, Yamamoto T, Goldstein JL, Brown MS. Increased mRNA for low density lipoprotein receptor in livers of rabbits treated with 17 alpha-ethinyl estradiol. *Proc Natl Acad Sci USA* 1986;83:792−6.

109 Eriksson M, Berglund L, Rudling M, Henriksson P, Angelin B. Effects of estrogen on low density lipoprotein metabolism in males: short-term and long-term studies during hormonal treatment of prostatic carcinoma. *J Clin Invest* 1989;84:802−10.

110 Denke MA, Grundy SM. Hypercholesterolemia in the elderly: resolving the treatment dilemma. *Ann Intern Med* 1990;112:780−92.

111 Nora JJ, Lortscher RM, Spangler RD, Bilheimer DW. Familial hypercholesterolemia with "normal" cholesterol in obligate heterozygotes. *Am J Med Genet* 1985;22: 585−91.

112 Bilheimer DW, East C, Grundy SM, Nora JJ. Clinical studies in a kindred with a kinetic LDL receptor mutation causing familial hypercholesterolemia. *Am J Med Genet* 1985;22:593−8.

113 Hobbs HH, Leitersdorf E, Leffert CC *et al.* Evidence for a dominant gene that suppresses hypercholesterolemia in a family with defective low-density lipoprotein receptors. *J Clin Invest* 1989;84:656−64.

114 Vega GL, Hobbs HH, Grundy SM. Low density lipoprotein kinetics in a family having defective LDL receptors in which hypercholesterolemia is suppressed. *Arteriosclerosis* 1991;11:578−85.

115 Grundy SM, Vega GL. Plasma cholesterol responsiveness to saturated fatty acids. *Am J Clin Nutr* 1988;47:822−4.

116 Vega GL, Grundy SM. *In vivo* evidence for reduced binding of low density lipoproteins to receptors as a cause of primary moderate hypercholesterolemia. *J Clin Invest* 1986;78:1410−14.

117 Innerarity TL, Weisgraber KH, Arnold KS *et al.* Familial defective apolipoprotein B-100: low density lipoproteins with abnormal receptor binding. *Proc Natl Acad Sci USA* 1987;84:6919−23.

118 Weisgraber KH, Innerarity TL, Newhouse YM *et al.* Familial defective apolipoprotein B-100: enhanced binding of monoclonal antibody MB47 to abnormal low density lipoproteins. *Proc Natl Acad Sci USA* 1988;85:9758−62.

119 Soria LF, Ludwig EH, Clarke HRG *et al.* Association between a specific apolipoprotein B mutation and familial defective apolipoprotein B-100. *Proc Natl Acad Sci USA* 1989;86:587−91.

120 Innerarity TL, Mahley RW, Weisgraber KH *et al.* Familial defective apolipoprotein B-100: A mutation of apolipoprotein B that causes hypercholesterolemia. *J Lipid Res* 1990;31:1337−49.

121 Tybjaerg-Hansen A, Gallagher J, Vincent J *et al.* Familial defective apolipoprotein B-100: detection in the United Kingdom and Scandinavia, and clinical characteristics of ten cases. *Atherosclerosis* 1990;80:235−42.

122 Rauh G, Schuster H, Fischer J *et al.* Familial defective apolipoprotein B-100: haplotype analysis of the arginine (3500)−glutamine mutation. *Atherosclerosis* 1991;88:219−26.

123 Utermann G, Pruin N, Steinmetz A. Polymorphism of apolipoprotein E. III. Effect of a single polymorphic gene locus on plasma lipid levels in man. *Clin Genet* 1979;15: 63−72.

124 Ehnholm C, Lukka M, Kuusi T, Nikkila E, Utermann G. Apolipoprotein E polymorphism in the Finnish population: gene frequencies and relation to lipoprotein concentrations. *J Lipid Res* 1986;27:227−35.

125 Weisgraber KH, Rall SC Jr, Mahley RW. Human E apoprotein heterogeneity: cysteine−arginine interchanges in the amino acid sequence of the apo-E isoforms. *J Biol Chem* 1981;256:9077−83.

126 Chait A, Albers JJ, Brunzell JD. Very low density lipoprotein over-production in genetic forms of hypertriglyceridaemia. *Eur J Clin Invest* 1980;10:17−22.

127 Janus ED, Nicoll AM, Turner PR, Magill P, Lewis B. Kinetic basis of the primary hyperlipidaemias: studies of apolipoprotein B turnover in genetically-defined subjects. *Eur J Clin Invest* 1981;10:161−71.

128 Kissebah AH, Alfarsi S, Adams PW. Integrated regulation of very low density lipoprotein triglyceride and apolipoprotein-B kinetics in man: normolipemic subjects, familial hypertriglyceridemia, and familial combined hyperlipidemia. *Metabolism* 1981;30:856−68.

129 Kissebah AH, Alfarsi S, Evans DJ. Low density lipoprotein metabolism in familial combined hyperlipidemia: mechanism of the multiple lipoprotein phenotypic expression. *Arteriosclerosis* 1984;4:614−24.

130 Kesaniemi YA, Grundy SM. Overproduction of low density lipoproteins associated with coronary heart disease. *Arteriosclerosis* 1983;3:40−6.

131 Vega GL, Illingworth DR, Grundy SM, Lindgren FT, Connor WE. Normocholesterolemic tendon xanthomatosis with overproduction of apolipoprotein B. *Metabolism* 1983;32:118−25.

Chapter 5
High-density Lipoproteins

JOHN P. KANE

High-density lipoproteins (HDL) and the risk of arteriosclerotic heart disease

Attention had been directed at the etiologic role of the apolipoprotein (apo) B-containing lipoproteins in atherogenesis for fully two decades before observations in prospective studies in Honolulu [1], Framingham [2], and Tromsø [3] suggested an independent inverse correlation of HDL cholesterol levels with risk of coronary heart disease. In the Framingham study, the risk for men with HDL cholesterol levels in the lowest quintile (<35 mg/dl) was over four times as great as among men in the top quintile (>54 mg/dl). The effect was also striking in women. Those in the lowest quintile (HDL cholesterol <45 mg/dl) experienced a risk over three times that seen in the highest quintile (HDL cholesterol >60 mg/dl) [4]. Analysis of data on patients in the Framingham and Lipid Research Clinics Prevalence Mortality Follow-up Studies (LRCF) [5–7] and the control patients from two large randomized intervention trials, the Coronary Primary Prevention Trial (CPPT) [8,9] and the Multiple Risk Factor Intervention Trial (MRFIT), have yielded a consistent pattern of independent inverse correlation with risk [10]. In the LRCF study, in which mortality only was assessed, increments of 1 mg/dl in HDL cholesterol were associated with decreases of 3.7% and 4.7% in death from coronary disease in men and women, respectively. In the other three studies, the decrement of risk was 2% per mg HDL cholesterol for men. In the Framingham study, women had a decrement of about 3%. In striking contrast with low-density lipoprotein (LDL) cholesterol, the predictive value of HDL cholesterol does not decline with increasing age. In none of the large prospective studies has HDL cholesterol been associated with increased overall mortality.

Data supporting the inverse risk relationship of HDL cholesterol and coronary disease have been forthcoming from a number of other studies as well [11–16]. Notable, however, are several studies in which such a relationship could not be discerned [17–20]. The British Regional Heart Study [19] involved measurement of total cholesterol and non-HDL cholesterol in the nonfasting state. This composite variable proved to be correlated directly with coronary risk and inversely with HDL cholesterol, such that its inclusion in a logistic regression model excluded a significant risk contribution from HDL cholesterol itself. Subsequent covariance analysis of these data using total cholesterol yielded a significant inverse correlation between HDL cholesterol and risk [10], suggesting that non-HDL cholesterol values may reflect the influence of determinants of the transfer of cholesteryl esters during alimentary lipemia or some other unanticipated factor related to coronary risk. Another study at odds with the inverse risk relationship is the US–USSR collaborative study among men 40–59 years of age [20]. It is noteworthy that the HDL cholesterol levels were about 10 mg/dl higher among the Russians and were correlated with ethanol intake. These data suggest that qualitative differences among HDL particle populations may be highly significant with regard to protection against atherosclerosis.

Taken together, the epidemiologic data provide reasonably consistent support for the inverse risk hypothesis, based on total HDL cholesterol. However, it is well established that there is an inverse correlation of HDL cholesterol with plasma triglycerides, reflecting the progressive replacement of cholesteryl esters in HDL by triglycerides as plasma triglyceride levels rise [21]. Furthermore, some studies have demonstrated an increased risk of coronary disease in patients with hypertriglyceridemia independent of other lipoproteins [22–27]. This relationship appears to be somewhat stronger in women [28,29]. Thus, the inverse relationship of HDL cholesterol levels with risk may be due in part to factors acting upon levels of HDL lipoproteins in plasma *per se*, whereas others are clearly affecting qualitative changes in HDL. It is indeterminate at this time whether the incremental risk associated with hypertriglyceridemia is mediated through the atherogenic potential of very low-density lipoproteins (VLDL) or intermediate-density lipoproteins (IDL), or via changes in HDL composition and function, which are a consequence of elevated plasma triglyceride levels.

HDL actually comprise at least several particle species. It is thus reasonable to suppose that the relative or absolute amounts of individual species in plasma might correlate better with coronary risk than does total HDL cholesterol. A number of studies have been directed at the testing of this hypothesis [30]. Most have been retrospective. Thus, potentially confounding factors, such as the initiation of β-adrenergic blockade, physiologic changes attendant to myocardial infarction, and alterations in diet make the interpretation of such studies difficult. Furthermore, most studies have been confined to separation of HDL populations by ultracentrifugation. Because the major fractions as separated, HDL_2 and HDL_3, are highly polydisperse and are clearly modified structurally by the technique itself, such information is of limited interpretability. In some such studies [31,32], HDL_2 was the better indicator of risk, but in the NHLBI in-house intervention study, HDL_3 levels were the only significant correlate [33]. Similarly, efforts have been extended to determine whether HDL apolipoproteins might be a better discriminator of risk. Most of these studies have been comparisons of survivors of myocardial infarction, or individuals who have angiographically defined disease, with controls. In the aggregate, these studies have not yielded a clear superiority of apo A-I levels over HDL cholesterol as predictors of risk [30]. Though apo A-II levels were also measured in many of these studies, in only one was it found to be a better discriminant than levels of apo A-I or HDL cholesterol [34]. Similarly, several studies have failed to identify apo D as a better discriminant than apo A-I or HDL cholesterol, though apo D levels in HDL isolated by ultracentrifugation were found to be decreased in male survivors of myocardial infarction [35]. In a small comparison of survivors of myocardial infarction and controls, the distribution of apo E between VLDL and HDL was found to be a better predictor of disease than levels of either HDL cholesterol or apo A-I [36].

Although there is clearly a relationship between plasma levels of total HDL cholesterol and the risk of atherogenesis, the biologic basis of the association is not clear. Because HDL play critical roles in the centripetal transport of cholesterol, it is attractive to postulate that high levels of HDL particles in blood will facilitate the uptake or processing of cholesterol in the retrieval pathway. However, this hypothesis remains unproven at this time. Other functions of HDL may play significant parts in the inhibition of atherogenesis. These include possible trophic effects on endothelium [37,38], inhibition of hydroperoxidation of LDL lipids and of oxidative modification of apo B [39,40], modification of the compositions of apo B-containing lipoproteins by exchange and transfer, including effects on postprandial lipemia [41–43], and enhancement of the production of prostaglandin by endothelium [44]. The biologic mechanisms by which HDL may influence atherogenesis are discussed in the following sections.

Structure of HDL

Although HDL were the first lipoproteins to be separated from plasma [45], we have less precise knowledge of their structure and speciation than we do of the other major lipoproteins. However, two general concepts now emerging are expected to provide the basis for great advances in our understanding of these lipoproteins.

1   Preparative ultracentrifugation, which for over 40 years has been the classical means of isolating HDL, disrupts the structures of HDL particles and fails to isolate other particles containing apo A-I, because they lie outside the classical density intervals assigned to HDL. Studies on HDL isolated by other means, chiefly immunosorption but also electrophoresis in nondenaturing gels, reveals a distribution of discrete, paucidisperse species, which must have stoichiometric compositions that are closely defined.

2   The distribution of HDL particle species in blood is a function of thermodynamic determinants involving lipid–lipid, lipid–protein, and probably protein–protein associations, and kinetic determinants associated with the function of enzymes such as lipoprotein lipase, lecithin cholesterol acyltransferase (LCAT), and hepatic lipase, as well as catalyzed transfer and exchange of lipids among particle species. Thus, the species distribution of HDL is linked to the metabolism of chylomicrons and the apo B_{100}-containing lipoproteins, as well as to the production and removal of HDL components *per se*. A corollary of this concept is that processes such as esterification and lipid transfer will continue in a blood sample after removal from the donor, running down thermodynamic gradients. It is also implicit that HDL speciation would be expected to change during postprandial lipemia. Thus, for accurate ascertainment of the species distribution in circulating blood, metabolic processes which can proceed spontaneously in plasma must be arrested in the sample until individual particle species can be assayed or isolated.

The structural organization of HDL can be viewed from the standpoint of the ordered lipids they contain [46]. The simplest of such structures are discoidal particles containing phospholipid and some unesterified cholesterol organized as mixed bilayers, with associated apo A-I, apo A-IV, apo E, or apo D. Apo A-I is disposed at the circumferential edges of the disks [46,47]. A major contribution to the lipid binding of these proteins comes from the interaction of amphipathic helices with phospholipid. Sequences that form amphipathic helices are found in varying numbers of 22-mer repeats in the members of the gene family encompassing the exchangeable apos A-I, A-IV, C-II, C-III, and E, all of which associate with native HDL [47]. These α-helices, which begin with prolyl residues, present hydrophobic, and zwitterionic, hydrophilic faces, which interact with the lipid and aqueous phases, respectively [48–50]. A number of observations suggest that other sequences with helix-forming potential serve as hinge domains, allowing the proteins to accommodate increases in the size and shape of the lipoprotein particles [51,52].

Spherical HDL particles of larger diameter are formed by the interlamellar accumulation of hydrophobic lipids, chiefly cholesteryl esters. Triglycerides also enter the lipoprotein core regions to varying degrees, depending on the total plasma triglyceride content and perhaps other determinants [46]. A major protein component of these particles, second only to apo A-I, is apo A-II. This small apoprotein (7 kDa) has a relatively high affinity for HDL lipids and contains a single free sulfhydryl group, which is capable of forming homodimers, and heterodimers with apo E-III or apo E-II. Apo E-IV lacks cysteine and hence cannot form heterodimers. The ability to form heterodimers with apo A-II may account for the greater tendency of apo E-III and E-II to associate with HDL than is the case with apo E-IV [53].

Analytical and preparative ultracentrifugation have classically been capable of separating two major, polydisperse populations of HDL: HDL_2, with a particle mass ranging from 238 to 386 kDa; and HDL_3, with particle masses from 148 to 186 kDa [54]. Numerous studies have demonstrated differences in the content of these fractions in ultracentrifuged plasma from men and women, and changes attendant to manipulation of diet or the administration of drugs or hormones such as estrogens. Further refinement in analytical ultracentrifugation [46] has contributed to the belief that more than two species of HDL exist, though centrifugal techniques appear incapable of isolating all the native species of HDL. Though unable to serve as the basis for isolation of individual particle species of HDL, electrophoresis in nondenaturing gels has revealed as many as eight discrete bands [55,56]. That several species exist which have discriminating particle diameters has been established by gradient gel electrophoresis [57]. The inference may be drawn from studies in transgenic animals that the apolipoproteins themselves contain determinants of the particle distribution of HDL. When human apo A-I is expressed in mice the distribution of HDL particle diameters changes toward a pattern associated with a high ratio of apo A-I to apo A-II [58,59].

Systematic measurement of the loss of HDL constituents during ultracentrifugation indicates that progressive sedimentation of apo A-I takes place which is not attributable to the high ionic strength of the medium, to shear, or to interaction with the tube wall [60]. This observation led to the development of a technique of minimally denaturing immunosorption (selected affinity immunosorption) for the sequestration of all HDL particles in their native states [61]. This technique involves the selection of an eluant-defined, pauciclonal population of antibodies, which will liberate sorbed lipoprotein particles quantitatively during brief exposure to a minimally perturbing eluant such as dilute acetic acid, or bicarbonate. Apo A-I-containing particles isolated in this fashion contain a higher ratio of protein to lipid and are more heterogeneous with respect to particle diameter than HDL prepared by ultracentrifugation [61]. Isoelectric focusing and electrophoresis in nondenaturing gel systems reveal the presence of up to eight discrete bands in these preparations. Two-dimensional gels of proteins associated with immunosorbed particles containing apo A-I reveal more protein species than those from ultracentrifuged HDL [62], with some differences between those associated with particles containing apo A-I only and those that contain apo A-I and apo A-II [62]. Transblot and sequence analysis of the proteins associated with HDL prepared by selected affinity immunosorption has revealed all the recognized exchangeable lipoproteins, apo D, and LCAT. In addition, however, there are a number of proteins with recognized functions, which were not previously known to associate with HDL [63] (ST. Kunitake, C. Carrilli, A. Protter, K. Lau, J. Kane, unpublished data). These include haptoglobin, fibrin, both subunits of the SP 40/40 sulfated glycoprotein, and the binding protein for complement component 4 (C4BP). The C4BP protein is now known to be identical to the proline-rich protein identified previously in plasma [64,65] (unpublished sequence data, C. Pullinger and J. Kane). The SP 40/40 protein is identical to a protein (apo J) that was described as a constituent of HDL [66]. Further, following the observation that HDL bind transition metals, two subspecies of HDL that contain ceruloplasmin and transferrin, respectively, have been isolated [67]. These fractions exert potent inhibition of the oxidation of LDL *in vitro*.

The speciation of HDL must be determined in part by the association of HDL particles with proteins, which occur at low abundance in the lipoprotein population [68]. Thus, it can be calculated that apo C-I [68], transferrin, ceruloplasmin, and the SP 40/40 sulfated glycoprotein [66] occur in HDL in such low abundance that only a fraction of the particles can bear a single copy. Ultracentrifugal and gel electrophoretic analysis, coupled with separation by immunoaffinity against apo A-I and apo A-II sequentially, lends further support to the existence of subspecies of HDL [69]. Application of vertical spin ultracentrifugation and gradient gel electrophoresis to immunoisolated HDL has detected a number of subspecies [52]. From the apparent Stokes radii of the particles, estimated by gradient gel electrophoresis and composition of the particles, it was postulated that HDL particles exist in a quantized series with respect to surface area, in which particles are defined by the number of copies of apo A-I or surrogates, such as apo A-II and apo C-II, which they contain, and upon the alternative association of a hinged helical domain. This is in apparent agreement with the quantized behavior of apo A-I in its interaction with dimyristoyl phosphatidylcholine [70].

Perhaps one of the most clearly defined HDL species to emerge in recent research has been the 65 kDa pre-β-HDL [71]. When apo A-I-containing lipoproteins are subjected to agarose gel electrophoresis after being sequestered from human plasma by selected affinity immunosorption, a clear dichotomy into populations with pre-β- and α-mobilities occurs [71]. Compositional analysis shows the particles with pre-β-mobility to contain about 80% protein. Free and unesterified cholesterol and phospholipid comprise the remainder. Studies of particle size on FPLC and gradient gels indicate a mass compatible with two copies of apo A-I and attendant lipid. Studies employing two-dimensional electrophoresis of radiolabeled HDL reveal three spots in the pre-β-zone [72]. FPLC analysis, however, shows that the particle species with dimeric apo A-I accounts for over 90% of the pre-β-HDL mass in the plasma of fasting humans (S. Kunitake, J. Kane, unpublished results). Between 3 and 20% of the apo A-I in blood is in these pre-β-HDL particles [71,73]. Specific endoprotease attack and circular dichroic analysis demonstrate different conformational dispositions of apo A-I in pre-β- and α-HDL species, respectively [74]. Also the affinity of pre-β-HDL particles for binding sites on hepatic membranes is about two orders of magnitude lower than for species of α-mobility [75].

In the following section, the structural characteristics of HDL will be discussed in the context of metabolic processes in which they participate.

HDL metabolism

The major protein species in HDL appear to be secreted by both intestine and liver. However, the particulate form in which they are secreted from hepatocytes and intestinal epithelium is not entirely clear. Discoidal forms are recognized in single-pass liver perfusates to which LCAT inhibitors have been added to prevent esterification of free cholesterol [76] and in intestinal lymph [77]. Whether any apo A-I or apo E is secreted in this form remains indeterminate at this time, because discoidal particles are not readily discerned among the lipoproteins which can be harvested from Golgi preparations [78]. An alternative model which accounts for some, if not all, *de novo* secretion of HDL constituents is the emergence of large nascent VLDL (liver) or chylomicrons (intestine), which have a high concentration of phospholipids in their surface monolayers, and which bear apo A-I and other exchangeable apolipoproteins [78]. Both apo A-I and A-II are secreted as proproteins, which undergo hydrolysis to their mature forms by specific endo-proteases [79, 80]. The observation that the secretion of murine apo A-I is suppressed in transgenic animals expressing human A-I protein infers feedback regulation of expression [59].

Nascent VLDL appear to be enriched in phosphatidylethanolamine and have little apo E on the particles [81]. Apo A-I-containing lipoproteins in rat liver perfusates contain appreciable triglyceride, when oleate is supplied, supporting the hypothesis that the precursor of HDL is a nascent VLDL that contains apo A-I [82]. A very rapid exchange of phospholipid for unesterified cholesterol occurs as nascent VLDL and chylomicrons come in contact with blood, attended by release of apo A-I, which organizes or becomes incorporated into discoidal HDL particles. These then evolve into spherical particles as LCAT activity produces cholesteryl esters, which then seek the hydrophobic core regions of the particles.

A contribution to HDL mass comes as well from peripheral tissues. Some discoidal particles appear to be secreted by macrophages as a means of mobilizing cholesterol [83]. These particles are accompanied by apo E, some of which is synthesized and secreted by macrophages. Additional cholesterol enters the HDL pool via small particles of pre-β-mobility, which contain apo A-I and which are excellent substrates for esterification by LCAT [84–86]. These particles acquire unesterified cholesterol from cell membranes [87]. Whereas it was posited originally that binding of HDL to cell membranes played a direct role in transfer of membrane cholesterol, the process probably involves desorption into the aqueous medium followed by binding to the HDL species involved [88–91]. Binding of HDL to a specific membrane protein, however, has been reported to increase the mobilization of cholesterol from some interior compartment to the plasma membrane in smooth-muscle cells and fibroblasts [89]. This process does not appear to involve endocytosis of the bound HDL [92]. However, others have not found correspondence between binding of HDL and efflux [91,93]. The rate of cholesterol efflux from cells appears to reflect the cell content of unesterified cholesterol [94]. A distinct process involving net egress of cholesterol from macrophages by endocytosis and subsequent retroendocytosis of HDL has also been reported [94].

The centripetal transport of cholesterol via HDL was first postulated by Glomset [95]. More recent work *in vitro* has demonstrated the key roles of esterification of cholesterol by LCAT, and catalyzed transfer of cholesteryl esters to acceptor lipoproteins [96,97]. Esterification reduces the local chemical potential of free cholesterol, maintaining the gradient along which cholesterol continues to move from tissue sites. Two pathways for the movement of cholesteryl esters to liver appear to exist: cholesteryl esters transferred to apo B-containing lipoproteins are endocytosed with those particles in liver by receptor-mediated processes involving the LDL and putative chylomicron remnant receptors [97]. HDL also appear to interact with liver, yielding cholesteryl esters to the hepatocyte. It is also possible that HDL, which contain apo E, may be endocytosed in liver by the LDL receptor. There is much greater flux along this pathway in certain hyperlipidemic states than in normal individuals. The initial source of free cholesterol may determine which pathway will be followed [98].

In the transfer pathway, continuous remodeling of HDL particles appears to take place [82]. Lipolysis of triglycerides in VLDL and chylomicrons by lipoprotein lipase provides a continuous flux of free cholesterol and phospholipid attendant to remodeling of the surface monolayers of those lipoproteins. There is also a flux of phospholipids from cells to plasma HDL [99,100]. The transfer of cholesteryl esters from HDL to triglyceride-rich lipoproteins and LDL involves exchange of triglycerides into HDL mediated by cholesteryl ester transfer protein (CETP) [101]. The functional importance of CETP is supported by the observation that transgenic animals expressing the protein have reduced levels of cholesterol in HDL [102,103]. Hepatic lipase then hydrolyzes the triglycerides of HDL and some portion of the phospholipid in the complexes, creating smaller, more dense particles that are improved donors for further transfer of cholesteryl esters.

There is a marked stimulation of transfer of phospholipid from chylomicrons to HDL and cholesteryl esters from HDL to chylomicrons in alimentary hyperlipidemia [104,105]. Transfer of cholesteryl esters is enhanced in part by redistribution of CETP during the hydrolysis of chylomicron triglycerides [104]. It is likely that at least one other transfer catalyzing protein is involved in the transformation of HDL in plasma. Phospholipid transfer protein appears to be responsible for facilitating the movement of phospholipids among lipoproteins [106]. Several other putative transfer proteins are under investigation at this time.

The process by which HDL particles transport cholesterol directly to the hepatocyte remains much less clear than the pathway in which cholesteryl esters are transferred to acceptor lipoproteins, which themselves are taken up by receptor-mediated endocytosis. It is possible that several mechanisms participate. However, the markedly greater uptake of sterol than of HDL protein suggests that the predominant pathway involves the separation of sterol from HDL complexes, probably during a binding event [107–109]. Cholesteryl ester transfer protein appears to facilitate transfer of esters to hepatocytes [110]. A number of additional putative uptake mechanisms are under investigation [111–113]. However, results of radiation inactivation studies suggest that the binding site for HDL on hepatocytes may not be a protein [114].

Factors that determine HDL levels in plasma

Metabolic determinants

Increased activity of lipoprotein lipase correlates with higher levels of HDL cholesterol in plasma [115]. Likewise, exercise training, which increases activity of lipoprotein lipase, is generally accompanied by increases in plasma levels in HDL cholesterol levels [116]. In contrast, the activity of hepatic lipase appears to be inversely related to HDL cholesterol levels in plasma [117–119]. Levels of HDL cholesterol are higher in premenopausal females than in males. It is noteworthy that the activity of the enzyme is substantially lower in women than in men, and is reduced by estrogens. Thus, the differential in hepatic lipase may contribute to the higher levels of HDL cholesterol found in women.

Diet and HDL

In most cross-sectional studies, there is an inverse relationship of HDL cholesterol levels with body weight and with obesity [120,121]. Long-term weight loss tends to increase HDL cholesterol levels [122–126]. In general, high fat intakes are associated with higher levels of HDL cholesterol [126,127], and reduction of the intake of fat by one-third among individuals consuming a typical American diet results in a substantial reduction of HDL cholesterol levels [128–131]. This effect is associated with decreased transport rates for HDL apolipoproteins [132]. At relatively lower levels of total fat intake (25%) of calories, the fatty acid composition of the diet appears to have little effect. However, in individuals consuming 30–40% of total calories as fat, some studies have found reductions in HDL cholesterol with major substitution of ω-6 fatty acids for saturates [129,133–137]. In contrast, mono-unsaturates have little effect on HDL cholesterol, despite reductions in LDL cholesterol levels [138]. The effects of ω-3 fatty acids on HDL cholesterol levels have been varied, and may depend greatly on the lipoprotein phenotype of the subjects. In some studies, increases of significant magnitude have been observed [139–141]; in others, decreases [142,143]. Both in epidemiologic studies and in human nutritional experiments, dietary cholesterol has small and variable effects on HDL cholesterol levels; however, significant individual variation may occur. However, cholesterol feeding at 1−1.5 g daily does increase the fraction of HDL that contains apo E [144]. Increased intake of carbohydrates is associated with lower levels of HDL cholesterol. Because carbohydrate is in general substituted for fat, this is equivalent to a reduced fat intake. Most types of soluble or insoluble dietary fiber have little effect on HDL cholesterol level [145]. Epidemiologic surveys tend to find increases in HDL cholesterol with even moderate alcohol intake [146,147]. It is likely that the increased secretion of VLDL [148] and therefore increased intravascular lipolysis of triglyceride is a major contributing factor in this effect [149].

Drugs and HDL

A number of drugs are known to lower levels of HDL cholesterol. Although the control of hypertension is thought to be an essential element in the multifactorial prevention of coronary disease, many antihypertensive agents [150], including diuretics [151] and nondiuretic agents [152], can bring about significant reductions in HDL cholesterol levels, which may vitiate some of the benefit of normalizing arterial pressure. In the case of diuretics, the reduction of HDL cholesterol levels is associated with increased levels of triglycerides in plasma. Even some centrally active sympatholytic agents have this property [153,154]. Also, many, but not all, β-adrenergic blocking agents cause significant reductions in HDL cholesterol. The greatest effect seems to be associated with agents lacking intrinsic sympathomimetic activity, including propranolol and metoprolol [151,152,155,156]. By contrast, the agents that have significant intrinsic sympathomimetic activity have either no effect on HDL or may even induce substantial increases [156,157]. Pindolol, for instance, can increase HDL cholesterol levels by 10−20%. This interesting theme relating sympathomimetic activity to HDL cholesterol levels can be traced still further, in that β agonists such as terbutaline have also been shown to induce increases in HDL cholesterol [158].

Reductions in HDL cholesterol levels usually occur in individuals taking probucol. This is accompanied by reductions in the apo A-I content of plasma. Recent findings indicate that the reduced level of HDL cholesterol is chiefly a reflection of increased efficiency of transfer of cholesteryl esters from HDL resulting from increased levels of cholesteryl ester transfer protein. This presents the possibility that the reduction of HDL cholesterol may be beneficial with respect to reverse transport [159,160].

Progestins may have either neutral or negative effects on HDL cholesterol levels. Recent observations suggest that the extent of lowering of HDL cholesterol is a direct reflection of the androgenic potential of individual progestigens [161].

No doubt the most effective agent in increasing levels of HDL cholesterol in plasma is niacin [162,163]. A portion of this effect is attributable to its marked activity in lowering plasma triglyceride levels, based on the inverse relationship of HDL cholesterol and plasma triglycerides discussed above. Its action on plasma triglycerides appears to be due to a decrease in VLDL triglyceride export, either via a decrease in the flux of fatty acids to liver from peripheral adipocytes or by specific action on VLDL production or secretion. Niacin also induces an increase in HDL apoprotein mass, chiefly reflecting a decrease in catabolism. In some subjects, HDL cholesterol levels may increase 60% or more on daily doses of $4-6$ g of niacin. Fractionation of HDL on gradient gels reveals a marked increase in the larger diameter particles (HDL_{2b}) when hyperlipidemic subjects are receiving niacin [164]. Smaller but also significant increases in HDL cholesterol levels are observed during the administration of the fibric acid derivatives clofibrate and gemfibrozil [165]. Again, a portion of the effect is attributable to lowering of triglyceride levels, probably by stimulation of removal mechanisms. Again, however, there is an increase in HDL protein mass.

Estrogens induce increases in total HDL mass, mediated through increases in the number of larger HDL_2 particles [166], changes that correlate with protective effects on the coronary vessels [167]. As discussed above, a major mechanism appears to be a substantial reduction in hepatic lipase activity. However, increased synthesis of apo A-I is also involved [166]. Another class of drugs that increases synthetic rates of apo A-I are phenytoin and related anticonvulsants [168,169]. The increase principally occurs among the HDL_2 particle population. Recent data suggest that these agents may decrease risk of coronary disease [169]. Significant increases in HDL cholesterol have been also observed in women but not in men during treatment with cimetidine [170,171]. This is accompanied by reduction of levels of sex hormone binding globulin (SHBG). It can be concluded that the effect is not due to the receptor blockade, because ranitidine is without effect on HDL. Furthermore, the lack of effect of cimetidine on plasma triglycerides indicates that the observed effect is probably not due to exchange of lipids between HDL and triglyceride-rich lipoproteins [170].

Smoking and HDL levels

From an epidemiologic standpoint cigarette smoking is a significant determinant of HDL cholesterol levels in both men and women [172–

176]. Though it is likely that smoking also contributes in other ways to the causation of coronary artery disease, the decrements in HDL cholesterol which occur with the consumption of 20–40 cigarettes daily could contribute materially to risk, based on the general relationship of HDL cholesterol to coronary risk in the population. The decrement in both men and women is from 4 to 8 mg/dl in heavy smokers. It has been pointed out that this may be masked to some extent by the fact that smokers tend to ingest more ethanol then do nonsmokers.

Genetics of HDL

The clearest evidence for genetic determinacy of HDL levels to date comes from studies in inbred mouse strains [177–179]. A single gene locus (*Ath-1*) modulates the response of HDL to high-fat diets and is a major determinant of risk of atherosclerosis [180,181]. In mice, an important determinant cosegregates with the apo A-II gene locus, which regulates the production rate of apo A-II [179]. This results in changes in the stoichiometry of apo A-I and apo A-II in HDL, and in the lipid content of the particles. Because levels of message are comparable in strains which do, and do not, bear the mutation, it was hypothesized that the different rates of apo A-II production reflected differences in translational efficiency. Proof of this hypothesis has been forthcoming from study of rates of translation *in vitro*

Clinical observation has provided much of the inferential support for significant genetic control of HDL levels in humans, to date. Clearly, hypoalphalipoproteinemia tends to be familial, often with what appears to be dominant transmission. A major underlying mechanism may involve increased catabolic rates for apo A-I and A-II in individuals with low levels of HDL cholesterol, whether or not they have hyper-triglyceridemia [182]. It is probable that multiple loci and alleles are involved in regulation of HDL levels in the population at large [179, 183–191] though major effects of a single gene are perceived within some kindreds. In the Lipid Research Clinic Family Study some evidence was found for a major gene effect on HDL levels, which did not conform to a clear Mendelian transmission pattern, though analysis was impaired by the small number of individuals in the kindreds studied [183]. A study of a large number of monozygous and dizygous twins has revealed interaction of familial factors with exogenous determinants [192]. The effects of alcohol and exercise tended to be confounded by familial factors, whereas the effects of smoking, body mass, and exogenous estrogens appear to be independent of familial influence.

The gene for apo A-I is located in a cluster with the genes for apo C-

III and apo A-IV [193,194] on chromosome 11, whereas the gene for apo A-II is located on chromosome 1 [195]. A number of restriction fragment length polymorphisms (RFLP) have been identified at both loci. A *Pst*I RFLP at the A-I locus has been associated with HDL cholesterol levels [196]. The *Pst*I polymorphism was also associated with plasma levels of apo A-I in a sample of British men [197]. A single base substitution has been described in the 5′ flanking region of the A-I–C-III–A-IV complex, located close to CACAT and TAAAATA sequences, which correlates with higher concentrations of apo A-I and HDL cholesterol levels in plasma, again in British males [198]. All such observations must be considered tentative at this time, and likely to be influenced strongly by ethnicity.

Major genetic disorders of HDL

Two of the most striking disorders affecting HDL result from abnormalities of LCAT and CETP, respectively. Several other genetic disorders are based on abnormalities of constituent proteins of HDL. Another, Tangier disease, remains enigmatic, but is characterized by abnormally rapid catabolism of HDL.

LCAT deficiency is manifested clinically in the homozygous state. LCAT activity is very low though the protein may be detectable immunochemically in plasma. The biochemical effect of LCAT deficiency centers on the accumulation of unesterified cholesterol in plasma, organized in abnormal lamellar lipoproteins and in an excess of small HDL particles resembling pre-β-HDL [199]. Secondary abnormalities occur in all other lipoproteins, largely due to accumulation of amphipathic lipids [200,201]. Clinical features include characteristic corneal opacities, glomerulopathy, neuropathy, and the presence of abnormal erythrocytes (target cells) which tend to hemolyze readily. Premature atherosclerosis has been observed in a number of patients. A related disorder ("fish eye disease") is characterized by corneal infiltrates and selective inability to esterify cholesterol in HDL [202,203].

Deficiency of CETP is often accompanied by high levels of HDL cholesterol in the presence of normal LCAT activity [204–205]. The relative absence of atherosclerosis in the few patients described to date raises the question as to whether the role of transfer of esters from HDL to acceptor lipoproteins is critical to centripetal transport in humans. It is possible that proteins other than CETP also function to catalyze transfer of cholesterol esters.

A number of sequence anomalies of apo A-I are now known [206]. The most metabolically significant disorders of the A-I locus detected so far are: a major rearrangement which causes deficiency of both apo A-I and apo C-III [207], a condition associated with premature coronary artery disease; and a mutation that introduces a cystine into the sequence of apo A-I (A-I Milano), which has major effects on HDL particles, mediated at least in part by the formation of disulfide-linked homodimers and heterodimers involving apo E [207,208].

Tangier disease is characterized clinically by the accumulation of cholesteryl esters in many tissues including the tonsils, lymph nodes, cornea, spleen, and intestinal mucosa [209]. Peripheral neuropathy has been observed in some patients. HDL levels in plasma are extremely low and the content of apo A-I may be as low as 2–3 mg/dl. Levels of LDL cholesterol are often as low as 20 mg/dl. The LDL have an unusually high content of triglycerides which leads to alterations in the conformation of apo B_{100} [72]. There are also abnormalities of chylomicron metabolism. There is a relative increase in the ratio of proapolipoprotein A-I to mature apo A-I in plasma [210] and the fractional catabolic rates of apo A-I and apo A-II are increased [211]. Though heterozygotes may be discernible by having lower levels of HDL cholesterol than normal, they do not seem to develop any of the clinical stigmata associated with the disorder. Coronary artery disease has appeared in some patients in middle age and beyond, but there appears to be no striking trend toward premature atherosclerosis in Tangier disease.

Strategies directed at retarding atherosclerosis by increasing the HDL content of plasma

Whether increasing levels of HDL cholesterol in plasma will inhibit atherogenesis remains speculative because evidence is lacking in humans that increasing the content of HDL in plasma *per se* will inhibit atherosclerosis or induce regression. In one study the repeated infusion of HDL into rabbits appeared to modify the atherogenic process significantly [212]. Considerable support for this concept comes from the observation that transgenic overexpression of human apolipoprotein A-I protects against atherosclerosis in a strain of mice susceptible to diet induced atherogenesis [213]. Perhaps the most impressive inference in humans comes from the results of the Helsinki study in which analysis on a proportional hazards model showed the increase in HDL cholesterol to be a more significant contributor to the outcome than changes which occurred in LDL [214]. Again, as described above, the reciprocal relationship of triglycerides between VLDL and HDL begs the question whether changes in VLDL or HDL may be the primary process involved. Further inferential support for a strategy directed at HDL comes from the observation that the administration of estrogen to postmenopausal women has a favorable impact on the development of coronary disease [167]. Also, in both the Familial Atherosclerosis Treatment Study (FATS) and Class II trial changes in HDL cholesterol contributed independently to the outcome [215]. In the SCOR intervention study, there was a similar trend [216].

The structural and functional properties of the particle species of HDL will have to be elucidated in detail before an HDL strategy can be fully exploited. It is probable that certain species of HDL have no protective function. Therefore it is possible that some situations in which total HDL cholesterol level is high may afford little protection [217]. Similarly, an increased rate of transfer of cholesteryl esters from HDL to acceptor lipoproteins may lower HDL cholesterol levels but have a beneficial effect on recovery of cholesterol from peripheral sites [217]. This area of lipoprotein research clearly holds enormous promise of potential therapeutic venues in the prevention of coronary disease. The recent demonstrations of regression of human coronary lesions with aggressive drug therapy of atherogenic hyperlipidemia [215,216,218] suggest that a comprehensive multifactorial intervention coupling HDL-directed strategies with others directed at reducing levels of LDL and preventing oxidative modification of lipoproteins may provide a broadly effective means of inhibiting or reversing atherosclerosis.

References

1 Rhoads GG, Gulbrandsen CL, Kagan A. Serum lipoproteins and coronary heart disease in a population study of Hawaii Japanese men. *N Engl J Med* 1976;294: 293–8.
2 Gordon T, Castelli W, Hjortland M, Kannel W, Dawber T. High density lipoprotein as a protective factor against coronary heart disease: the Framingham Study. *Am J Med* 1977;66:707–14.
3 Miller NE, Thelle DS, Førde OH, Mjøs OD. The Tromsø heart study: high-density lipoprotein and coronary heart-disease: a prospective case-control study. *Lancet* 1977;i:964–8.
4 Wilson PWF, Abbott RD, Castelli WP. High density lipoprotein cholesterol and mortality. The Framingham Heart Study. *Arteriosclerosis* 1988;8:737–41.
5 Committee TLRCPE. Plasma lipid distribution in selected North American Populations: The Lipid Research Clinics Program Prevalence Study. *Circulation* 1979;60:427–39.
6 Gordon DJ, Ekelund LG, Karon JM *et al.* Predictive value of the exercise tolerance test for mortality in North American men: The Lipid Research Clinics Mortality Follow-Up Study. *Circulation* 1986;74:252–61.
7 Jacobs DR, Mebane IL, Bangdiwala SI, Criqui MH, Tyroler HA. High density lipoprotein cholesterol as a predictor of cardiovascular disease mortality in men and women: The Follow-up Study of the Lipid Research Clinics Prevalence Study. *Am J Epidemiol* 1990;131:32–47.

8 Program TLRC. The Coronary Primary Prevention Trial: design and implementation. *J Chron Dis* 1979;32:609−31.

9 Program LRC. The Lipid Research Clinics Coronary Primary Prevention Trial results. I. Reduction in incidence of coronary heart disease. *JAMA* 1984;251:351−64.

10 Gordon DJ, Probstfeld JL, Garrison RJ *et al*. High density lipoprotein cholesterol and cardiovascular disease. Four prospective American studies. *Circulation* 1989;79:8−14.

11 Brunner D, Weisbort J, Mashulam N *et al*. Relation of serum total cholesterol and high-density lipoprotein cholesterol percentage to the incidence of definite coronary events. Twenty-year follow-up of the Donolo-Tel-Aviv prospective coronary artery disease study. *Am J Cardiol* 1987;59:1271−6.

12 Livshits G, Weisbort J, Meshulam N, Brunner D. Multivariate analysis of the twenty-year follow-up of the Donolo-Tel Aviv Prospective Coronary Artery Disease Study and the usefulness of high density lipoprotein cholesterol percentage. *Am J Cardiol* 1989;63:676−81.

13 Goldbourt U, Medalie JH. High density lipoprotein cholesterol and incidence of coronary heart disease—the Israeli ischemic heart disease study. *Am J Epidemiol* 1979;109:296−308.

14 Assmann G, Schulte M. *The PROCAM Trial—Prospective Cardiovascular Muenster Trial*. Hedingen/Zuerich: Panscientia Verlag, 1986.

15 Enger SC, Hjerman T, Foss OP. High density lipoprotein cholesterol and myocardial infarction and sudden coronary death: a prospective case-control study in middle-aged men of the Oslo study. *Artery* 1979;5:170−81.

16 Goldbourt U, Holtzman E, Neufield HN. Total and high density lipoprotein cholesterol in the serum and risk of mortality: evidence of the threshold effect. *Br Med J* 1985;290:1239−43.

17 Wiklund O, Wilhelmsen L, Elmfeldt D *et al*. Alpha-lipoprotein cholesterol concentration in relation to subsequent myocardial infarction in hyper-cholesterolemic men. *Atherosclerosis* 1980;37:47−53.

18 Keys A, Karvonen MJ, Punsar S *et al*. HDL serum cholesterol and 24-year mortality of men in Finland. *Int J Epidemiol* 1984;13:428−35.

19 Pocock SJ, Shaper AG, Phillips AN, Walden M, Whitehead TP. High density lipoprotein cholesterol is not a major risk factor for ischemic heart disease in British men. *Br Med J* 1986;292:515−19.

20 Levy RI, Klimov AN. High density lipoprotein cholesterol (HDL-C) and mortality in USSR and US middle age men: the Collaborative US−USSR Mortality Follow-Up Study. *Circulation* 1987;76(Suppl IV):IV-167.

21 Myers LH, Phillips NR, Havel RJ. Mathematical evaluation of methods for estimation of the concentration of the major lipid components of human serum lipoproteins. *J Lab Clin Med* 1976;88:491−505.

22 Carlson LA, Böttiger LE. Risk factors for ischaemic heart disease in men and women. Results of the 19-year follow-up of the Stockholm Prospective Study. *Acta Med Scand* 1985;218:207−11.

23 Åberg H, Lithell H, Selinius I, Hedstrand H. Serum triglycerides are a risk factor for myocardial infarction but not for angina pectoris: results from a 10-year follow-up of Uppsala Primary Prevention Study. *Atherosclerosis* 1985;54:89−97.

24 Lapidus L, Bengtsson C, Lindqvist O, Sigurdsson JA, Rybo E. Triglycerides—main lipid risk factor for cardiovascular disease in women? *Acta Med Scand* 1985;217:481−9.

25 Castelli WP. The triglyceride issue: a view from Framingham. *Am Heart J* 1986;112:432−7.

26 Barbir M, Wile D, Trayner I, Aber VR, Thompson GR. High prevalance of hypertriglyceridaemia and apolipoprotein abnormalities in coronary artery disease. *Br Heart J* 1988;60:397−403.

27 Nikkilä M, Koivula T, Niemelä K, Sisto T. High density lipoprotein cholesterol and

triglycerides as markers of angiographically assessed coronary artery disease. *Br Heart J* 1990;63:78–81.

28 Austin MA. Plasma triglyceride as a risk factor for coronary heart disease. The epidemiologic evidence and beyond. *Am J Epidemiol* 1989;129:249–59.

29 Avins AL, Haber RJ, Hulley SB. The status of hypertriglyceridemia as a risk factor for coronary heart disease. *Clin Lab Med* 1989;9:153–68.

30 Miller NE. Associations of high-density lipoprotein subclasses and apolipoproteins with ischemic heart disease and coronary atherosclerosis. *Am Heart J* 1987;113:589–97.

31 Miller NE, Hammett F, Saltissi S *et al*. Relation of angiographically defined coronary artery disease to plasma lipoprotein subfractions and apolipoproteins. *Br Med J* 1981;282:1741.

32 Wallentin L, Sundin B. HDL_2 and HDL_3 lipid levels in coronary artery disease. *Atherosclerosis* 1985;59:131.

33 Levy RI, Brensike JF, Epstein SE *et al*. The influence of changes in lipid values induced by cholestyramine and diet on progression of coronary artery disease: results of the NHLBI Type II Intervention Study. *Circulation* 1984;69:335.

34 Fager G, Wiklund O, Olofsson S-O, Wilhelmsen L, Bodjers G. Multivariate analysis of serum apolipoproteins and risk factors in relation to acute myocardial infarction. *Arteriosclerosis* 1981;1:273.

35 James RW, Martin B, Pometta D, Grab B, Suenram A. Apoprotein D in a healthy male population and in male myocardial infarction patients and their male first degree relatives. *Atherosclerosis* 1986;60:49.

36 Bittolo BG, Cazzolato G, Saccardi M, Kostner GM, Avogaro P. Total plasma apo E and high density lipoprotein apo E in survivors of myocardial infarction. *Atherosclerosis* 1984;53:69.

37 Tauber J-P, Cheng J, Gospodarowicz D. Effect of high and low density lipoproteins on proliferation of bovine vascular endothelial cells. *J Clin Invest* 1980;66:697–706.

38 Darbon JM, Tournier JF, Tauber JP, Bayard F. Possible role of protein phosphorylation in the mitogenic effect of high density lipoproteins on cultured vascular endothelial cells. *J Biol Chem* 1986;261:8002–8.

39 Klimov AN, Kozhemiakin LA, Pleskov UM, Andreeva LI. Antioxidant effect of high-density lipoproteins in peroxidation of low-density lipoproteins. *Bull Eksper Biologii I Med* 1987;103:550.

40 Ohta T, Takata K, Horiuchi S, Morino Y, Matsuda I. Protective effect of lipoproteins containing apoprotein A-I on Cu^{2+}-catalyzed oxidation of human low density lipoproteins. *FEBS Lett* 1989;257:435–8.

41 Patsch JR, Karlin JB, Scott LW, Smith LC, Gotto AM Jr. Inverse relationship between blood levels of high density lipoprotein subfraction 2 and magnitude of postprandial lipemia. *Proc Natl Acad Sci USA* 1983;80:1449–53.

42 Kashyap ML, Barnhart RL, Srivastava LS *et al*. Alimentary lipemia: plasma high-density lipoproteins and apoproteins CII and CIII in healthy subjects. *Am J Clin Nutr* 1983;37:233–43.

43 Zilversmit DB. Atherogenesis: a postprandial phenomenon. *Circulation* 1979;60:473–85.

44 Spector AA, Scanu AM, Kaduse TL *et al*. Effect of human plasma lipoproteins on prostacyclin production by cultured endothelial cells. *J Lipid Res* 1985;26:288–99.

45 Macheboeuf MA. Recherches sur les phosphoaminolipides et les sterides du serum et du plasma sanguins. *Bull Soc Chim Biol* 1929;11:268.

46 Small DM. HDL system: A short review of structure and metabolism. *Atherosclerosis Rev* 1987;16:1–8.

47 Luo C-C, Li W-H, Moore MN, Chan L. Structure and evolution of the apolipoprotein multigene family. *J Mol Biol* 1986;187:325–40.

48 Kanellis P, Romans AY, Johnson BJ *et al*. Studies of synthetic peptide analogs of the

amphipathic helix: effect of charged amino acid topography on lipid affinity. *J Biol Chem* 1980;255:11464−72.

49 Anantharamaiah GM, Jones JL, Brouillette CG *et al*. Studies of synthetic peptide analogs of the amphipathic helix. *J Biol Chem* 1985;260:10248−55.

50 Segrest JP, Chung BH, Brouillette CG, Kanellis P, McGahan R. Studies of synthetic peptide analogs of the amphipathic helix: Competitive displacement of exchangeable apolipoproteins from native lipoproteins. *J Biol Chem* 1983;258:2290−5.

51 Brouillette CG, Jones JL. Ng T *et al*. Structure of the high density lipoproteins: Studies of apo A-I:PC recombinants by high field proton NMR, gradient gel electrophoresis and electron microscopy. *Biochemistry* 1984;23:359−67.

52 Cheung MC, Segrest JP, Albers JJ *et al*. Characterization of high density lipoprotein subspecies: structural studies by single vertical spin ultracentrifugation and immunoaffinity chromatography. *J Lipid Res* 1987;28:913−29.

53 Weisgraber KH. Apolipoprotein E distribution among plasma lipoproteins: role of the cystine−arginine interchange at residue 112. *J Lipid Res* 1990;31:1503−11.

54 Nelson GJ. *Blood Lipids and Lipoproteins: Quantitation, Composition, and Metabolism*. New York: Robert E. Krieger, 1979.

55 Utermann G. Disc-electrophoresis patterns of human serum high density lipoproteins. *Clin Chim Acta* 1972;36:521.

56 Janecki J, Fijalkowska A. A simple method of quantitative estimation of the subfractions of human small molecular diameter lipoproteins. *J Clin Chem Clin Biochem* 1979;17:789.

57 Blanche PJ, Gong EL, Forte TM, Nichols AV. Characterization of human high density lipoproteins by gradient gel electrophoresis. *Biochim Biophys Acta* 1981;665:408−19.

58 Chajek-Chaul T, Hayek T, Welsh A, Breslow JL. Expression of the human apolipoprotein A-I gene in transgenic mice alters high density lipoprotein (HDL) particle size distribution and diminishes selective uptake of HDL cholesteryl esters. *Proc Natl Acad Sci* 1991;88:6731−7.

59 Rubin EM, Ishida BY, Clift SM, Krauss RM. Expression of human apolipoprotein A-I in transgenic mice results in reduced plasma levels of murine apolipoprotein AI and the appearance of two new high density lipoprotein size subclasses. *Proc Natl Acad Sci USA* 1991;88:434−8.

60 Kunitake ST, Kane JP. Factors affecting the integrity of high density lipoproteins in the ultracentrifuge. *J Lipid Res* 1982;23:936−40.

61 McVicar JP, Kunitake ST, Hamilton RL, Kane JP. Characteristics of human lipoproproteins isolated by selected-affinity immunosorption of apolipoprotein A-I (high density lipoproteins). *Proc Natl Acad Sci USA* 1984;81:1356−60.

62 James RW, Hochstrasser D, Tissot J-D *et al*. Protein heterogeneity of lipoprotein particles containing apolipoprotein A-I without apolipoprotein A-II and apolipoprotein A-I with apolipoprotein A-II isolated from human plasma. *J Lipid Res* 1988;29:1557−71.

63 Carrilli CT, Kunitake ST, Protter AA, Kane JP. Protein characterization of HDL purified by selected affinity immunoabsorption. *Arteriosclerosis* 1990;10:808a.

64 Sata T, Havel RJ, Kotite L, Kane JP. New protein in human blood plasma, rich in proline, with lipid-binding properties. *Proc Natl Acad Sci USA* 1976;73:1063−7.

65 Matsuguchi T, Okamura S, Aso T, Sata T, Niho Y. Molecular cloning of the cDNA for proline-rich protein (PRP): identity of PRP as C4b binding protein. *Biochem Biophys Res Commun* 1989;165:138−44.

66 de Silva HV, Stuart WD, Duvic CR *et al*. A 70-kDa apolipoprotein designated apoJ is a marker for subclasses of human plasma high density lipoproteins. *J Biol Chem* 1990;265:13240−7.

67 Kunitake ST, Jarvis MR, Hamilton RL, Kane JP. Binding of transition metals by apolipoprotein A-10-containing plasma lipoproteins. Inhibition of oxidation of low density lipoproteins. *Proc Natl Acad Sci USA* 1992;89.

68 Kane JP. Speciation of HDL. *Adv Exp Med Biol* 1986;201:29—35.

69 Cheung MC, Wolf AC, Lum KD, Tollefson JH, Albers JJ. Distribution and localization of lecithin:cholesterol acyltransferase and cholesteryl ester transfer activity in A-I-containing lipoproteins. *J Lipid Res* 1986;27:1135—44.

70 Brouillette CG, Jones JL, Ng TC *et al.* Structural studies of apolipoprotein A-I/phosphatidylcholine recombinants by high-field proton NMR, nondenaturing gradient gel electrophoresis, and electron microscopy. *Biochemistry* 1984;23:359—67.

71 Kunitake S, La Sala K, Kane J. Apoprotein A-I-containing lipoproteins with pre-beta electrophoretic mobility. *J Lipid Res* 1985;26:549—53.

72 Francone OL, Gurakar A, Fielding C. Distribution and functions of lecithin: cholesterol acyltransferase and cholesteryl ester transfer protein in plasma lipoproteins. *J Biol Chem* 1989;264:7066—72.

73 Ishida BY, Frohlich J, Fielding CJ. Prebeta-migrating high density lipoprotein: quantitation in normal and hyperlipemic plasma by solid phase radioimmunoassay following electrophoretic transfer. *J Lipid Res* 1987;28:778—86.

74 Kunitake ST, Young SG, Chen GC *et al.* Conformation of apolipoprotein B-100 in the low density lipoproteins of Tangier disease. *J Biol Chem* 1990;265:20739—46.

75 Mendel CM, Kunitake ST, Kane JP. Discrimination between subclasses of human high density lipoproteins by the HDL binding sites of bovine liver. *Biochim Biophys Acta* 1986;875:59—68.

76 Hamilton RL, Williams MC, Fielding CJ, Havel RJ. Discoidal bilayer structure of nascent high density lipoproteins from perfused rat liver. *J Clin Invest* 1976;58: 667—80.

77 Glickman RM, Magun AM. High density lipoprotein formation by the intestine. *Methods Enzymol* 1986;129:519—36.

78 Hamilton RL, Moorehouse A, Havel RJ. Isolation and properties of nascent lipoproteins from highly purified rat hepatocytic Golgi fractions. *J Lipid Res* 1991;32: 529—43.

79 Edelstein C, Scanu AM. Extracellular posttranslational proteolytic processing of apolipoproteins. In *Biochemistry and Biology of Plasma Lipoproteins* (eds AM Scanu, A Spector). New York: Marcel Dekker, 1986:53.

80 Gordon JI, Sims HF, Edelstein C, Scanu AM, Strauss AW. Human proapolipoprotein A-II is cleaved following secretion from Hep G2 cells by a thiol protease. *J Biol Chem* 1984;259:15556.

81 Hamilton RL, Fielding PE. Nascent very low density lipoproteins from rat hepatocytic Golgi fractions are enriched in phosphatidylethanolamine. *Biochem Biophys Res Commun* 1989;160:162—7.

82 Marsh JB, Diffenderfer MR. Isolation of nascent high-density lipoprotein from rat liver perfusates by immunoaffinity chromatography: effects of oleic acid infusions. *Metabolism* 1991;40:26—30.

83 Basu SK, Goldstein JL, Brown MS. Independent pathways for secretion of cholesterol and apolipoprotein E by macrophages. *Science* 1983;219:871—3.

84 Fielding CJ. Early events in the transfer of cell-derived cholesterol to human plasma—the role of prebeta-migrating high density lipoprotein species. In *High Density Lipoproteins and Atherosclerosis II* (ed. NE Miller). Amsterdam: Excerpta Medica, 1989:257—62.

85 Kunitake S, La Sala K, Mendel C, Chen G, Kane J. Some unique properties of apo A-I containing lipoproteins with pre-beta electrophoretic mobility. In *Proceedings of the Workshop on Lipoprotein Heterogeneity* (ed. K Lippel). Rockville: NIH, 1987:419—28.

86 Francone OL, Guraker A, Fielding C. Distribution and functions of lecithin:cholesterol acyltransferase and cholesteryl ester transfer protein in plasma lipoproteins. *J Diol Chem* 1989;264:7066—72.

87 Castro GR, Fielding CJ. Early incorporation of cell-derived cholesterol into pre-β-migrating high-density lipoprotein. *Biochemistry* 1988;27:25—9.

88 Rothblat GH, Phillips MC. Mechanism of cholesterol efflux from cells. *J Biol Chem* 1982;257:4775—82.

89 Slotte JP, Oram JF, Bierman EL. Binding of high density lipoproteins to cell receptors promotes translocation of cholesterol from intracellular membranes to the cell surface. *J Biol Chem* 1987;262:12904−7.

90 Phillips MC, Rothblat GH. Cholesterol flux between high density lipoproteins and cells. *Atherosclerosis Rev* 1987;16:57−86.

91 Mendel CM, Kunitake ST. Cell-surface binding sites for high density lipoproteins do not mediate efflux of cholesterol from human fibroblasts in tissue culture. *J Lipid Res* 1988;29:1171−8.

92 Oram JF, Johnson CJ, Brown TA. Interaction of high density lipoprotein with its receptor on cultured fibroblasts and macrophages. *J Biol Chem* 1987;262:2405−10.

93 Karlin JB, Johnson WJ, Benedict CR *et al*. Cholesterol flux between cells and high density lipoprotein: lack of relationship to specific binding of the lipoprotein to the cell surface. *J Biol Chem* 1987;262:12557−64.

94 DeLamatre J, Wolfbauer G, Phillips MC, Rothblat GH. Role of apolipoproteins in cellular cholesterol efflux. *Biochim Biophys Acta* 1986;875:419−28.

95 Glomset JA. The plasma lecithin:cholesterol acyltransferase reaction. *J Lipid Res* 1968;9:155−67.

96 Fielding PE, Fielding CJ, Havel RJ, Kane JP, Tun P. Cholesterol net transport, esterification, and transfer in human hyperlipidemic plasma. *J Clin Invest* 1983; 71:449−60.

97 Fielding CJ. Factors affecting the rate of catalyzed transfer of cholesteryl esters in plasma. *Am Heart J* 1987;113:532−7.

98 Miida T, Fielding CJ, Fielding PE. Mechanism of transfer of LDL-derived free cholesterol to HDL subfractions in human plasma. *Biochemistry* 1990;29:10469−74.

99 Stein Y, Glangeaud MC, Fainaru M, Stein O. The removal of cholesterol from aortic smooth muscle cells in culture and Landschutz ascites cells by fractions of human high density apolipoprotein. *Biochim Biophys Acta* 1975;380:106−18.

100 Bielicki JK, Johnson WJ, Glick JM, Rothblatt GH. Efflux of phospholipids from fibroblasts with normal and elevated levels of cholesterol. *Biochim Biophys Acta* 1991;1084: 7−11.

101 Tall AR. Plasma lipid transfer proteins. *J Lipid Res* 1986;27:361−7.

102 Agellon LB, Walsh A, Hayek T *et al*. Reduced high density lipoprotein cholesterol in human cholesteryl ester transfer protein transgenic mice. *J Biol Chem* 1991;266:10796−801.

103 Walsh A, Ito Y, Breslow JL. Apolipoprotein AI gene expression in transgenic mice. *Biotechnology* 1991;16:227−35.

104 Tall AR. Metabolism of postprandiol lipoproteins. *Meth Enzymol* 1985;129:469−82. *J Clin Invest* (in press).

105 Castro GR, Fielding CJ. Effects of postprandial lipemia on plasma cholesterol metabolism. *J Clin Invest* 1985;75:874−82.

106 Tollefson JH, Ravnik S, Albers JJ. Isolation and characterization of a phospholipid transfer protein (LTP-II) from human plasma. *J Lipid Res* 1988;29:1593−602.

107 Pittman RC, Knecht TP, Rosenbaum MS, Taylor JCA. A nonendocytotic mechanism for the selective uptake of high density lipoprotein-associated cholesterol esters. *J Biol Chem* 1987;262:2443−50.

108 Glass C, Pittman RC, Weinstein DB, Steinberg D. Dissociation of tissue uptake of cholesterol ester from that of apoprotein A-I of rat plasma high density lipoprotein: selective delivery of cholesterol ester to liver, adrenal, and gonad. *Proc Natl Acad Sci USA* 1983;80:5435−9.

109 Stein Y, Dabash Y, Hollander G, Halperin G, Stein O. Metabolism of HDL-cholesteryl ester in the rat, studied with a nonhydrolyzable analog, cholesteryl linoleyl ether. *Biochim Biophys Acta* 1983;752:98−105.

110 Granot E, Tabas I, Tall AR. Human plasma cholesteryl ester transfer protein enhances the transfer of cholesteryl ester from high density lipoproteins into cultured HepG^2 cells. *J Biol Chem* 1987;262:3182−7

111 Tozuka M, Fidge N. Purification and characterization of two high-density-lipoprotein-

binding proteins from rat and human liver. *Biochem J* 1989;261:239–44.

112 Kambouris AM, Roach PD, Calvert GD, Nestel PJ. Retroendocytosis of high density lipoproteins by the human hepatoma cell line, HepG2. *Arteriosclerosis* 1990;10:582–90.

113 Schouten D, Kleinherenbrink-Stins MF, Brouwer A *et al*. Characterization *in vitro* of interaction of human apolipoprotein E-free high density lipoprotein with human hepatocytes. *Arteriosclerosis* 1990;10:1127–35.

114 Mendel CM, Kunitake ST, Kane JP, Kempner ES. Radiation inactivation of binding sites for high density lipoproteins in human fibroblast membranes. *J Biol Chem* 1988;263:1314–19.

115 Nikkila EA, Taskinen M, Kekki M. Relationship of plasma high-density lipoprotein cholesterol to lipoprotein-lipase activity in adipose tissue and skeletal muscle of man. *Atherosclerosis* 1978;29:497–501.

116 Kiens B, Lithell H. Lipoprotein metabolism influenced by training-induced changes in human skeletal muscle. *J Clin Invest* 1989;83:558–64.

117 Kuusi TP, Saarinen P, Nikkila EA. Evidence for the role of hepatic endothelial lipase in the metabolism of plasma high density lipoprotein₂ in man. *Atherosclerosis* 1980;36:589–93.

118 Tikannen MJ, Nikkila EA, Kuusi T, Sipinen S. Different effects of two progestins on plasma high density lipoprotein (HDL₂) and postheparin plasma hepatic lipase activity. *Atherosclerosis* 1981;40:365–9.

119 Applebaum-Bowden D, McLean P, Steinmetz A *et al*. Lipoprotein, apolipoprotein, and lipolytic enzyme changes following estrogen administration in postmenopausal women. *J Lipid Res* 1990;30:1895–906.

120 Glueck CJ, Taylor HL, Jacobs D *et al*. Plasma high-density lipoprotein cholesterol. Associations with measurements of body mass. The Lipid Research Clinics Program Prevalence Study. *Circulation* 1980;62(Suppl 4):62.

121 Knuiman JT, West CE, Burema J. Serum total and high density lipoprotein cholesterol concentrations and body mass index in adult men from 13 countries. *Am J Epidemiol* 1982;116:631.

122 Zimmerman J, Kaufmann NA, Fainaru M. Effect of weight loss in moderate obesity on plasma lipoprotein and apolipoprotein levels and on high density lipoprotein composition. *Arteriosclerosis* 1984;4:115.

123 Friedman CI, Fako JM, Patel ST *et al*. Serum lipoprotein responses during active and stable weight reduction in reproductive obese females. *J Clin Endocrinol Metab* 1982;55:258.

124 Wolf RN, Grundy SM. Influence of weight reduction on plasma lipoproteins in obese patients. *Arteriosclerosis* 1983;3:160.

125 Follick MJ, Abrams DB, Smith TW, Henderson O, Herbert PN. Contrasting short- and long-term effects of weight loss on lipoprotein levels. *Arch Intern Med* 1984;144:1571.

126 Knuiman JT, West CE, Katan MB, Hautvast JGAJ. Total cholesterol and high density lipoprotein cholesterol levels in populations differing in fat and carbohydrate intake. *Arteriosclerosis* 1987;7:612–19.

127 Knuiman JT, Westenbrink S, van der Heyden L. Determinants of total and high density lipoprotein cholesterol in boys from Finland, the Netherlands, Italy, the Philippines and Ghana with special reference to diet. *Hum Nutr Clin Nutr* 1983;37C:237.

128 Gonen B, Patsch W, Kuisk L, Schonfeld G. The effect of short-term feeding of a high carbohydrate diet on HDL subclasses in normal subjects. *Metabolism* 1981;30:1125.

129 Schaefer EJ, Levy RI, Ernst ND, Van Sant FD, Brewer HB. The effects of low cholesterol, high polyunsaturated fat, and low fat diets on plasma lipid and lipoprotein cholesterol levels in normal and hypercholesterolemic subjects. *Am J Clin Nutr* 1981;34:1758.

130 Kashyap ML, Barrnhart RL, Srivastava LS. Effects of dietary carbohydrate and fat on plasma lipoproteins and apolipoproteins C-II and C-III in healthy men. *J Lipid Res* 1982;23:877.

131 Ehnholm C, Huttunen JK, Pietinen P. Effect of a diet low in saturated fatty acids on plasma lipids, lipoproteins, and HDL subfractions. *Arteriosclerosis* 1984;4:265.

132 Brinton EA, Eisenberg S, Breslow JL. A low-fat diet decreases high density lipoprotein (HDL) cholesterol levels by decreasing HDL apolipoprotein transport rates. *J Clin Invest* 1990;85:144−51.

133 Tan MH, Dickinson MA, Albers JJ *et al*. The effect of a high cholesterol and saturated fat diet on serum high-density lipoprotein-cholesterol, apoprotein A-1, and apoprotein E levels in normolipidemic humans. *Am J Clin Nutr* 1980;33:2559−65.

134 Ernst N, Fisher M, Bowen P, Schaefer EJ, Levy RI. Changes in plasma lipids and lipoproteins after a modified fat diet. *Lancet* 1980;ii:111.

135 Shepherd J, Packard CJ, Patsch JR, Gotto JAM, Taunton OD. Effects of dietary polyunsaturated and saturated fat on the properties of high density lipoprotein and the metabolism of apolipoprotein A-I. *J Clin Invest* 1978;60:1582−92.

136 Turner JD, Le N-A, Brown WV. Effect on changing dietary fat saturation on low-density lipoprotein metabolism in man. *Am J Physiol* 1981;241:E57.

137 Mattson FH, Grundy SM. Comparison of effects of dietary saturated, monounsaturated, and polyunsaturated fatty acids on plasma lipids and lipoproteins in man. *J Lipid Res* 1985;26:194−202.

138 Grundy SM. Comparison of monounsaturated fatty acids and carbohydrates for lowering plasma cholesterol. *N Engl J Med* 1986;314:745−8.

139 Sanders TAB, Vickers M, Kaines AP. Effect on blood lipids and haemostasis of a supplement of cod liver oil, rich in eicosapentaenoic and docosahexaenoic acids, in healthy young men. *Clin Sci* 1981;61:317.

140 Sanders TAB, Roshaanai F. The influence of different types of n-3-polyunsaturated fatty acids on blood lipids and platelet function in healthy volunteers. *Clin Sci* 1983;64:91.

141 Hay CRM, Durber AP, Saynor R. Effect of fish oil on platelet kinetics in patients with ischaemic heart disease. *Lancet* 1982;i:1269.

142 Nestel PJ, Connor WE, Reardon MF *et al*. Suppression by diets rich in fish oil of very low density lipoprotein production in man. *J Clin Invest* 1984;74:82.

143 Illingworth DR, Harris WS, Connor WE. Inhibition of low density lipoprotein synthesis by dietary omega-3 fatty acids in humans. *Arteriosclerosis* 1984;4:270.

144 Mahley RW, Innerarity TL, Bersot TP, Lipson A, Margolis S. Alterations in human high-density lipoproteins, with or without increased plasma-cholesterol, induced by diets high in cholesterol. *Lancet* 1978;ii:807.

145 Hillman LC, Peters SG, Fisher CA, Pomare EW. The effects of the fiber components pectin, cellulose and lignin on serum cholesterol levels. *Am J Clin Nutr* 1985;42:207.

146 Gordon T, Ernst N, Fisher M, Rifkind BM. Alcohol and high-density lipoprotein cholesterol. *Circulation* 1981;64(Suppl 3):63.

147 Phillips NR, Havel RJ, Kane JP. Levels and interrelationships of serum and lipoprotein cholesterol and triglycerides. Association with adiposity and the consumption of ethanol, tobacco, and beverage containing caffeine. *Arteriosclerosis* 1981;1:13−24.

148 Wolfe BM, Havel RJ, Marliss EB *et al*. Effects of a three-day fast and of ethanol on splanchnic metabolism of free fatty acids, amino acids, and carbohydrates in healthy young men. *J Clin Invest* 1976;57:329−40.

149 Belfrage B, Berg P, Hagerstrand I *et al*. Alterations of lipid metabolism in healthy volunteers during long-term ethanol intake. *Eur J Clin Invest* 1977;7:127−31.

150 Chobanian AV. Hypertension, antihypertensive drugs, and atherogenesis: mechanisms and clinical implications. *J Clin Hypertens* 1986;3(Suppl):148S−157S.

151 Ames R. The effects of antihypertensive drugs on serum lipids and lipoproteins. I. Diuretics. *Drugs* 1986;32:260−78.

152 Ames R. The effects of antihypertensive drugs on serum lipids and lipoproteins. II. Non-diuretic drugs. *Drugs* 1986;32:335−57.

153 Ames R, Hill P. Antihypertensive therapy and the risk of coronary heart disease. *J Cardiovasc Pharmacol* 1982;4:S206−S212.

154 Leon AS, Agre J, McNally C *et al*. Blood lipid effects of antihypertensive therapy: a

double-blind comparison of the effects of methyldopa and propranalol. *J Clin Pharmacol* 1984;24:209–17.

155 Cutler R. Effects of antihypertensive agents on lipid metabolism. *Am J Cardiol* 1983;51:628–31.

156 Lehtonen A. Effect of beta blockers on blood lipid profile. *Am Heart J* 1985;109: 1192–6.

157 Pasotti C, Capra A, Fiorella G, Vibelli C, Chierchetti SM. Effects of pindolol and metoprolol on plasma lipids and lipoproteins. *Br J Clin Pharmacol* 1982;13: 435S–430S.

158 Hooper PL, Woo W, Visconti L, Pathak DR. Terbutaline raises high-density-lipoprotein-cholesterol levels. *N Engl J Med* 1981;305:1455–7.

159 McPherson R, Hogue M, Milne RW, Tall AR, Marcel YL. Increase in plasma cholesteryl ester transfer protein during probucol treatment. Relation to changes in high density lipoprotein composition. *Arterioscler Thromb* 1991;11:476–81.

160 Sirtori CR, Sirtori M, Caalabresi L, Ranchaschini G. Changes in high density lipoprotein subfraction distribution and increased cholesteryl ester transfer after probucol. *Am J Cardiol* 1988;62:73B–75B.

161 Van Der Vange N, Kloosterboer HJ, Haspels AA. Effects of seven low dose combined oral contraceptives on high density lipoprotein subfractions. *Br J Obstet Gynaecol* 1987;94:559–67.

162 Carlson LA, Olsson AG, Orö L, Rössner S, Walldius G. Effects of hypolipidemic regimes on serum lipoproteins. In *Atherosclerosis III* (eds G Schettler, A Weizel). New York: Springer-Verlag, 1974:768.

163 Kane JP, Malloy MJ. When to treat hyperlipidemia. *Adv Intern Med* 1988;33:143–64.

164 Johansson J, Carlson LA. The effects of nicotinic acid treatment on high density lipoprotein particle size subclass levels in hyperlipidaemic subjects. *Atherosclerosis* 1990;93:207–16.

165 Kane JP, Malloy MJ. Treatment of hyperlipidemia. *Annu Rev Med* 1990;41:471–82.

166 Schaefer EJ, Foster DM, Zech LA *et al.* The effects of estrogen administration on plasma lipoprotein metabolism in premenopausal females. *J Clin Endocrinol Metab* 1983;57:262–7.

167 Bush TL, Barrett-Connor E, Connor LD *et al.* Cardiovascular mortality and noncontraceptive use of estrogen in women: Results from the Lipid Research Clinics Program Follow-up Study. *Circulation* 1987;75:1102–9.

168 Luoma PV. Enzyme inducers. In *Pharmacological Control of Hyperlipidemia* (eds R Fears, RI Levy, J Shepherd, CJ Packard, NE Miller). Barcelona: Prous Science Publishers, 1986:365–76.

169 Nikkilä M, Kaste M, Enholm C, Viikari J. Increase of serum high-density lipoproteins in phenytoin users. *Br Med J* 1978;ii:90.

170 Grainger SL, Nanjee MN, Thompson RPH, Miller NE. Effects of cimetidine and ranitidine on plasma high-density lipoprotein subclasses in humans. *Pharmacology* 1988;36:420–6.

171 Miller NE, Lewis B. Cimetidine and HDL-cholesterol. *Lancet* 1983;i:529–30.

172 Rifkind BM. High-density lipoprotein cholesterol and coronary artery disease: survey of the evidence. *Am J Cardiol* 1990;66:3A-6.

173 Criqui MH, Wallace RB, Heiss G *et al.* Cigarette smoking and plasma high-density lipoprotein cholesterol: the Lipid Research Clinics Program Prevalence Study. *Circulation* 1980;62:70–6.

174 Wilson PNF, Garrison RJ, Abbott RD, Castelli WP. Factors associated with lipoprotein cholesterol levels: the Framingham Study. *Arteriosclerosis* 1983;3:272–81.

175 Heiss G, Johnson NJ, Reiland S *et al.* The epidemiology of plasma high-density lipoprotein cholesterol levels: the Lipid Research Clinics Program Prevalence Study summary. *Circulation* 1980;62:116–36.

176 Willett W, Hennekens CH, Castelli W *et al.* Effects of cigarette smoking on fasting

triglyceride, total cholesterol, and HDL-cholesterol in women. *Am Heart J* 1983;105:417−21.

177 Lusis AJ, LeBoeuf RC. Genetic control of plasma lipid transport: mouse model. *Methods Enzymol* 1986;128:877−94.

178 Lusis AJ. Genetic factors affecting blood lipoproteins: the candidate gene approach. *J Lipid Res* 1988;29:397−429.

179 Doolittle MH, LeBoeuf RC, Warden CH, Bee LM, Lusis AJ. A polymorphism affecting apolipoprotein A-II translational efficiency determines high density lipoprotein size and composition. *J Biol Chem* 1990;27:16380−8.

180 Paigen B, Mitchell D, Reve K, Morrow A, Lusis AJ, LeBoeuf RC. *Ath-1*, a gene determining atherosclerosis susceptibility and high density lipoprotein levels in mice. *Proc Natl Acad Sci USA* 1987;84:3763−7.

181 LeBoeuf RC, Doolittle MH, Montcalm A, Martin DC, Reve K, Lusis A. Phenotypic characterization of the *Ath-1* gene controlling high density lipoprotein levels and susceptibility to atherosclerosis. *J Lipid Res* 1990;31:91−102.

182 Brinton EA, Eisenberg S, Breslow JL. Increased apo A-I and apo A-II fractional catabolic rate in patients with low high density lipoprotein-cholesterol levels with or without hypertriglyceridemia. *J Clin Invest* 1991;87:536−44.

183 Bucher KD, Kaplan EB, Namboodiri KK *et al*. Segregation analysis of low levels of high-density lipoprotein cholesterol in the collaborative lipid research clinics program family study. *Am J Hum Genet* 1987;40:489−502.

184 Namboodiri KK, Green PP, Kaplan EB *et al*. Family aggregation of high density lipoprotein cholesterol. *Atherosclerosis* 1983;3:616−25.

185 Iselius L, Lalouel JM. Complex segregation analysis of hyperalphalipoproteinemia. *Metabolism* 1982;31:521−3.

186 Rao DC, Lalouel JM, Suarez BK *et al*. A genetic study of hyperalphalipoproteinemia. *Am J Med Genet* 1983;15:195−203.

187 Siervogel RM, Morrison JA, Kelly K *et al*. Familial hyper-alpha-lipoproteinemia in 26 kindreds. *Clin Genet* 1980;17:13−25.

188 Vergani C, Bettale G. Familial hypoalphalipoproteinemia. *Clin Chim Acta* 1981;114:45−52.

189 Byard PJ, Borecki IB, Glueck CJ *et al*. A genetic study of hypoalphalipoproteinemia. *Genet Epidemiol* 1984;1:43−51.

190 Hasstedt SJ, Albers J, Cheung MC *et al*. The inheritance of high density lipoprotein cholesterol and apolipoproteins A-1 and A-II. *Atherosclerosis* 1984;51:21−9.

191 Borecki IB, Rao DC, Third JLHC, Laskarzewski PM, Glueck CJ. A major gene for primary hypoalphalipoproteinemia. *Am J Hum Genet* 1986;38:373−81.

192 Cohn BA, Brand RJ, Hulley SB. Correlates of high density lipoprotein cholesterol in women by the method of co-twin control. *Am J Epidemiol* 1989;129:988−99.

193 Cheung P, Kao FT, Law ML *et al*. Localization of a structural gene for human apolipoprotein AI on the long arm of human chromosome 11. *Proc Natl Acad Sci USA* 1984;81:508−11.

194 Karathanasis SK. Apolipoprotein multigene family: tandem organisation of apolipoprotein AIV, AI and CIII genes. *Proc Natl Acad Sci USA* 1985;82:6374−8.

195 Knott TJ, Eddy RL, Robertson ME *et al*. Chromosomal localisation of the human apoprotein CI gene and of a polymorphic apoprotein AII gene. *Biochem Biophys Res Commun* 1984;125:299−306.

196 Ordovas JM, Schaefer EJ, Salem D *et al*. Apolipoprotein A-I gene polymorphism associated with premature coronary artery disease and familial hypoalphalipo-proteinaemia. *N Engl J Med* 1986;314:671−7.

197 Kessling AM, Rajput-Williams J, Bainton D *et al*. DNA polymorphisms of the apolipoprotein AII and AI−CIII−AIV genes: a study in men selected for differences in high-density-lipoprotein cholesterol concentration. *Am J Hum Genet* 1988;42:458−67.

198 Jeenah M, Kessling A, Miller N, Humphries S. G to A substitution in the promoter

region of the apolipoprotein AI gene is associated with elevated serum apolipoprotein AI and high density lipoprotein cholesterol concentrations. *Mol Biol Med* 1990;7: 233–41.

199 Norum KR, Gjone E, Glomset JA. Familial lecithin:cholesterol acyltransferase deficiency, including Fish Eye Disease. In *The Metabolic Basis of Inherited Disease* (eds CR Scriver, AL Beaudet, WS Sly, D Valle). New York: McGraw-Hill, 1989:1181–94.

200 Glomset JA, Applegate K, Forte T *et al.* Abnormalities in lipoproteins of d = 1.006 g/ml in familial lecithin:cholesterol acyltransferase deficiency. *J Lipid Res* 1980;21:1116.

201 Glomset JA, Norum KR, Nichols AV *et al.* Plasma lipoproteins in familial lecithin: cholesterol acyltransferase deficiency: effects of dietary manipulation. *Scand J Clin Lab Invest* 1975;35:142–3.

202 Holmquist L, Carlson LA. a-Lecithin:cholesterol acyltransferase deficiency. *Acta Med Scand* 1987;222:23–6.

203 Holmquist L, Carlson LA. Inhibitory effect of normal high density lipoproteins on lecithin:cholesterol acyltransferase activity in Fish Eye Disease plasma. *Acta Med Scand* 1987;222:15–21.

204 Inazu A, Brown ML, Hesler CB *et al.* Increased high density lipoprotein levels caused by a common cholesteryl ester transfer protein gene mutation. *N Engl J Med* 1990; 323:1234–8.

205 Brown ML, Inazu A, Hesler CB *et al.* Molecular basis of lipid transfer protein deficiency in a family with increased high-density lipoproteins. *Nature* 1989;342: 448–51.

206 Schonfeld G. The genetic dyslipoproteinemias—nosology update 1990. *Atherosclerosis* 1990;81:81–93.

207 Gualandri V, Franceschini G, Sitori CR *et al.* AI$_{Milano}$ apoprotein identification of the complete kindred and evidence of a dominant genetic transmission. *Am J Hum Genet* 1985;37:1083–97.

208 Franceschini G, Calabresi L, Tosi C *et al.* Apolipoprotein AI. *J Biol Chem* 1990;265;12224–31.

209 Assmann G, Schmitz G, Brewer HB. Familial high density lioprotein deficiency: Tangier Disease. In *The Metabolic Basis of Inherited Disease* (eds CR Scriver, AL Beaudet, WS Sly, D Valle). New York: McGraw-Hill, 1989;1267–82.

210 Brewer HB Jr, Fairwell T, Meng MS, Kay L, Ronan R. Human proapoA-I$_{Tangier}$: Isolation of proapoA-I$_{Tangier}$ and amino acid sequence of the peptide. *Biochem Biophys Res Commun* 1983;113:934.

211 Schaeffer EJ, Blum CB, Levy RJ *et al.* Metabolism of high density apolipoproteins in Tangier disease. *N Engl J Med* 1978;299:905.

212 Badimon JJ, Badimon L, Fuster V. Regression of atherosclerotic lesions by high density lipoprotein plasma fraction in the cholesterol-fed rabbit. *J Clin Invest* 1990;85:1234–41.

213 Rubin EM, Krauss RM, Spomgler EA, Verstuyft JG, Clift SM. Inhibition of early athero-genesis in transgenic mice by human apolipoprotein A-I. *Nature* 1991;353:265–7.

214 Manninen V, Elo MO, Frick MH *et al.* Lipid alterations and decline in the incidence of coronary heart disease in the Helsinki heart study. *JAMA* 1988;260:641–51.

215 Brown G, Albers JJ, Fishe LD. Regression of coronary artery disease as a result of intensive lipid lowering therapy in men with high levels of apolipoprotein B. *N Engl J Med* 1990;323:1289–98.

216 Kane JP, Malloy MJ, Ports TA *et al.* Regression of coronary atherosclerosis during treatment of familial hypercholesterolemia with combined drug regimens. *JAMA* 1990;264:3007–12.

217 Miller NE. Raising high density lipoprotein cholesterol. *Biochem Pharmacol* 1990;40:403–10.

218 Cashin-Hemphill L, Mack WJ, Pogoda JM *et al.* Beneficial effects of colestipol–niacin on coronary atherosclerosis. A 4 year follow-up. *JAMA* 1990;264:3013–17.

Chapter 6

Triglyceride-rich Lipoprotein Structure, Function, and Metabolism: Role in Coronary Heart Disease

WILLIAM A. BRADLEY & SANDRA H. GIANTURCO

Introduction

Lipoproteins are macromolecular, quasispherical assemblies of lipids and apoproteins that transport water-insoluble lipids through the aqueous milieu of plasma in their lipophilic cores [1]. Lipoprotein cores contain varying amounts of cholesteryl ester and triglyceride, and water-insoluble vitamins, drugs, and carcinogens, such as α-tocopherol, probucol, benzopyrene, and butter-fat yellow [2]. This chapter focuses on a unique class of lipoproteins, the triglyceride-rich lipoproteins (TGRLP), and discusses their structure and function, their assembly and metabolism, and their involvement in the pathogenesis of atherosclerosis and thrombosis. Unlike other lipoproteins that are cholesterol enriched (intermediate-density lipoproteins (IDL), low-density lipoproteins (LDL), and high-density lipoproteins (HDL)), the TGRLP are so named because triglyceride is their major component, usually greater than 50% by weight.

TGRLP have received less attention than LDL or HDL, both scientifically and in the popular press, since the levels of LDL-C and HDL-C are considered to be important in determining risk for cardiovascular disease. In this chapter we present current evidence that TGRLP may be an important and independent contributor to coronary heart disease (CHD).

Structure

TGRLP are the most heterogeneous class of lipoproteins. There are two sites of assembly, the intestine and the liver. TGRLP from the intestine that transport dietary (exogenous) lipids are called chylomicrons and are normally present only in the postprandial state. TGRLP from the liver are known as very low-density lipoproteins (VLDL) and are always present. Most studies in the past have centered on TGRLP from fasted subjects since ultracentrifugation, the usual method of TGRLP isolation, did not separate TGRLP of different metabolic origins. Within each of the general classifications of intestinal and hepatic TGRLP is a myriad of lipoprotein particles of different sizes, densities, compositions, and apoprotein content. Some of these physical and chemical differences have functional consequences, discussed below.

Table 6.1 identifies the major subspecies of TGRLP as defined by their flotation characteristics, used for their isolation in the ultracentrifuge. Using density gradient ultracentrifugation, it is possible to subfractionate TGRLP into more homogeneous populations. Most often three general subfractions of fasting VLDL (S_f 100–400, S_f 60–100, and S_f 20–60) from normal and hyperlipidemic individuals have been studied [3]. Subfractionation allows a more valid comparison of TGRLPs from different types of subjects as to their biologic function *in vitro*. Comparable TGRLP subclasses from different subjects are at least more similar in composition than unfractionated "total" TGRLP ($d < 1.006\,g/ml$), since the distribution of particles among subclasses changes from individual to individual. In general, however, the distribution of VLDL particles is skewed to the smaller VLDL S_f 20–60 in normolipemic, fasted individuals and to the larger VLDL S_f >60 in individuals with elevated triglycerides, i.e., individuals with hypertriglyceridemia.

Assembly in liver

VLDL are synthesized in hepatocytes [4] within the intracellular membrane compartments. Fatty acids used in triglyceride synthesis are from several sources. *De novo* synthesis occurs from acetyl-CoA produced by carbohydrate catabolism. Free fatty acids bound to plasma albumin are another source, and hydrolysis of lipids that are returned to the liver via lipoproteins provides yet another source. The cholesterol comes either from *de novo* synthesis in the liver or from returning plasma lipoproteins. Lipid synthesis for VLDL takes place exclusively on the cytoplasmic side of the endoplasmic reticulum (ER) membranes. The lipid moves to the lumen of the ER where apoprotein (apo) B_{100} and presumably apo E are added from the rough endoplasmic reticulum (RER). The nascent TGRLP then move to the Golgi apparatus for glycosylation of the proteins, before transport to the plasma membrane and finally secretion into the space of Disse [5]. Apo B is required for secretion of nascent VLDL particles. Apo B_{100}, the major apoprotein of VLDL, is a large, glycosylated protein (4536 amino acid residues; molecular weight 512 000) [6,7], synthesized in the hepatocytes and secreted on VLDL. Apo B_{100} is not only necessary for the secretion of the VLDL but is also a determinant for the recapture of VLDL catabolic products (S_f 20–60 remnants, IDL, and LDL) via the LDL receptor-

Table 6.1 Triglyceride-rich lipoproteins. Comparison of physical characteristics with cholesterol-rich apo B-containing lipoproteins

TRIGLYCERIDE-RICH LIPOPROTEINS **153**

Lipoprotein (S_f)*	Density range† (g/ml)	Average hydration density‡ (g/ml)	Molecular weight‡	Size (nm)	Composition (% wt)	
					Protein	Lipid
Chylomicrons (S_f >400)	>1.006	0.93	$0.5-300 \times 10^8$	75-450	1-2	98-99
VLDL	>1.006					
(S_f 100-400)		0.95	$20-50 \times 10^6$	48.9 ± 2.2§, range (40-75)	5.3 ± 0.49¶	95
(S_f 60-100)		0.97	$10-20 \times 10^6$	38.0 ± 3.4§, range (34-40)	8.4 ± 1.1¶	91.6
(S_f 20-60)		0.98	$5-10 \times 10^6$	32.7 ± 3.4§, range (30-34)	11.9 ± 1.4¶	88.1
IDL (S_f 12-20)	$d = 1.006-1.019$	1.01	$3-5 \times 10^6$	27-30	19	81
LDL (S_f 0-12)	$d = 1.019-1.063$	1.03	2.2×10^6	21-27‖	21	79

* S_f, flotation rate, obtained by analytical ultracentrifugation [3] in an NaCl medium of 1.063 g/ml.
† Density range interval used classically to isolate major classes of lipoprotein.
‡ Average hydration densities and molecular weights from [3].
§ From [57]: sized by electron microscopy of phosphotungstate-stained lipoproteins.
¶ Adapted from [57].
‖ LDL heterogeneity: four major subclasses (LDLI, diameter 26.6-27.2 nm; LDLII A and B, diameter 25.4-26.5 nm; LDLIII A and B, diameter 24.4-25.4 nm; LDLIV A and B, diameter 21.8-24.3 nm).

mediated pathway by the liver. We will return to the determinants of receptor-mediated uptake of TGRLP by cells later in this chapter.

Assembly in intestine

Chylomicrons are assembled in enterocytes of the intestine [8]. They are secreted into the intestinal lymphatic capillaries, transported through the mesenteric lymphatic vessels, and enter the bloodstream via the thoracic duct at the great veins in the neck.

During the synthesis of the nascent chylomicrons in the enterocyte, both fatty acids and 2-monoacylglycerols are delivered to the enterocytes as bile salt micelles. Although the glycerol-3-phosphate pathway exists in the enterocyte, the more energy-efficient monoacylglycerol pathway is the major route by which triglycerides are produced. The triglycerides synthesized closely resemble the dietary fat absorbed. After synthesis, presumably in the smooth endoplasmic reticulum (SER), triglycerides migrate through the cisternae of the ER system to the RER, akin to VLDL assembly in the hepatocyte.

Small amounts of consumed dietary cholesterol are esterified and must be hydrolyzed before absorption. Some of the cholesterol is then esterified by enterocyte acyl CoA:cholesterol acyltransferase (ACAT) to produce cholesteryl oleate and linoleate primarily.

Phospholipid, cholesteryl esters, and protein are added to triglycerides at the junction of the smooth and rough ER to produce a nascent chylomicron. Recent data suggest that some apoprotein and lipid are added as late as in the Golgi [9,10]. These nascent chylomicrons are transported along microtubules to the Golgi apparatus for glycosylation before transport to the plasma membrane for release (exocytosis) into the intestinal lymphatics.

The major apoproteins of nascent chylomicrons are apo B_{48}, apo A-I, and apo A-IV. Apo B_{48} is the major apo B species found in isolated jejunal enterocytes from adult humans [11], although a recent report using a radiolabeling technique and monoclonal antibodies specific to apo B_{100} indicated that human intestine can synthesize small amounts of apo B_{100} [12]. Apo B_{48} is translated from a uniquely, post-transcriptionally edited mRNA [11,13] in which a cytosine (C) is converted to uracil (U) at codon CAA (specifying Gln 2153 in apo B_{100}) creating an in-frame stop codon. This mRNA synthesizes a protein (molecular weight 248 000) which is half the molecular weight of the normal apo B_{100} gene product and which is essential for secretion of the chylomicrons from the enterocyte. Apo A-I and apo A-IV, also associated with nascent chylomicrons, are synthesized in the enterocyte and their synthesis is increased in response to fat feeding [14,15]. Apo Cs and apo E do not appear to be synthesized by the intestine but associate with chylomicrons in the lymphatics; these apoproteins probably filter from plasma into the mesenteric lymph.

Metabolism

Dietary (exogenous) TGRLP

Upon entering the bloodstream, chylomicrons immediately change from their "nascent" or lymphatic form and will be considered in this chapter as "plasma chylomicrons" or, as commonly referred to, "chylomicron remnants" or postprandial TGRLP. The common marker of origin of postprandial TGRLP is their apo B_{48} protein component. Immediately within the bloodstream there is a rapid exchange of chylomicron surface components with circulating plasma lipoprotein components. These surface components are replaced by an exchange and gain of apolipoproteins, particularly apo Cs and apo E [16–19]. Most plasma chylomicrons then continue their journey through various capillary beds where the chylomicron triglyceride is hydrolyzed by the action of lipoprotein lipase.

Lipoprotein lipase action is described in detail in several excellent reviews [20–22]. The lipase itself is anchored noncovalently to the capillary endothelial cell plasma membrane via a phosphatidyl inositol glycosaminoglycan (GAG)-chain, probably heparan sulfate proteoglycan [21,23]. Lipoprotein lipase has an essential cofactor, apo C-II [24,25]. This requirement is dramatically demonstrated in patients who are lacking apo C-II and thus develop an exaggerated hypertriglyceridemia [26], which is reversible upon transfusion of apo C-II.

Clearance rates of plasma chylomicron triglycerides are very rapid with half-lives of 1–5 minutes in normal subjects [27]. The resulting chylomicron remnants are depleted in triglycerides and reduced in size: the triglyceride decreases from about 90% to about 70%; the cholesteryl ester content increases from about 1% up to 10% of the particle weight. It is thought that as the cholesterol:phospholipid ratio of these particles approaches a molar ratio of 1.0, the action of lipase is inhibited [28,29]. Additionally, the chylomicron remnants may become cholesteryl ester enriched partially by the action of cholesteryl ester transfer protein during their lipolysis [30].

The chylomicron remnants are subsequently removed from the circulation by uptake via hepatic parenchymal cells, but not Kupffer cells [31–33], most likely through receptor-mediated processes.

Receptors potentially responsible for uptake include the LDL receptor [34,35], a putative apo E receptor (or chylomicron remnant receptor) [36], and the LDL receptor-related protein (LRP) [37–39]. Chylomicron remnants may be initially sequestered in the space of Disse [40,41]. The receptor-mediated uptake of chylomicron remnants in the liver is most likely mediated by apo E which is acquired primarily in the plasma compartment. Apo E is not a required protein for receptor-mediated uptake of TGRLP in cells of reticuloendothelial origin (discussed below) [42,43].

Once the chylomicron remnants are removed by the hepatocytes, they are internalized, and the cholesteryl esters hydrolyzed in lysosomes. The liberated cholesterol has several fates. Cholesterol inhibits cholesterogenesis [44] by suppression of 3-hydroxy-3-methylglutaryl-coenzyme A (HMG-CoA) reductase, the rate-limiting enzyme in cholesterol biosynthesis. Cholesterol can be: (i) stored as ester after reesterification; (ii) used for the synthesis of bile acids, which is the major exit route from the body; or (iii) repackaged into VLDL and secreted back into the bloodstream.

Both past and recent data suggest an alternate site of catabolism for chylomicrons and their remnants. Monocyte/macrophage-derived foam cells occur in bone marrow, spleen, liver, and xanthomas of humans with fasting chylomicronemia, indicating that uptake of intestinally derived TGRLP by monocyte/macrophages occurs *in vivo* [45,46]. Recent animal studies indicate that in some animal species, including the marmoset, bone marrow and splenic macrophages take up chylomicrons [41]. Infusion of apo E accelerates hepatic uptake of chylomicron remnants but not uptake of chylomicrons by bone marrow. This suggests that apo E is likely not involved in macrophage uptake of chylomicrons, although it is involved in hepatic uptake of remnants.

Thus, after the absorption of (exogenous) dietary fats, chylomicrons are assembled in the intestine, transported through the plasma where much of the triglyceride is hydrolyzed for energy and storage, cholesteryl esters are gained, and the plasma-modified chylomicron remnants delivered to the liver, where the remaining constituent fats are either removed from the body or reused.

Endogenous (hepatically derived) TGRLP (VLDL)

Nascent VLDL enter the bloodstream with their characteristic complement of apoproteins, apo B_{100}, apo E, and apo C. In plasma VLDL gain additional apo C and, particularly in hypertriglyceridemic subjects, probably apo E. Thus, VLDL provide the body with a pathway by which the liver can dispose of excess triglyceride (derived from lipogenesis, from chylomicron metabolism, and from free fatty acids delivered by albumin). VLDL, like their intestinal cousins, are acted upon by lipoprotein lipase and apo C-II to hydrolyze the triglyceride, albeit at a slower rate. As large VLDL are hydrolyzed, remnants of decreasing size are formed. These can be separated by density gradient ultracentrifugation into subfractions with different physical and metabolic properties [3,47]. As will be discussed later (see p. 162), the apo E content of these particles is one determinant of their ability to interact with the LDL receptor and to be removed directly from plasma without conversion to smaller particles. Those VLDL that are not directly taken up by cells are further hydrolyzed, losing the major complement of their triglyceride and becoming increasingly cholesteryl ester enriched until finally LDL particles remain. In humans it is thought that the majority, if not all, of the circulating LDL is formed by this process. The possibility of direct secretion of some LDL by the liver remains an open question, albeit an important one. The products of VLDL lipolysis (small VLDL S_f 20−60, IDL, and LDL) exit the plasma compartment primarily via LDL receptor-mediated uptake in the liver, most likely by parenchymal cells. Once delivered to the liver the triglyceride and cholesteryl ester are either reutilized, stored, or cholesteryl ester is hydrolyzed to cholesterol which enter pathways for bile acid synthesis and is excreted from the body. What happens when such systems go awry is the next topic.

Pathogenesis: role of TGRLP in coronary heart disease

Epidemiologic evidence for the role of TGRLP in coronary artery disease and myocardial infarction

Several early epidemiologic studies indicated that triglyceride was a risk factor for coronary artery disease. A review of these studies in 1980 [48] had a major impact on the philosophy of the treatment of hyperlipidemia in the USA. This review dismissed triglycerides as an independent risk factor, even though not all studies reviewed in that article supported this conclusion, for two stated reasons. First, in some but not all studies, multivariate analyses indicated that triglyceride did not remain a significant independent risk factor when HDL-C was controlled even when triglyceride was a significant univariate risk factor. Second, it was stated that there were no animal studies and no studies that demonstrated biologic mechanisms suggest a role for triglyceride in atherogenesis. That triglyceride could not be atherogenic remains a commonly held view, not only because of the discrepancies between univariate and multivariate analyses of risk, but probably because large amounts of cholesterol, not triglyceride, accumulate in atherosclerotic lesions. Cholesterol and triglyceride are both components of lipoproteins. TGRLP contain more total cholesterol per particle than LDL, so uptake of one TGRLP by a cell delivers more cholesterol than one LDL particle. Abnormal TGRLP that accumulate in hypertriglyceridemic subjects have specific receptor-mediated uptake mechanisms not available to normal TGRLP [42,49–58]. Triglyceride, unlike cholesterol, can be readily catabolized by cells or by lipoprotein lipase in the arterial wall, providing biologic mechanisms for the disposal of triglyceride which are not available to cholesterol. Therefore, it is not surprising that, while triglyceride and cholesterol may both enter the arterial wall during atherogenesis, only cholesterol is found to accumulate significantly in lesions.

The epidemiologic associations between plasma triglyceride and CHD have been reviewed recently [59]. In this comprehensive review Austin points out that although the association between plasma triglyceride and CHD is not completely consistent, there is a strong overall trend that suggests a relationship. Austin [59] emphasizes that the statistical properties of triglyceride as a risk factor must be considered. Importantly, and not always realized, there is often large variation in the measurement of triglyceride with greater intraindividual, as well as interindividual, variation in triglyceride than in cholesterol. Therefore, attempts to correlate triglyceride with other lipid measurements, which are inherently more accurately measured and less variable, with risk, leads to an underestimation of the actual triglyceride effect in disease when using multivariate analysis.

In 18 prospective studies reviewed in this report [59] from 1965 until 1991 that used a range of endpoints from angina and myocardial infarction to CHD-associated death, plasma triglyceride levels alone were found to correlate significantly with occurrence of CHD in 15 studies. Even when adjusted for either total cholesterol or LDL-C, in nine of 16 endpoints, plasma triglyceride levels remained significantly correlated. Finally, in the five prospective studies in which HDL-C was controlled, one study continued to show an association of CHD with plasma triglyceride.

In 17 case-controlled and cross-sectional studies (see Austin review, [59]) triglyceride alone was associated with CHD in all but one study. In those cases controlling for total cholesterol or LDL-C, six out of six studies continued to demonstrate a triglyceride-associated risk. In the four studies which controlled for HDL-C, three out of four studies indicated that triglyceride remains significantly correlated with CHD in men.

To date, epidemiologic associations between triglyceride and CHD indicate a strong trend [59]. In most studies univariate analyses demonstrate a significant relation with a variety of endpoints. When multivariate analyses are carried out triglyceride remains significantly associated when LDL-C, total cholesterol, or HDL-C are controlled in many, but not all, studies. However, in studies in which HDL-C is controlled triglyceride has remained significant the least. This apparent dilemma may be due to the inherent variation in plasma triglyceride levels (thus lowering its statistical significance and underestimating its association with CHD) and to the strong inverse relationship between HDL-C and plasma triglyceride [59].

Triglyceride is likely an important risk factor in CHD and the majority of plasma triglycerides are found associated with TGRLP. This suggests that TGRLP are potentially atherogenic and perhaps thrombogenic, as described later, at least in hypertriglyceridemic subjects at increased coronary artery disease risk. In the remainder of this chapter we will review some of the current data which suggest potential cellular mechanisms whereby certain TGRLP can be atherogenic (and/or thrombogenic) both in hypertriglyceridemic and normal subjects.

Mechanistic evidence for the role of TGRLP in atherosclerosis in hypertriglyceridemia

Several types of hypertriglyceridemia are associated with premature atherosclerosis and the accumulation of lipid-filled macrophages (foam cells) throughout the body [45]. Macrophages play a key role in atherogenesis, forming many of the foam cells found in arterial plaques [60–63]. Chylomicrons and large VLDL from certain hypertriglyceridemic subjects are the only *native* human lipoproteins known to produce massive, rapid, receptor-mediated lipid accumulation in macrophages *in vitro*, causing them to resemble foam cells histologically [42,52,54,55,64–68]. The lipid which accumulates in macrophages after receptor-mediated uptake of a lipoprotein *in vitro* reflects the lipid composition of the lipoprotein [52,64]. Initially, triglyceride is the predominant lipid which accumulates in macrophages exposed to TGRLP from certain hypertriglyceridemic subjects; however, hypertriglyceridemic TGRLP also can induce a 27-fold increase in cholesteryl ester even in short term (4-hour) incubations [55].

Foam cells occur *in vivo* in subjects with persistent chylomicrons (hyperlipoproteinemia Types 1, 3, 5), with exaggerated postprandial response (Type 4, low HDL levels), and with persistent chylomicron remnants (Type 3) [45] suggesting that postprandial TGRLP induce foam-cell formation. Diabetic subjects with fasting chylomicrons develop human monocyte/macrophage-derived foam cells in eruptive xanthomas that are filled with more triglyceride than cholesteryl ester [46], as seen *in vitro*. When plasma triglyceride levels are normalized after insulin therapy, chylomicrons disappear and foam-cell triglyceride is rapidly lost, leaving cholesteryl ester as the predominant lipid [46]. A similar sequence might occur in developing arterial foam cells following receptor-mediated uptake of postprandial TGRLP: initial triglyceride and cholesteryl ester engorgement (triglyceride ≫ cholesteryl ester) followed by selective hydrolysis and removal of triglyceride, leaving cholesteryl ester as the predominant lipid. Indeed, recent *in vitro* studies indicate that murine J774 macrophages accumulate three to 10 times more cholesteryl ester in long-term incubations with hypertriglyceridemic VLDL [68] than previously reported in short-term incubations in P388D$_1$ cells, another murine macrophage line [55].

Zilversmit originally proposed that both hepatic and intestinal TGRLP might be atherogenic, that atherogenesis may be a postprandial phenomenon, and that TGRLP and their lipolytic remnants are atherogenic because they can contribute their lipids to the artery wall [69,70]. Thus, premature atherosclerosis would develop even in persons with normal fasting lipoprotein profiles if their postprandial TGRLP were atherogenic. The magnitude and duration of postprandial lipemia have recently been studied in detail. When a bolus fat load is ingested, it induces an increase in plasma triglyceride levels and changes in all plasma lipoproteins, especially in the TGRLPs, that are evident for at least 14 hours. The type of fat consumed chronically affects the postprandial response, with saturated fat producing a greater postprandial lipemia relative to diets rich in ω-6 or ω-3 fatty acids; the type of fat in the acute load has a less pronounced effect [71]. The postprandial response in any given individual is remarkably reproducible, as long as diet, weight, and physical activity remain constant [72,73]. Individuals respond reproducibly to a fat load with single, double, or triple postprandial triglyceride peak(s) [74]. Several factors affect the postprandial response, at least postprandial lipemia, as well as atherosclerosis risk. These factors included fasting HDL and triglyceride levels [72–75], type of primary hyperlipidemia [73,76], apo E phenotypes [77,78], age, and gender, with older subjects having greater postprandial triglyceride increases than younger subjects [74]. Although the magnitude and duration of postprandial lipemia are controlled by the aforementioned factors, the postprandial TGRLP are relatively short-lived. Because of the short half-life of TGRLP in plasma, particularly postprandial TGRLP, in order to be atherogenic, rapid, probably receptor-mediated uptake would have to occur. Though postprandial TGRLP may have a short

Table 6.2 Summary of the interactions of apo B-containing lipoproteins with lipoprotein receptors of macrophages

Lipoproteins	Lipoprotein receptors			
	LDLR	MφTGRLPR	AcLDLR	LRP
Normal (fasted) TGRLP				
VLDL S_f 100–400	−	−	−	NR
S_f 60–100	−	−	−	NR
S_f 20–60	+	−	−	NR
HTG (fasted) TGRLP				
VLDL S_f 100–400	+	+/−	−	NR
S_f 60–100	+	+/−	−	NR
S_f 20–60	+	+/−	−	NR
Normal (postprandial) TGRLP				
ppTGRLP S_f >400	+/−	+	−	NR
ppTGRLP S_f 100–400	+	−	−	NR
S_f 60–100	+	−	−	NR
S_f 20–60	+	−	−	NR
HTG (postprandial) TGRLP				
ppTGRLP S_f >400	+	+	−	NR
S_f 100–400	+	+	−	NR
S_f 60–100	+	+/−	−	NR
S_f 20–60	+	+/−	−	NR
IDL S_f 12–20	+	−	−	NR
LDL S_f 0–12	+	−		+
Ac-LDL	−	−	+	NR
Ox-LDL	−	+	+	NR
β-VLDL	+	+/−	−	+/−
β-VLDL + apo E*	+	NR	−	+
N-VLDL S_f 100–400 + apo E*	+	−	−	NR

LDLR, low-density lipoprotein receptor; LRP, LDL receptor-related protein; Ac-LDL, acetylated LDL; Ox-LDL, oxidized LDL; AcLDLR, acetyl LDL (R is a scavenger R); TGRLP, triglyceride-rich lipoproteins; VLDL, very low-density lipoproteins; HTG, hypertriglyceridemia; ppTGRLP, postprandial TGRLP; ±, not all patients' lipoproteins bind; +, binds; −, does not bind; NR, not reported.
* Apo E incubated with lipoprotein.

plasma half-life [27], in a chronic postprandial state (a normal living state) a constant insult of these potentially atherogenic particles might still have a major role in foam-cell formation. The following will examine the role of lipoprotein receptors in the rapid, receptor-mediated uptake of TGRLP.

MACROPHAGE LIPOPROTEIN RECEPTORS

Receptors that could be involved in foam-cell formation induced by TGRLP and postprandial TGRLP include the LDL receptor, a distinct macrophage receptor that binds certain hypertriglyceridemic VLDL and chylomicrons and, possibly, the LRP [79] (Table 6.2). It is unlikely that the acetyl LDL receptor [64] which binds oxidized LDL [80] is involved in TGRLP uptake by macrophages, since chylomicrons and hypertriglyceridemic VLDL fail to bind to this receptor [52].

Chylomicrons are thought not to bind to LDL receptors [34], but do bind to receptors on macrophages [52,55,81,82]. Chylomicron remnants, in contrast to chylomicrons, bind to LDL receptors [34,35]. LRP has a specificity and Ca^{2+} requirement similar to the LDL receptor; rat LRP binds rabbit and rat LDL even better than β-VLDL, chylomicrons, and chylomicron remnants [38]. Apo E-enriched β-VLDL [83] and apo E phospholipid complexes [39] also bind to LRP. LRP is especially prevalent in hepatic endosomal membranes [38] but is also present in skin fibroblasts [83] and $P388D_1$ macrophages [39] and therefore appears to have a more general distribution, like the LDL receptor, and unlike the distinct macrophage receptor for TGRLP which is restricted to reticuloendothelial cells.

THE LDL RECEPTOR

This is expressed primarily in the liver, but it is present on all cells of the body [84]. LDL receptor activity of human monocyte/macrophages diminishes upon adherence of monocytes, and declines further during differentiation into macrophages [85–88]. In the human monocytic THP-1 cell line, LDL receptor activity of monocytes disappears after phorbol ester-induced differentiation into macrophages [89,90]. LDL receptor activity can be induced in THP-1 monocytes as well as most cell types by preincubation in lipoprotein-deficient medium, i.e., in the presence of low concentrations of exogenous sterol.

LDL RECEPTOR BINDING DETERMINANTS

Apo B mediates the binding of LDL [84], IDL (S_f 12–20), and $VLDL_3$ (S_f 20–60) [91,92] to the LDL receptor. Only these small lipoproteins (S_f 0–60) from normal subjects bind specifically to the LDL receptor of fibroblasts [49,51] or of human monocytic cells [93]. In hypertriglyceridemia, however, VLDL S_f >60 also bind to the LDL receptor [49,51,53,54]. The abnormal binding of hypertriglyceridemic VLDL S_f >60 to the LDL receptor is mediated by apo E, not apo B [53,91,92, 94,95]. TGRLP S_f >60 bind to the LDL receptor only if intact apo E of a specific conformation is present [53]. This conformation has been shown to have two distinct properties: susceptibility to thrombin-specific cleavage in the intact lipoprotein, and recognition by a monoclonal antibody, 1D7, which binds to the domain of apo E including residues 129–169. The apo B of large TGRLP S_f >60 does not bind to the LDL receptor; presumably the apo B of these large particles does not have the correct conformation to bind [91,92,96–98]. The LDL receptor-accessible apo E is present in hypertriglyceridemic VLDL S_f >60 but not in normal VLDL [91]. Incorporation of apo E into normal VLDL S_f >60 permits LDL receptor-mediated uptake [51,95].

MACROPHAGE TGRLP RECEPTOR

An alternate macrophage receptor binds abnormal TGRLP from certain hypertriglyceridemic subjects and some postprandial TGRLP independent of apo E [42,54,55]. This receptor also binds rabbit β-VLDL with relative low affinity, accounting for the observed competition with human hypertriglyceridemic VLDL and the previous use of the name β-VLDL receptor [55]. Early studies in murine macrophages suggested that a "β-VLDL receptor" distinct from the LDL receptor existed [99]. However, anti-LDL receptor antibodies block most, of the uptake of β-VLDL by macrophages preincubated to induce LDL receptor activity, indicating that β-VLDL bind primarily to LDL receptors when they are expressed [35,42,100,101], binding that is mediated by apo E. Residual receptor-mediated uptake of β-VLDL that is not via the LDL receptor is likely via the TGRLP macrophage receptor. Uptake of human abnormal TGRLP devoid of apo E by the macrophage TGRLP receptor pathway is not inhibited by anti-LDL receptor antibodies that inhibit the LDL receptor-mediated uptake of β-VLDL in the same cells [42]. The macrophage TGRLP receptor is distinct from the LDL receptor immunochemically, in ligand specificity, in cellular distribution, in regulation, and in molecular weight of the candidate receptor proteins [42]. Hypertriglyceridemic VLDL (S_f 100–400) that contain apo B_{100}, apo B_{48} or fragmented apo B (produced by protease processing), and plasma "chylomicrons" (B_{48} with or without B_{100}) bind to the macrophage receptor independent of apo E and, unlike normal VLDL, produce massive triglyceride and cholesteryl ester engorgement and foam-cell morphology after uptake. The macrophage receptor is expressed in murine macrophages, in normal human monocyte/macrophages, in the human THP-1 monocytic cell line, and in endothelial cells but not in fibroblasts [42,58].

The primary role of the alternate macrophage receptor *in vivo* may be disposal of abnormal TGRLP (including postprandial TGRLP) when normal catabolic routes are saturated, to protect other arterial cells from the potentially deleterious effects of uptake. Since this receptor is not downregulated by cholesterol loading [42], foam-cell formation would ensue when accumulation rates exceed lipid disposal.

TGRLP coagulation factors and thrombosis

Meade and colleagues [102] suggested that elevation of specific coagulation factors and fibrinogen are associated with cardiovascular mortality. In the Northwick Park Heart Study of 1511 white males out of a total study group of nearly 3500 men and women, plasma cholesterol and triglyceride levels correlated positively with activated factor VII (factor VIIc) [103]. Moreover, plasma levels of factor VIIc decreased as lipid concentrations decreased [104,105] and hypertriglyceridemia is associated with hypercoagulability [105]. In 18 severely hypertriglyceridemic patients, factor Xc was significantly elevated compared with normolipemics. Drug therapy that lowered triglyceride levels resulted in consistent lowering of plasma levels of factor VIIc and factor Xc. Elkeles and coworkers [104] also noted a decrease in factor VIIc, factor VIIIc, and factor Xc and increased fibrinolytic activity in hypertriglyceridemic subjects on a fat-modified diet that lowered plasma triglyceride levels. Mitropoulos *et al.* [103,111] demonstrated that factor VIIc/VIIt is dramatically elevated in plasma of pregnant women, which they attributed to increased conversion of factor VIIc to the two-chain (α-VII$_a$) form in the presence of lipoprotein particles of $S_f > 20$ (i.e., TGRLP), which are elevated in pregnancy. Both factor VII and factor X, as well as factor II (prothrombin) have been found to associate with TGRLP *in vitro* [106,107; Bradley, unpublished observations]. Furthermore, Vukovitch and colleagues [108] reported that von Willebrand factor/factor VIII also are associated with chylomicrons and VLDL in postprandial plasma.

More recent epidemiologic studies further indicate that factor VII coagulant activity (VIIc) is a strong predictor of CHD [109]. Again, factor VIIc correlates positively with TGRLP (chylomicrons and VLDL). Two mechanisms for this relationship have been considered. One mechanism suggests that large TGRLP ($S_f > 20$) are involved in the conversion of native single chain factor VII to its fully activated two-chain species, α-VII$_a$ [110,111]. A second proposed mechanism is that factor VIIc associates with TGRLP, resulting in a reduced fractional catabolism of factor VIIc [106,112]. To clarify this point, Miller *et al.* [113] fed nine adults a standardized diet and followed the effect of postprandial triglyceridemia on factor VIIc. A persistent, positive influence of plasma triglyceride concentration on increased factor VIIc at peak lipemia (160 minutes) but not at later timepoints was demonstrated, suggesting that TGRLP were causing an increase in factor VIIc activity.

Other possible interactions of coagulation factors with TGRLP have been suggested. In hypertriglyceridemia and postprandially, VLDL S_f >60 and chylomicrons contribute significantly to the total plasma phospholipid pool (about 35% in TGRLP). The TGRLP phospholipid surface may serve as an alternate binding site for vitamin K-dependent proteins that have an affinity for phospholipid in the presence of Ca^{2+} through an interaction with γ-carboxyglutamic acid (Gla) residues. Indeed, hypertriglyceridemic VLDL S_f >60 contain the Gla-protein, prothrombin, when isolated under conditions that preserve Ca^{2+}-dependent interactions, i.e., without added chelators [107]. Bajaj et al. [114] demonstrated that VLDL, alone among the lipoproteins, serves as a phospholipid source for the conversion of prothrombin to thrombin by factor X_a. Most intriguing, coagulation factors have been shown to degrade specific apolipoproteins of VLDL. Thrombin, for example, degrades apo E [53,91,107,117,118] and apo B [91,115−117] in intact lipoproteins at specific peptide bonds. Moreover, protease activity associated with large VLDL produces thrombin-like fragments of the apoproteins [118]. This proteolytic processing of the hypertriglyceridemic VLDL S_f >60 abolishes its binding to the LDL receptor, but can enhance uptake by the macrophage receptor, accelerating foam-cell formation *in vitro* [42,54,55]. Coagulation factors may contribute to the atherogenicity of TGRLP if this process occurs *in vivo*.

Total VLDL (*d* <1.006 fraction) rapidly enhanced the expression of procoagulant activity in human peripheral blood monocytes [119,120] with a 6.7-fold increase in thromboplastin activity consistent with increased surface expression of tissue factor. This was not considered a direct effect on monocyte tissue factor, but indirect due to an interaction with leukocytes. VLDL are heterogeneous and subspecies can have very different properties in terms of cellular receptor interactions or *in vivo* metabolism [56]. The mechanism of the induced tissue factor expression in peripheral blood monocytes by VLDL was therefore complicated by the heterogeneity (both in lipoproteins and cells) of the system.

The association of coagulation factors, particularly factors VII, X, and II, with TGRLP is now well documented and may be involved in both atherosclerosis and thrombosis by a variety of mechanisms. In the future the following questions need to be addressed. (i) What determines interaction of coagulation factors with TGRLP, what governs factor activation, and what are the consequences on apoprotein structure? (ii) What is the role of protease processing of TGRLP by coagulation factors on the atherogenicity of TGRLP? (iii) Do hypertriglyceridemic TGRLP by virtue of binding to specific receptors on endothelial cells affect the activity of tissue factor or thrombomodulin, key endothelial cell regulators of clotting? (iv) What are the mechanisms of TGRLP modulation of endothelial cell net fibrinolytic activity (see below)? (v) Do hypertriglyceridemic TGRLP of subjects with documented myocardial infarction show greater evidence of protease processing, coagulation factor interaction, and enhanced atherogenic and thrombogenic activity than do TGRLP from healthy normolipemic or hypertriglyceridemic subjects? Such potential links between thrombolytic and atherogenic processes are only now under study and may begin to enhance our understanding of these complex, highly regulated mechanisms and eventually our approach to treating the disorders involved.

Hypertriglyceridemia, TGRLP, and fibrinolysis

Central to fibrinolysis is the proenzyme, plasminogen. Plasminogen is converted to its active form, plasmin, by tissue plasminogen activator (t-PA), the major physiologic plasminogen activator. It is plasmin which hydrolyzes fibrin, thus causing clot disintegration or fibrinolysis. The activity of t-PA is highly regulated by the fast acting inhibitor, plasminogen activator inhibitor-1 (PAI-1). Deficient fibrinolytic activity can cause increased thrombotic events in patients. Decreased fibrinolysis due to increased PAI-1 levels occurs in obesity [121], in diabetes (non-insulin dependent) [122], and in hypertriglyceridemia [123,124]. Increased PAI-1 levels in young males with recurring myocardial infarction correlated with high significance to their total plasma triglyceride levels [123]. Hypertriglyceridemic VLDL subfractions specifically perturb the rapid release of t-PA and urokinase-type plasminogen activator (u-PA=UK) [125] normally associated with endothelial cells. Hypertriglyceridemic VLDL subfractions induced significant PAI-1 release into the media of human umbilical vein endothelial cells in a dose-dependent manner, which may be a function of expressed LDL receptor activity [126]. Thus, large hypertriglyceridemic TGRLP appear to perturb the balance of endothelial cell fibrinolytic expression in a rapid and complex fashion. This combination of increased antifibrinolytic activity and increased procoagulant activity, described previously, associated with large TGRLP may lead, under certain circumstances, to a potentially dangerous thrombotic state in specific subjects.

Summary and conclusions

TGRLP are dynamic, heterogeneous, macromolecular complexes which undergo a myriad of reactions, including lipolysis, lipid exchange, uptake by specific cell surface receptors in the periphery and liver, interaction with components of the coagulation cascade, and (interaction with) fibrinolytic balance. TGRLP carry most of the plasma triglyceride and can, in hypertriglyceridemia, carry a major fraction of the total cholesterol (large TGRLP contain more than five times more cholesterol per lipoprotein particle than one LDL). TGRLP, both endogenous and exogenous (dietary), have the potential to contribute to atherogenic processes through direct receptor-mediated interactions with cells of the arterial wall, potentially causing macrophages to fill with lipid (both triglyceride and cholesterol) leading to foam-cell formation. This is a chronic process which may take decades to cause narrowing of the lumen in coronary vessels. TGRLP may also participate in more acute aspects of CHD, particularly in accelerating thrombotic events by either increasing factor VII activity or perturbing fibrinolytic balance (in inducing elevated PAI-1 levels) or perhaps both. In any event, elevated blood triglyceride in the form of TGRLP can no longer be dismissed as a contributor to CHD. Additional studies into the mechanisms of TGRLP interaction with the vessel wall, with coagulation factors, and with fibrinolytic components are necessary in order to develop rational therapeutic approaches to this all too common finding, elevated plasma triglyceride levels.

References

1 Bradley WA, Gotto AM Jr. Structure of intact human plasma lipoproteins. In *Disturbances in Lipid and Lipoprotein Metabolism* (eds JM Dietschy, AM Gotto Jr, J Ontko). Bethesda, MD: American Physiology Society, 1978:111–37.

2 Chen TC, Bradley WA, Gotto AM Jr, Morrisett JD. Binding of the chemical carcinogen, p-dimethylaminoazobenzine, by human low density lipoproteins. *FEBS Lett* 1979;104:236–40.

3 Lindgren FT, Jensen LC, Hatch RT. The isolation and quantitative analysis of serum lipoproteins. In *Blood Lipids and Lipoproteins: Quantitation, Composition, and Metabolism* (ed. GL Nelson). New York: Wiley Interscience, 1972:181–274.

4 Havel RJ. Approach to the patient with hyperlipidemia. *Med Clin North Am* 1982;66: 319–33.

5 Havel RJ, Kane JP. Disorders of the biogenesis and secretion of lipoproteins containing the B apolipoproteins. In *The Metabolic Base of Inherited Disease* (eds CS Scriver, AL Beaudet, WS Sly, D Valle). New York: McGraw-Hill, 1989:1139–64.

6 Yang CY, Chen SH, Gianturco SH *et al*. Sequence, structure, receptor-binding domains and external repeats of human apolipoprotein B-100. *Nature* 1986;323:738–42.

7 Knott TJ, Pease RJ, Powell LM *et al*. Complete protein sequence and identification of structural domains of human apolipoprotein B. *Nature* 1986;323:734–8.

8 Redgrave TG. Formation and metabolism of chylomicrons. *Int Rev Physiol* 1983;28: 103–30.

9 Howell KE, Palade GE. Heterogeneity of lipoprotein particles in hepatic Golgi fractions. *J Cell Biol* 1982;92:833–45.

10 Bamberger MJ, Lane MD. Possible role of the Golgi apparatus in the assembly of very low density lipoprotein. *Proc Natl Acad Sci USA* 1990;87:2390–4.

11 Powell LM, Wallis SC, Pease RJ *et al.* A novel form of tissue specific RNA-processing produces apolipoprotein B-48 in intestine. *Cell* 1987;50:831–40.

12 Levy E, Rochette C, Londono I *et al.* Apolipoprotein B-100: Immunolocalization and synthesis in human intestinal mucosa. *J Lipid Res* 1990;31:1937–46.

13 Chen SH, Habib G, Yang C-Y *et al.* Apolipoprotein B-48 is a product of a messenger RNA with an origin specific in frame stop codon. *Science* 1987;238:363–6.

14 Glickman RM, Green PHR. The intestine and source of apoAI. *Proc Natl Acad Sci USA* 1977;74:1569–73.

15 Green PHR, Glickman RM, Riley JW, Quinet E. Human apolipoprotein A-IV. Intestinal origin and distribution in plasma. *J Clin Invest* 1980;65:911–16.

16 Havel RJ, Kane JP, Kashyap ML. Interchange of apolipoprotein between chylomicron and high density lipoproteins during alimentary lipemia in man. *J Clin Invest* 1973; 52:32–8.

17 Imaizumi K, Fainaru M, Havel RJ. Composition of proteins of mesenteric lymph chylomicrons in the rat and alterations produced upon exposure of chylomicrons to blood serum and serum proteins. *J Lipid Res* 1978;19:712–22.

18 Redgrave T, Small DM. Quantitation of the transfer of surface phospholipid from chylomicrons to the high density lipoprotein fraction during the catabolism of chylomicrons in the rat. *J Clin Invest* 1979;64:162–71.

19 Robinson SF, Quarfordt SH. Chylomicron apoprotein alteration after plasma exposure. *Biochim Biophys Acta* 1978;541:492–503.

20 Jackson RL. Lipoprotein lipase and hepatic lipase. In *The Enzymes* (ed. PD Boyer). New York: Academic Press, 1984:6.

21 Olivecrona T, Bengtsson-Olivecrona UG. Lipoprotein and hepatic lipase. *Curr Opin Lipidol* 1990;1:222–30.

22 Kern PA. Lipoprotein lipase and hepatic lipase. *Curr Opin Lipidol* 1991;2:162–9.

23 Cisor LA, Hooguwuf AJ, Cupp M, Rapport CA, Bensadoin A. Secretion and degradation of lipoprotein lipase in cultured adipocytes. *J Biol Chem* 1989;264:1767–74.

24 Havel RJ, Shore VG, Shore B, Bier DM. Role of specific glycopeptides of human serum lipoproteins in the activation of lipoprotein lipase. *Circ Res* 1970;27:595–600.

25 LaRosa JC, Levy RI, Herbert P, Lux SE, Fredrickson DS. A specific apoprotein activator for lipoprotein lipase. *Biochem Biophys Res Commun* 1970;41:57–62.

26 Breckenridge WC, Little JA, Steiner G, Chow A, Poapst M. Hypertriglyceridemia associated with deficiency of apolipoprotein CII. *N Engl J Med* 1978;298:1265–73.

27 Grundy SM, Mok HYI. Chylomicron clearance in normal and hyperlipidemic man. *Metabolism* 1976;11:1225–39.

28 Fielding CJ. Human lipoprotein lipase. Inhibition of activity by cholesterol. *Biochim Biophys Acta* 1970;218:221–6.

29 Fielding CJ, Rentson JB, Fielding PE. Metabolism of cholesterol-enriched chylomicrons. Catabolism of triglyceride by lipoprotein lipase of perfused heart and adipose tissues. *J Lipid Res* 1978;19:705–11.

30 Castro GR, Fielding CJ. Effects of postprandial lipemia on plasma cholesterol metabolism. *J Clin Invest* 1985;75:874–82.

31 Lippiello PM, Dijkstra J, van Galen M, Scherphof G, Waite BM. The uptake and metabolism of chylomicron-remnant lipids by nonparenchymal cells in perfused liver and by Kupffer cells in culture. *J Biol Chem* 1981;256:7454–60.

32 Nilsson A, Zilversmit DB. Distribution of chylomicron cholesteryl ester between parenchymal and Kupffer cell of rat liver. *Biochim Biophys Acta* 1971;248:137–42.

33 Redgrave T. Formation of cholesteryl-ester rich particulate lipid during metabolism of chylomicrons. *J Clin Invest* 1970;49:465–71.

34 Floren CH, Albers, JJ, Kudchadkar BJ, Bierman EL. Receptor-dependent uptake of human chylomicron remnants by cultured skin fibroblasts. *J Biol Chem* 1981;256:425–33.

35 Ellsworth JL, Kraemer FB, Cooper AD. Transport of β-VLDL and chylomicron

remnants by macrophages is mediated by the LDL receptor pathway. *J Biol Chem* 1987;262:2316−25.

36 Mahley RW, Hui DY, Innerarity TL, Beisiegel U. Chylomicron remnant metabolism. Role of hepatic lipoprotein receptors in mediating uptake. *Arteriosclerosis* 1989; 9(Suppl):I14−I18.

37 Kowal RC, Herz J, Weisgraber KH *et al.* Opposing effects of apolipoproteins E and C on lipoprotein binding to low density lipoprotein receptor-related protein. *J Biol Chem* 1990;265:10771−9.

38 Lund H, Takahashi K, Hamilton RL, Havel RJ. Lipoprotein binding and endosomal itinerary of the low density lipoprotein receptor-related protein in rat liver. *Proc Natl Acad Sci USA* 1989;86:9318−22.

39 Beiseigel U, Weber W, Ihrke G, Herz J, Stanley KK. The LDL-receptor-related protein, LRP is an apolipoprotein E binding protein. *Nature* 1989;341:162−4.

40 Stein O, Stein Y, Goodman DS, Fidge NH. The metabolism of chylomicron cholesteryl ester in rat liver. A combined radiographic-electron microscopic and biochemical study. *J Cell Biol* 1969;43:410−31.

41 Mahley RW, Hussain MM. Chylomicron and chylomicron remnant catabolism. *Curr Opin Lipidol* 1991;2:170−6.

42 Gianturco SH, Lin AH-Y, Hwang S-LC *et al.* A distinct murine macrophage receptor for human triglyceride-rich lipoproteins. *J Clin Invest* 1988;82:1633−43.

43 Gianturco SH, Lin AH-Y, Ramprasad MP, Song R, Bradley WA. Monocyte− macrophage receptor pathway for abnormal triglyceride-rich lipoproteins. In *Drugs Affecting Lipid Metabolism X* (eds AM Gotto Jr, LC Smith). Amsterdam: Elsevier, 1990: 261−4.

44 Nervi FO, Weis HJ, Dietschy JM. The kinetic characteristics of inhibition of hepatic cholesterogenesis by lipoproteins of intestinal origin. *J Biol Chem* 1975;250:4145−51.

45 Fredrickson DS, Goldstein JL, Brown MS. The familial hyperlipoproteinemias. In *The Metabolic Basis of Inherited Diseases*, 4th edn (eds JG Stanbury, MF Wyngaarden, DS Fredrickson). New York: McGraw-Hill, 1978:604−55.

46 Parker F, Bagdade JD, Odland GF, Bierman EL. Evidence for the chylomicron origin of lipids accumulating in diabetic eruptive xanthomas: A correlative lipid biochemical, histochemical, and electron microscopic study. *J Clin Invest* 1970;49:2172−87.

47 Gianturco SH, Bradley WA. The role of apolipoprotein processing in receptor recognition. In *Methods in Enzymology* (eds J Segrest, JJ Albers). Orlando: Academic Press, 1986;129:319−44.

48 Hulley SB, Rosenman RH, Bawol RD, Brand RJ. Epidemiology as a guide to clinical decisions: The association between triglyceride and coronary heart disease. *N Engl J Med* 1980;302:1383−9.

49 Gianturco SH, Gotto AM Jr, Jackson RL *et al.* Control of 3-hydroxy-3-methylglutaryl-CoA reductase activity in cultured human fibroblasts by very low density lipoproteins of subjects with hypertriglyceridemia. *J Clin Invest* 1978;61:320−8.

50 Gianturco SH, Eskin SG, Navarro LT *et al.* Abnormal effects of hypertriglyceridemic very low density lipoproteins on 3-hydroxy-3-methylglutaryl-CoA reductase activity and viability of cultured bovine aortic endothelial cells. *Biochim Biophys Acta* 1980; 618:143−52.

51 Gianturco SH, Brown FB, Gotto AM Jr, Bradley WA. Receptor-mediated uptake of hypertriglyceridemic very low density lipoproteins by normal human fibroblasts. *J Lipid Res* 1982;23:984−93.

52 Gianturco SH, Bradley WA, Gotto AM Jr, Morrisett JD, Peavy DL. Hypertriglyceridemic very low density lipoproteins enhance triglyceride synthesis and accumulation in mouse peritoneal macrophages. *J Clin Invest* 1982;70:168−78.

53 Gianturco SH, Gotto AM Jr, Hwang S-LC *et al.* Apolipoprotein E mediates uptake of S_f 100−400 hypertriglyceridemic very low density lipoproteins by the low density lipoprotein receptor pathway in normal human fibroblasts. *J Biol Chem* 1983;258: 4526−33.

54 Gianturco SH, Gotto AM Jr, Bradley WA. Hypertriglyceridemia: Lipoprotein receptors and atherosclerosis. *Adv Exp Med Biol* 1985;183:45–71.

55 Gianturco SH, Brown SA, Via DP, Bradley WA. The β-VLDL receptor pathway in murine P388D1 cells. *J Lipid Res* 1986;27:412–20.

56 Gianturco SH, Bradley WA. Structural and functional heterogeneity in very low density lipoproteins from normal and hypertriglyceridemic subjects. In *Proceedings of the Workshop on Lipoprotein Heterogeneity* (ed. K Lippel). Bethesda: National Institutes of Health, NIH Publication No. 87–2646, 1987:75–87.

57 Gianturco SH, Packard CJ, Shepherd J et al. Abnormal suppression of 3-hydroxy-3-methylglutaryl-CoA reductase activity in cultured human fibroblasts by hypertriglyceridemic very low density lipoprotein subclasses. *Lipids* 1980;15:456–63.

58 Gianturco SH, Bradley WA. Lipoprotein-mediated cellular mechanisms for atherosclerosis in hypertriglyceridemia. *Semin Thromb Hemost* 1988;14:164–8.

59 Austin MA. Plasma triglyceride and coronary heart disease. *Arterioscler Thromb* 1991;11:2–14.

60 Fowler S, Shio H, Haley NJ. Characterization of lipid-laden aortic cells from cholesterol-fed rabbits. IV. Investigation of macrophage-like properties of aortic cell populations. *Lab Invest* 1979;41:372–8.

61 Gerrity RG. The role of the monocyte in atherogenesis. I. Transition of blood-borne monocytes into foam cells in fatty lesions. *Am J Pathol* 1981;103:181–90.

62 Gerrity RG. The role of the monocyte in atherogenesis. II. Migration of foam cells from atherosclerotic lesions. *Am J Pathol* 1981;103:191–200.

63 Faggiotto A, Ross R. Studies of hypercholesterolemia in the nonhuman primate II. Fatty streak conversion to fibrous plaque. *Arteriosclerosis* 1984;4:341–56.

64 Goldstein JL, Brown MS. Lipoprotein metabolism in the macrophage: Implications for cholesterol deposition in atherosclerosis. *Annu Rev Biochem* 1983;52:223–61.

65 Ostlund-Lindqvist AM, Guftafson S, Lindquist P, Witztum JL, Little JA. Uptake and degradation of human chylomicrons by macrophages. Role of lipoprotein lipase. *Arteriosclerosis* 1983;3:433–40.

66 Bersot TP, Innerarity TL, Mahley RW, Havel RJ. Cholesteryl ester accumulation in mouse peritoneal macrophages induced by β-migrating very low density lipoproteins from patients with atypical dysbetalipoproteinemia. *J Clin Invest* 1983;72:1024–33.

67 Bersot TP, Innerarity TL, Pitas RE et al. Fat feeding in humans induces lipoproteins of density less than 1.006 that are enriched in apolipoprotein [a] and that cause lipid accumulation in macrophages. *J Clin Invest* 1986;77:622–30.

68 Huff MW, Evans AJ, Sawyez CG, Wolfe BM, Nestel PJ. Cholesterol accumulation in J774 macrophages induced by triglyceride rich lipoproteins. Comparison of very low density lipoprotein from subjects with type III, IV and V hyperlipoproteinemias. *Arterioscler Thromb* 1991;11:221–3.

69 Zilversmit DB. A proposal linking atherogenesis to the interaction of endothelial lipoprotein lipase with triglyceride rich lipoproteins. *Circ Res* 1973;6:633–8.

70 Zilversmit DB. Atherogenesis: A postprandial phenomenon. *Circulation* 1979;60:473–85.

71 Weintraub MS, Zechner R, Brown A, Eisenberg S, Breslow JL. Dietary polyunsaturated fats of the ω-6 and ω-3 series reduce postprandial lipoprotein levels. *J Clin Invest* 1988;82:1884–93.

72 Patsch JR, Karlin JB, Scott LW, Smith LC, Gotto AM Jr. Inverse relationship between blood levels of high density lipoprotein subfraction 2 and magnitude of postprandial lipemia. *Proc Natl Acad Sci USA* 1983;80:1449–53.

73 Weintraub MS, Eisenberg S, Breslow JL. Different patterns of postprandial lipoprotein metabolism in normal type IIa, type III, and type IV hyperlipoproteinemic individuals. *J Clin Invest* 1987;79:1110–19.

74 Cohn JS, McNamara JR, Cohn SD, Ordovas JM, Schaefer EJ. Postprandial plasma lipoprotein changes in human subjects of different ages. *J Lipid Res* 1988;29:469–79.

75 Cohn JS, McNamara JR, Cohn SD, Ordovas JM, Schaefer EJ. Plasma apolipoprotein

changes in the triglyceride-rich lipoprotein fraction of human subjects fed a fat-rich meal. *J Lipid Res* 1988;29:925–36.

76 Genest J, Sniderman A, Cianflone K *et al.* Hyperapobetalipoproteinemia. *Arteriosclerosis* 1986;6:297–304.

77 Gregg RE, Gabelli C, Brewer HB. Regulation of the metabolism of apo-B containing lipoproteins by apolipoprotein E and the low density lipoprotein and remnant lipo- protein receptors. In *Proceedings of the Workshop on Lipoprotein Heterogeneity* (ed. K Lippel). Bethesda: National Institutes of Health, NIH Publication No. 87–2646, 1987:237–47.

78 Weintraub MS, Eisenberg S, Breslow JL. Dietary fat clearance in normal subjects is regulated by genetic variation in apolipoprotein E. *J Clin Invest* 1987;80:1571–7.

79 Herz J, Hamann U, Rogne S *et al.* Surface location and high affinity for calcium of a 500-kd liver membrane protein closely related to the LDL-receptor suggest a physiological role as lipoprotein receptor. *EMBO J* 1988;7:4119–27.

80 Steinbrecher UP, Zhang H, Lougheed M. Role of oxidatively modified LDL in atherosclerosis. *Free Radic Biol Med* 1990;9:155–68.

81 Van Lenten BJ, Fogelman AM, Hokom MM *et al.* Regulation of the uptake and degradation of β-very low density lipoprotein in human monocyte–macrophages. *J Biol Chem* 1983;258:5151–7.

82 Nestel PJ, Billington T, Bozelmans J. Metabolism of human plasma triacylglycerol- rich lipoproteins in rodent macrophages: Capacity for interaction at β-VLDL receptor. *Biochim Biophys Acta* 1985;837:314–24.

83 Kowal RC, Herz J, Goldstein JL, Esser V, Brown MS. Low density lipoprotein receptor-related protein mediates uptake of cholesteryl esters derived from apoprotein E-enriched lipoproteins. *Proc Natl Acad Sci USA* 1989;86:5810–14.

84 Goldstein JL, Brown MS. The low density lipoprotein pathway and its relations to atherosclerosis. *Annu Rev Biochem* 1977;46:897–930.

85 Fogelman AM, Schechter I, Seager J *et al.* Malondialdehyde alteration of low density lipoprotein leads to cholesteryl ester accumulation in human monocyte– macrophages. *Proc Natl Acad Sci USA* 1980;77:2214–18.

86 Fogelman AM, Haberland ME, Seager J, Hokom M, Edwards PA. Factors regulating the activities of the low density lipoprotein receptor and the scavenger receptor on human monocyte–macrophages. *J Lipid Res* 1981;22:1131–41.

87 Traber MG, Kayden HJ. Low density lipoprotein receptor activity in human monocyte-derived macrophages and its relation to atheromatous lesions. *Proc Natl Acad Sci USA* 1980;77:5466–70.

88 Knight BL, Soutar AK. Changes in the metabolism of modified and unmodified low- density lipoproteins during the maturation of cultured blood monocyte–macrophages from normal and homozygous familial hypercholesterolaemic subjects. *Eur J Biochem* 1982;125:407–13.

89 Hara H, Tanishita H, Yokoyama S, Tajima S, Yamamoto A. Induction of acetylated low density lipoprotein receptor and suppression of low density lipoprotein receptor on the cells of human monocytic leukemia cell line (THP-1 cell). *Biochem Biophys Res Commun* 1987;146:802–8.

90 Via DP, Pons L, Dennison DK, Fanslow AE, Bernini F. Induction of acetyl-LDL receptor activity by phorbol ester in human monocyte cell line THP-1. *J Lipid Res* 1989;30:1515–24.

91 Bradley WA, Hwang S-L-C, Karlin JB *et al.* Low density lipoprotein (LDL) receptor binding determinants switch from apolipoprotein E (apoE) to apoB during conversion of hypertriglyceridemic very low density lipoprotein (HTG-VLDL) to LDL. *J Biol Chem* 1984;259:14728–35.

92 Krul ES, Tikkanen MJ, Cole TG, Davie JM, Schonfeld G. Roles of apolipoproteins B and E in the cellular binding of very low density lipoproteins. *J Clin Invest* 1985; 75:361–9.

93 Sacks FM, Breslow JL. Very low density lipoproteins stimulate cholesteryl ester

formation in U937 macrophages. Heterogeneity and biologic variation among normal humans. *Arteriosclerosis* 1987;7:35–46.

94 Hui DY, Innerarity TL, Milne RW, Marcel YL, Mahley RW. Binding of chylomicron remnants and β-very low density lipoproteins to hepatic and exhepatic lipoprotein receptors. *J Biol Chem* 1984;259:15060–8.

95 Eisenberg S, Friedman G, Vogel T. Enhanced metabolism of normolipemic human plasma very low density lipoprotein in cultured cells by exogenous apolipoprotein E-3. *Arteriosclerosis* 1988;8:480–7.

96 Catapano AL, Jackson RL, Gilliam EB, Gotto AM Jr, Smith LC. Quantification of apoC-II and apoC-III of human very low density lipoproteins by analytical isoelectric focusing. *J Lipid Res* 1978;19:1047–52.

97 Schonfeld G, Patsch W, Pfleger B, Witztum JL, Weidman SW. Lipolysis produces changes in the immunoreactivity and cell reactivity of very low density lipoproteins. *J Clin Invest* 1979;64:1288–97.

98 Schonfeld G, Tikkanen MJ, Hahn K-S. In *Drugs Affecting Lipid Metabolism VIII*. (eds D Kritchevsky, WL Holmes, R Paoletti). New York: Plenum Press, 1985:135–57.

99 Goldstein JL, Ho YK, Brown MS, Innerarity TL, Mahley RW. Cholesteryl ester accumulation in macrophages resulting from receptor-mediated uptake and degradation of hypercholesterolemic canine β-very low density lipoproteins. *J Biol Chem* 1980;255:1839–48.

100 Koo C, Wernette-Hammond L, Innerarity TL. Uptake of canine β-VLDL by mouse peritoneal macrophages is mediated by a LDL receptor. *J Biol Chem* 1986;261:11194–201.

101 Koo C, Wernette-Hammond ME, Garcia Z *et al*. Uptake of cholesterol-rich remnant lipoproteins by human monocyte-derived macrophages is mediated by low density lipoprotein receptors. *J Clin Invest* 1988;81:1332–40.

102 Meade TW, North WR, Chakrabarti R *et al*. Haemostatic function and cardiovascular death: early results of a prospective study. Lancet 1980;i:1050–4.

103 Mitropoulos KA. Hypercoagulability and factor VII in hypertriglyceridemia. *Semin Thromb Hemost* 1988;14:246–52.

104 Elkeles RS, Chakrabarti R, Vickers M, Stirling Y, Meade TW. Effect of treatment of hyperlipidaemia on haemostatic variables. *Br Med J* 1980;2:973–4.

105 Simpson HCR, Meade TW, Stirling Y *et al*. Hypertriglyceridaemia and hypercoagulability. Lancet 1983;i:786–9.

106 DeSousa C, Soria C, Ayrault-Jarrier M *et al*. Association between coagulation factors VII and X with triglyceride-rich lipoproteins. *J Clin Pathol* 1988;41:940–4.

107 Bradley WA, Song J-N, Gianturco SH. Thrombin/prothrombin interactions with very low density lipoproteins. *Ann N Y Acad Sci* 1986;485:159–69.

108 Vukovitch T, Marktl M, Nemeth G. Heterogenicity of human factor VIII/VWF in lipemic plasma. *Thromb Res* 1985;38:215–23.

109 Meade TW, Mellows S, Brozovic M *et al*. Haemostatic function and ischaemic heart disease: principal results of the Northwick Park Heart Study. Lancet 1986;ii:533–7.

110 Mitropoulos KA, Martin JC, Reeves BEA, Esnouf MP. The activation of the contact phase of coagulation by physiologic surfaces in plasma: the effect of large negatively charged liposomal vesicles. *Blood* 1989;73:1525–33.

111 Mitropoulos KA, Martin JC, Burgess AI *et al*. The increased rate of activation of factor VII in late pregnancy can contribute to increased reactivity of factor VII. *Thromb Haemost* 1990;63:349–55.

112 DeSousa C, Bruckert E, Giral JP *et al*. Coagulation factor VII and plasma triglycerides. Decreased catabolism as a possible mechanism of factor VII hyperactivity. *Haemostasis* 1989;19:125–30.

113 Miller GJ, Martin JC, Mitropoulos KA *et al*. Plasma factor VII is activated by postprandial triglyceridaemia irrespective of dietary fat composition. *Atherosclerosis* 1991;86:163–71.

114 Bajaj SP, Harmony JAK, Martinez-Carrion M, Castellino FJ. Human plasma lipoproteins as accelerators of prothrombin activation. *J Biol Chem* 1976;251:5233−6.

115 Lee DM, Koren E, Singh S, Mok T. Presence of B-100 in rat mesenteric chyle. *Biochem Biophys Res Commun* 1984;123:1149−56.

116 Cardin AD, Witt KR, Chao J *et al.* Degradation of apolipoprotein B-100 of human plasma low density lipoproteins by tissue and plasma kallikreins. *J Biol Chem* 1984; 259:8522−8.

117 Cardin AD, Ranganathan S, Hirose N *et al.* Structural organization of apolipoprotein B-100 of human plasma low density lipoproteins. Comparison to B-48 of chylomicrons and very low density lipoproteins. *J Biol Chem* 1986;261:16744−8.

118 Bradley WA, Gilliam EB, Gotto AM Jr, Gianturco SH. Apoprotein-E degradation in human very low density lipoproteins by plasma protease(s): chemical and biological consequences. *Biochem Biophys Res Commun* 1982;109:1360−7.

119 Schwartz BS, Levy GA, Curtiss LK, Fair DS, Edgington TS. Plasma lipoprotein induction and suppression of the generation of cellular procoagulant activity *in vitro*. *J Clin Invest* 1981;67:1650−8.

120 Levy GA, Schwartz BS, Curtiss LK, Edgington T. Plasma lipoprotein induction and suppression of the generation of cellular procoagulant activity *in vitro*. *J Clin Invest* 1981;67:1614−22.

121 Vague P, Juhan-Vague I, Aillaud MF *et al.* Correlation between blood fibrinolytic activity, plasminogen activator inhibitor level, plasma insulin level, and relative body weight in normal and obese subjects. *Metabolism* 1986;35:250−3.

122 Auwerx J, Bouillon R, Collen D, Geboers J. Tissue-type plasminogen activator antigen and plasminogen activator inhibitor in diabetes mellitus. *Arteriosclerosis* 1988;8:68−72.

123 Hamsten A, Bjorn W, DeFaire U, Blomback M. Increased plasma levels of a rapid inhibitor of tissue plasminogen activator in young survivors of myocardial infarction. *N Engl J Med* 1985;313:1557−63.

124 Juhan-Vague I, Vague P, Alessi MC *et al.* Relationship between plasma insulin, triglyceride, body mass index and plasminogen activator-inhibitor-1. *Diabete Metab* 1987,13.331=8.

125 Booyse FM, Bruce R, Gianturco SH, Bradley WA. Normal but not hypertriglyceridemic very low density lipoprotein induces rapid release of tissue plasminogen activator from cultured human umbilical vein endothelial cells. *Semin Thromb Hemost* 1988; 14:175−9.

126 Sitko-Rahm A, Wiman B, Hamsten A, Nilsson J. Secretion of plasminogen activator inhibitor-1 from cultured human umbilical vein endothelial cells is induced by very low density lipoprotein. *Arteriosclerosis* 1990;10:1067−73.

Chapter 7
Lipoprotein(a) and Coronary Artery Disease

ANGELO M. SCANU

Historical perspective

Lipoprotein(a) or Lp(a), first reported in 1963 by Berg [1], is now recognized to be a genetic trait that a number of epidemiologic studies [2–5] have found associated with an increased prevalence of coronary artery disease (CAD). The structure of Lp(a) escaped investigation until the successful application of techniques of molecular biology that led to the unexpected finding that apolipoprotein(a) or apo(a), the specific marker of Lp(a), has a striking structural similarity to plasminogen, a key zymogen of the fibrinolytic system. This chapter will provide an updated account of the structural characteristics of Lp(a), and the current views concerning its potential pathogenic role in coronary heart disease (CHD) both from the atherogenic and thrombogenic viewpoints.

Structure of Lp(a) [2–7]

Lp(a) represents a class of lipoprotein particles having as a protein moiety the apo B_{100}–apo(a) complex (Fig. 7.1). Apo B_{100} in this complex is currently assumed to be structurally identical to apo B_{100} which is the apolipoprotein of authentic low-density lipoproteins (LDL). The current evidence indicates that the linkage of apo(a) likely involves cysteine 4190 located in the carboxyl end of apo B_{100}. In the cases where two copies of apo(a) are linked to apo B_{100}, cysteine 3190 is also expected to be involved. Apo(a) is a glycoprotein containing about 30% carbohydrate in weight with a polypeptide chain varying in size between 300 and 800 kDa. Recent studies have shown that it has a striking structural similarity to plasminogen although differing from it in several features (Table 7.1), namely: (i) absence of Kringles 1, 2 and 3; (ii) presence of 15–37 Kringle 4-like domains compared to the single Kringle 4 in plasminogen; (iii) inability of conversion into an active fibrinolytic enzyme owing to a genetically determined arg → cys substitution at the activation site. Thus, apo(a) is a giant zymogen with a high number of anchoring sites represented by the several Kringle 4 domain repeats (Fig. 7.2). Apo(a) is a water-soluble glycoprotein with

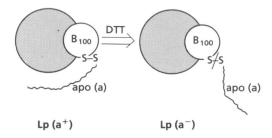

Fig. 7.1 Schematic representations of Lp(a) as a spherical particle containing apo B_{100} linked by a disulfide bridge to apo(a), the specific glycoprotein marker of Lp(a). Upon the action *in vitro* of a reducing agent like dithiothreitol (DTT), apo(a) is dissociated from the apo B_{100}-containing complex resulting in what is defined as Lp(a⁻). There is no evidence that apo B_{48}, the apo B mainly synthesized in the intestine, is involved in covalent linkage to apo(a).

Table 7.1 Properties of apo(a) and plasminogen

Parameter	Apo(a)	Plasminogen
Molecular weight (kDa)	280–800	≈90 000
Signal sequence	19 residues*	19 residues†
NH$_2$ terminus	Glu–Gln–Ser–His–Val–Val . . .	Glu–Pro–Leu–Asp–Asp–Tyr . . .
	Absent	Present
Kringle 1–3	13–37‡	1
Kringle 4, number	1	1
Kringle 5, number	Ser–Ile	Arg–Val
Activation site	4308–4309	561–562
Catalytic triad	Ser–His–Asp	Ser–His–Asp

* Apo(a):–Met–Glu–His–Lys–Glu–Val–Val–Leu–Leu–Leu–Leu–Leu–Phe–Leu–Lys– Ser–Ala–Ala–Pro.

† Plasminogen:–Met–Glu–His–Lys–Glu–Val–Val–Leu–Leu–Leu–Leu–Leu–Phe– Leu–Lys–Ser–Gly–Gln–Gly . . .

‡ Isoforms with higher or lower Kringle 4 number are theoretically possible but not yet documented.

little affinity for lipids; thus, affiliation with lipids in Lp(a) is via its attachment to apo B_{100}. This notion has emerged from *in vitro* studies showing that the apo B_{100}–apo(a) complex, once freed of its lipid complement by extraction with organic solvents, has lipophilic properties [8]. Depending upon the lipid matrix one can have either particles with LDL-like characteristics with a cholesteryl ester-rich core (CE-Lp(a)), or very low-density lipoprotein (VLDL)-like particles with a triglyceride (TG)-rich core (TG-Lp(a)) [5]. Because the size of apo(a) that is linked to apo B_{100} varies, the weight of the protein moiety in CE-Lp(a) and

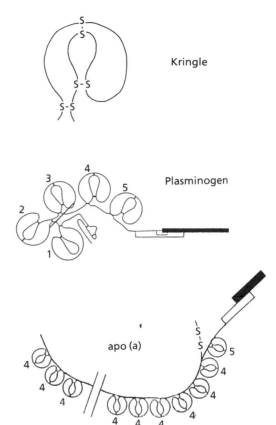

Fig. 7.2 The fundamental looped structure of a representative kringle characterized by three intrachain disulfide bridges. This structure contains from 80 to 100 amino acids. The amino acid sequence differs in the five kringles of plasminogen and are named from 1 to 5. Apo(a) contains up to 37 Kringle 4-like domains and 1 Kringle 5. Not all apo(a) Kringles are identical to each other. Moreover, there is no complete homology between apo(a) Kringle 4 and plasminogen Kringle 4.

TG-Lp(a) also varies. This is one of the reasons for their density and size heterogeneity of Lp(a). To sum up, Lp(a) is a variant of LDL in which apo B_{100} has been genetically modified by a covalent attachment to a plasminogen-like protein resulting in a lipoprotein structure with functional properties distinct from those of apo B_{100}.

Genetics of apo(a) [2–4]

The apo(a) gene is localized on the long arm of chromosome 6 adjacent to the plasminogen gene comprising several alleles likely deriving from the splicing of the apo(a) gene. Several apo(a) RNA transcripts have been identified in the liver and their size correlated with the size of the apo(a) isoforms. At this time, the generally accepted view is that the apo(a) gene is transmitted in an autosomal codominant mode operating on a polygenic background likely affected by environmental factors. A definitive answer must await the elucidation of the apo(a) gene, the exact determination of the actual number of apo(a) alleles, and the elucidation of the physical–chemical properties of the several apo(a) isoforms.

Lp(a) in species other than humans

The presence of Lp(a) has been demonstrated in the blood of apes and Old World monkeys [9–11] but not in New World monkeys [9] or species like dogs, rats, mice, or chickens. The presence in guinea pigs has recently been reported [12] but needs further validation. Rather surprising is the presence of Lp(a) in the plasma of the hedgehog, a hibernating animal rather low in the evolutionary scale [13]. This observation invites further studies on the structural properties of the Lp(a) of this animal species. The best information on Lp(a) is in rhesus monkey and baboons. The Lp(a) of the rhesus monkey has structural features very similar to humans, except for the absence of Kringle 5 and amino acid substitutions in the catalytic triad [14]. Otherwise the Lp(a) in the plasma of these animals recognizes the same degree of density heterogeneity as humans, as well as similar apo(a) polymorphism. There is also an immunologic cross-reactivity between human and simian apo(a). In the single monkey studies by Tomlinson *et al.* [14] a message of apo(a) was also found in the brain and in the testis which are organs not known to synthesize apo B_{100}, and probably not mature apo(a). The current information on the baboon is comparatively less extensive than that in the rhesus monkey; however, it is likely that the two structures are very similar to each other [11]. The rhesus monkey model has also provided evidence that the LDL receptor is not functionally involved in the metabolism of Lp(a) [10], while studies in the baboon have demonstrated a relationship between apo(a) transcripts and plasma apo(a) size [15].

Physiology of Lp(a) [4,6]

The liver is the major if not the only site of synthesis of Lp(a). The steps of this synthesis and assembly have not yet been well worked out. The preliminary evidence derived from studies in hepatocytes in culture indicates that apo B_{100} and apo(a) are synthesized separately and that their linkage occurs intracellularly, possibly at the site of the Golgi apparatus where the glycosylation step of apo(a) may also take place. That the complexation of the apo B_{100}–apo(a) complex occurs prior to cellular export is suggested by the fact that mature Lp(a) can be found in the nascent particles secreted into the culture medium. Free apo(a) has also been found in the medium which suggests that not all synthesized apo(a) is bound to apo B_{100} and that only under well defined conditions, possibly requiring a specific enzyme, does linkage occur. In the plasma, essentially all apo(a) is bound to apo B_{100} as a part of the Lp(a) complex. It is possible that any free apo(a) that enters the circulation undergoes hydrolysis by the action of proteolytic enzymes in the plasma. The factors that control the plasma levels of Lp(a) are not well established: synthesis has been suggested to contribute about 40% [3]; other factors may be at play, i.e., intravascular remodeling, redistribution, and catabolism. Although suggested by some workers [3] a functional role of the LDL receptor in the uptake and catabolism of Lp(a) appears to be improbable and therefore also the participation of the scavenger receptor; the involvement of either a receptor specific for Lp(a) or a nonreceptor-mediated pathway is suspected. Recent studies have shown that Lp(a) can traverse the vascular endothelium and remain intact [16–18]. Thus, it is possible that some Lp(a) degradation may occur in the subendothelial space following chemical modifications that render this lipoprotein a candidate for uptake by the scavenger receptor of resident macrophages (for more detail see Chapter 4). When plasma levels of Lp(a) are below 7 mg/dl Lp(a) protein or 30 mg/dl total Lp(a), no pathologic sequelae have been reported [6]. Currently, we do not know whether there is a good side of Lp(a). It has been suggested that by escaping uptake by the LDL receptor pathway Lp(a) may be involved in a selective delivery of cholesterol to sites where active cell division (i.e., tissue repair) takes place. It might also have a modulating role in the fibrinolytic process occurring at the endothelial surface (possibly in the process of conversion of plasminogen to fibrin).

One of the characteristics of Lp(a) is to vary almost 1000-fold in its plasma concentrations among individuals and to have a skewed distribution showing that about 80% of the population has normal plasma levels of Lp(a) [2–6]. This is true for whites; Afroamericans have considerably higher levels of Lp(a) with a bell-shape curve distribution. The reasons for this racial difference, which is also present in childhood, are not known.

Lp(a) as a cardiovascular pathogen

As already mentioned, based mainly on epidemiologic evidence (see [6] for review), only high plasma levels of Lp(a) are associated with an increased incidence of CAD. The LDL-like structure of Lp(a) makes one suspect that the atherogenic action occurs via the cholesterol content of its core and the prothrombogenic action through its plasminogen-like characteristics. These two putative mechanisms will be first examined separately although they may work in a synergistic way.

Lp(a) and atherogenicity [2,4,5]

A most attractive hypothesis is that Lp(a), by escaping uptake by the LDL receptor, is preferentially targeted to macrophages transforming them into foam cells, a first step towards the development of the atherosclerotic plaque. However, the current evidence does not support an interaction of native Lp(a) with the scavenger receptor. For this to occur, Lp(a) must undergo structural modifications by the action of either oxygen-free radicals, proteoglycans, glycosaminoglycans, or fibrin that would occur once Lp(a) traverses the vascular endothelium and accumulates in the subendothelial intima. In favor of this hypothesis are the data indicating that a large amount of material recognized by anti-Lp(a) antibodies accumulates in the subendothelial space of arterial vessels [16] or vein grafts [17]. This "filtration" theory implies that atherogenicity is proportional to plasma Lp(a) levels, a fact which, however, has not been universally documented.

Lp(a) thrombogenicity [4,18]

The thrombogenicity of Lp(a) derives from the structural similarity of apo(a) to plasminogen. Apo(a) has been shown to compete with plasminogen in *in vitro* and *ex vivo* systems. The competition can occur at the level of the fibrin(ogen) molecule as well as its fragments. Moreover, Lp(a) has been shown to competitively displace plasminogen from the plasminogen receptor in macrophages, endothelial cells, and platelets. This competition appears to involve the kringle region of apo(a), although the precise structural determinants for this competition have yet to be established. The competitive events are likely to occur at the endothelial surface where there is a finely regulated balance between fibrinolysis and antifibrinolysis. However, an association between Lp(a) and fibrin has also been documented in the arterial intima at the level of the atherosclerotic plaque and considered to contribute to the genesis and progression of this plaque [19]. A thrombogenic action by Lp(a) has not yet been clearly documented *in vivo*. It is possible, however, that Lp(a)-related events occur at focal points of the vascular endothelium and may not be readily detected at the level of whole plasma.

Clinical considerations (see [6] for review)

The studies suggesting that high plasma levels of Lp(a) have an atherothrombotic potential must be viewed with concern since 15–20% of the white population have high plasma levels of Lp(a), an incidence that is even higher in blacks. Much of this pathogenicity of Lp(a) is genetically determined and difficult to control, since our means to influence the plasma levels of Lp(a) are rather limited at this time. However, it is becoming apparent that the pathogenicity of Lp(a) increases in the presence of other risk factors, which include disorders like familial hypercholesterolemia, hypoalphalipoproteinemia, diabetes, obesity, hypertension, etc. Exogenous factors relating to lifestyle (i.e., cigarette smoking, sedentary life, stress, etc.) may also be contributory. Thus, in a preventive sense, we must work towards the control of these correctable risk factors and approach them early in life to effectively influence the establishment and the progression of the atherothrombotic process. Screening of children is indicated in families with a history of premature cardiovascular disease. Lp(a) exhibits an autosomal codominant mode of transmission and is expressed early in life. In subjects with high plasma levels of Lp(a), premarriage counseling is advisable.

Therapy

As already mentioned in the previous section, we are limited in our ability to significantly modify the plasma levels of Lp(a). This is particularly true for the CE-Lp(a) particles that have been shown to be refractory to dietary approaches and drug therapy. An exception is niacin, which in subjects with high levels of plasma Lp(a) may reduce these levels by about 30% [20]. The response, however, is not universal and one has to face the risk of the side-effects attending the prolonged use of this pharmacologic agent, which for this purpose has to be used in high dosage (i.e., 3–4 g daily). Clearly, we have to look forward to newer drugs designed to take into account the structure and biology of Lp(a). Attention must also be directed at the TG-Lp(a) particles since their plasma levels might be easier to manage, particularly in postprandial hypertriglyceridemia which is amenable to control by modulating fat and/or carbohydrate intake alone or in combination with drugs like fibrates or niacin.

Acknowledgments

The original research work by the author was supported by Program Project grant HL-18577 from the US Public Health Service. The author also gratefully acknowledges the valuable help of Ms Sue Hutchison in the preparation of the manuscript.

References

1 Berg K. A new serum type system in man—the Lp system. *Acta Pathol Microbiol Scand* 1963;59:369–82.
2 Scanu AM (ed.). *Lipoprotein(a)*. San Diego: Academic Press, 1990.
3 Utermann G. The mysteries of lipoprotein(a). *Science* 1989;246:904–10.
4 Scanu AM, Fless GM. Lp(a): Heterogeneity and biological relevance. *J Clin Invest* 1990;85:1709–15.
5 Scanu AM. Lipoprotein(a): A genetically determined cardiovascular pathogen in search of a function. *J Lab Clin Med* 1990;116:142–6.
6 Scanu AM, Scandiani L. Lipoprotein(a): Structure, biology and clinical relevance. In *Advances in Internal Medicine*, Vol. 36 (eds GH Stollerman, JT LaMont, JJ Leonard, MD Siperstein). St Louis: Mosby Year Book, 1991:249–70.
7 McLean JW, Tomlinson JE, Kuang W *et al.* cDNA sequence of human apolipoprotein(a) is homologous to plasminogen. *Nature* 1987;330:132–7.
8 Fless GM, Pfaffinger DJ, Eisenbart JD, Scanu AM. Solubility, immunochemical and lipoprotein binding properties of apoB100-apo(a), the protein moiety of lipoprotein(a). *J Lipid Res* 1990;31:909–17.
9 Makino K, Abe A, Maeda S *et al.* Lipoprotein(a) in nonhuman primates. Presence and characteristics of Lp(a) immunoreactive materials using antihuman Lp(a) serum. *Atherosclerosis* 1989;78:81–5.
10 Neven L, Khalil A, Pfaffinger D *et al.* Rhesus monkey model of familial hyper-cholesterolemia: relation between plasma Lp(a) levels, apo(a) isoforms and LDL-receptor function. *J Lipid Res* 1990;31:633–43.
11 Rainwater DL, Lanford RE. Production of lipoprotein(a) by primary baboon hepatocytes. *Biochim Biophys Acta* 1989;1003:30–5.
12 Rath M, Pauling L. Immunological evidence for the accumulation of lipoprotein(a) in the atherosclerotic lesion of the hypoascorbemic guinea pig. *Proc Natl Acad Sci USA* 1990;87:9388–9.
13 Laplaud PM, Beaubatie L, Rall SJ Jr, Luc G, Saboureau M. Lipoprotein(a) is the major apoB-containing lipoprotein in the plasma of a hibernator, the hedgehog. *J Lipid Res* 1988;29:1157–70.
14 Tomlinson JE, McLean JW, Lawn RM. Rhesus monkey apolipoprotein(a): sequence, evolution and site of synthesis. *J Biol Chem* 1989;264:5957–65.
15 Hixson JE, Britten S, Manis G, Rainwater DL. Apolipoprotein(a)apo(a)glycoprotein isoforms result from size differences in apo(a) mRNA in baboons. *J Biol Chem* 1989;264:6013–16.
16 Rath M, Niendorf A, Reblin T *et al.* Detection and quantification of lipoprotein(a) in the arterial wall of 107 coronary bypass surgery. *Arteriosclerosis* 1989;9:579–92.
17 Cushing GL, Gaubatz JW, Nava M *et al.* Quantitation and localization of apolipoprotein(a) and B in coronary artery bypass vein graft resected at operation. *Arteriosclerosis* 1989;9:593–603.
18 Loscalzo J. Lipoprotein(a): A unique risk factor for atherothrombotic disease. *Arteriosclerosis* 1990;10:672–9.
19 Beisiegel U, Niendorf A, Wolf C, Reblin T, Rath M. Lipoprotein(a) in the arterial wall. *Eur Heart J* 1990;11:174–83.
20 Carlson LA, Mansten A, Asplund A. Pronounced lowering of serum levels of lipo-protein Lp(a) in hyperlipidaemic subjects treated with nicotinic acid. *J Intern Med* 1989;226:271–6.

Chapter 8
Postprandial Lipoproteins and Atherosclerosis

BYUNG H. CHUNG & GEORGE A. TALLIS

Introduction

The link between cholesterol and atherosclerosis has been established by compositional analysis of atherosclerotic plaques and studies of animals on atherogenic diets [1,2]. Although epidemiologic studies have shown that the incidence of coronary heart disease (CHD) in humans is correlated with the level of serum total cholesterol or low-density lipoprotein (LDL) cholesterol [3], many patients with CHD have normal serum total cholesterol or LDL cholesterol. In most epidemiologic studies, the measurement of serum cholesterol and/or lipoproteins has been made in the fasting state because it is believed that these values give a more stable baseline than nonfasting levels. However, humans are predominantly in the postprandial lipemic state during the day as a result of regular meals. Thus, most epidemiologic studies have not considered the role of postprandial lipoproteins, which are not normally detected in the fasting state, in the development of atherosclerosis.

Postprandial chylomicrons are often considered to be cholesterol-poor particles. However, when the number of cholesterol molecules per chylomicron particle is compared with that of an LDL particle, chylomicrons contain about 30× more molecules of cholesterol than LDL (Table 8.1). Thus, the capacity of postprandial chylomicrons to deliver cholesterol to cells is considerable. The amount of cholesterol associated with postprandial lipoproteins and their remnants in the fasting state is relatively small when compared to plasma LDL cholesterol (less than 2% of LDL cholesterol), but the daily transport of cholesterol through postprandial lipoproteins is equal to or greater than the cholesterol flux through LDL because of the higher fractional catabolic rate of postprandial lipoproteins (Table 8.1). Since the postprandial lipoprotein response varies widely between human subjects [4–12], the amount of cholesterol transported daily by the postprandial lipoproteins will be much more variable than that transported by LDL. Zilversmit [13] suggested that the cholesterol associated with chylomicron remnants may be just as atherogenic as that carried by LDL.

Table 8.1 Comparison of composition and metabolic parameters of chylomicrons and/or chylomicron remnants with LDL

Parameters	Lipoproteins	
	Chylomicrons	LDL
*Composition (% of mass)**		
Triglycerides	86.0−92.0	7.0
Unesterified cholesterol	0.8−1.6	9.0
Esterified cholesterol	0.8−1.4	36.0
Phospholipids	6.0−8.0	22.0
Proteins	1.0−1.5	26.0
Molecular mass (Da)	$0.4-30 \times 10^9$	2.3×10^6
Particle diameter (nm)	60.0	9.6
Molecules of lipid per particle†		
Triglycerides	507 000	298
Unesterified cholesterol	25 840	475
Esterified cholesterol	27 700	1310
Metabolic parameters‡		
Plasma concentration (cholesterol)	2 mg/dl	130 mg/dl
Plasma pool size	0.06 g	4.0 g
Fractional clearance rate	100/day	0.5−1/day
Flux	6 g/day	2−4 g/day

* Adapted from [17] and [19].
† Adapted from [95].
‡ Adapted from [96].

There are no available prospective data relating the postprandial lipemic response to occurrence of CHD. Epidemiologic studies relating the level of postprandial lipoproteins to CHD have been hampered because the time of maximal appearance of postprandial lipoproteins in blood after ingestion of a meal is variable both within and between individuals; in addition, some subjects have more than one postprandial peak [10,12]. Therefore, it is necessary to take multiple samples in order to determine the peak level of postprandial lipoproteins. Furthermore, methods for the large-scale separation and quantitation of postprandial lipoproteins and their remnants are currently lacking.

Epidemiologic studies by Shekelle and Stamler [14] showed that a high intake of dietary cholesterol was correlated with CHD, but that this association was partially independent of the fasting serum cholesterol level. This suggests that dietary cholesterol and fat may influence the atherogenic process via transient postprandial lipoproteins. Case control studies [15,16] have shown that the levels and/or resident time of postprandial lipoproteins and their remnants were significantly higher in

CHD patients than in control subjects. This suggests that postprandial lipoproteins may be important in the development of atherosclerosis.

Synthesis and metabolism of postprandial lipoproteins

Chylomicrons are triglyeride-rich particles formed in the small intestine during lipid absorption. Dietary fat is hydrolyzed into free fatty acids and glycerol in the small intestine, and these hydrolytic products are absorbed by the intestinal epithelium and esterified to form triacylglycerol and phospholipids. Dietary cholesterol is esterified by acyl CoA:cholesteryl acyltransferase in the intestinal mucosa [17]. These lipids are then combined with specific apolipoproteins in the intestinal microsomes and secreted as chylomicrons [17].

Chylomicrons are heterogeneous spherical particles with a size range of 75.0−600.0 nm and a mean diameter of $\sim$ 120.0 nm [18]. They have a density less than 0.95 g/ml and a mass ranging from 0.4 $\times$ 10^9 to 30 $\times$ 10^9 Da [19]. Triglycerides are the major component of chylomicrons, comprising 86−92% by mass. Cholesterol, phospholipids, and protein comprise 1.0−8.0% of the total mass of chylomicrons (Table 8.1). Apolipoprotein species identified in postprandial chylomicrons include apo A-I, apo A-II, apo A-IV, apo B_{48}, apo C-I, apo C-II, and apo C-III [20]. Apo B_{48} is a unique marker protein for postprandial lipoproteins and is necessary for their secretion from intestinal mucosal cells [21]. Although it was thought that apo B_{100} in circulating blood was exclusively derived from the liver, there is some evidence that human small intestine can synthesize a small amount of apo B_{100} [22]. After secretion, chylomicrons acquire additional apoproteins (apo C-I, apo C-II, apo C-III, and apo E) from high-density lipoprotein (HDL) which displace phospholipid from the chylomicron surface to HDL [23]. This modification is critical in subsequent chylomicron metabolism. Apo C-II is a cofactor which activates lipoprotein lipase [24,25], whereas apo C-III probably inhibits premature removal of chylomicrons by the liver [26,27]. Chylomicron particles rapidly lose most of their triglyceride following lipolysis at the endothelial surface [28,29]. Free fatty acids generated from the hydrolysis of chylomicrons are bound by albumin [28]. Hydrolysis of chylomicron triglycerides by lipoprotein lipase results in production of excess surface components consisting mainly of phospholipids, unesterified cholesterol, and apo A and apo Cs. These surface remnants are cleared by HDL [30]. Following lipolysis and the loss of surface components, chylomicrons become chylomicron remnants which are less than 5% of the original chylomicron mass[17].

Remnants are depleted in triglycerides and relatively enriched in cholesteryl ester, phospholipids, and proteins [17]. The major apolipoproteins of the remnants are apo B_{48} and apo E [17].

Chylomicron remnants are rapidly removed by the liver after binding to a specific hepatic receptor which recognizes apo E [31]. Although newly formed chylomicrons also contain apo E, the binding of chylomicrons to the liver receptors is inhibited by apo Cs on the chylomicrons [31]. Loss of apo Cs during lipolysis constitutes one of the modifications that permits recognition of apo E by the chylomicron remnant receptor [31]. It is important to note that dietary cholesterol transported by chylomicrons is delivered almost exclusively to the liver and does not contribute directly to cholesterol in other plasma lipoproteins. However, delivery of chylomicron remnants to the liver can increase the level of circulating very low-density lipoprotein (VLDL) by stimulating hepatic synthesis of VLDL [32].

Factors affecting the magnitude and duration of postprandial lipemia

The postprandial lipemic response varies markedly both in normolipidemic subjects and in the different types of hyperlipidemia [4–12]. Factors such as age, gender, apo E phenotype, composition of background diet, drug treatment, exercise, and glycemic control in diabetics have been reported to influence the extent and duration of postprandial lipemia.

Fasting triglyceride, HDL cholesterol, and the activities of enzymes responsible for the clearance of postprandial lipoproteins and their remnants are correlated with the degree of postprandial lipemia [4,7,9,10,33,34]. The fasting triglyceride level is the most consistent predictor with correlation coefficients reported from 0.40 to 0.95 [4,7,10,33]. The postprandial lipemic response correlated negatively with the levels of HDL cholesterol [9,10] and apo C-III [10] in fasting serum. Patsch *et al.* [7,34] have shown that the HDL_2 subfraction is a better predictor than total HDL. The magnitude of postprandial lipemia correlated inversely with lipoprotein lipase activity [9,34] and positively with hepatic lipase activity [34] in postheparin serum from normolipidemic subjects.

Kashyap *et al.* [10] reported that the postprandial lipemic response was three to four times higher in males than females, but in the study of Cohn *et al.* [12] men had only a 30% higher postprandial triglyceride increase than women. The lower postprandial lipemic response in women may reflect a higher activity of lipoprotein lipase in adipose tissue and postheparin serum in women compared with men [34,35].

Increasing age is usually associated with an increase in the magnitude and duration of postprandial lipemia [12,36]. A decrease in lipoprotein lipase activity and a possible change in hepatic chylomicron remnant receptor function with increasing age have been suggested as possible explanations [36].

Weintraub *et al.* [9] have compared the postprandial lipemic response in various phenotypes of hyperlipidemia. This study found that patients with Type IIa hyperlipidemia had lower chylomicron response to a fat load than normolipidemic subjects, whereas patients with Type III and IV hyperlipidemia had a much greater (more than fivefold) chylomicron response than normolipidemics. The clearance of chylomicron remnants from the circulation was markedly delayed in patients with Type III hyperlipidemia when compared with normolipidemics, Type IIa, or Type IV hyperlipidemic subjects [9]. Weintraub *et al.* [37] have also shown that the rate of clearance of postprandial lipoproteins is regulated by genetic variation at the apo E locus. These investigators demonstrated that normolipidemic subjects with an E-III/E-II phenotype cleared chylomicron remnants at a much slower rate than subjects with an E-III/E-III phenotype, while subjects with E-IV/E-IV or E-IV/E-III phenotypes cleared the remnants at a somewhat faster rate than individuals with E-III/E-III phenotype. Cortner *et al.* [8] found that the half-life of chylomicron remnants in Type III hyperlipidemic patients with E-II/E-II phenotype was 40× or 12× longer, respectively, than either normal subjects or patients with endogenous hypertriglyceridemia. Individuals with an E-II/E-II phenotype and a normal fasting triglyceride had a chylomicron remnant half-life which was much shorter (10×) than that of the E-II/E-II individuals with an increased fasting triglyceride; however, this half-life was still two to four times longer than that of normal subjects [8]. Patients with homozygous familial hypercholesterolemia exhibited a normal chylomicron response to a fat load [37]. In contrast to the greatly reduced rate of LDL clearance, the removal of chylomicron remnants in these patients was normal [38], suggesting that the receptors responsible for clearing chylomicron remnants are genetically distinct from LDL receptors.

A number of recent studies have shown that the fat composition of the background diet influences the lipemic response to a fat load [39,40]. Weintraub *et al.* [39] showed that a background diet rich in n-6 polyunsaturated fat (vegetable oil) or n-3 polyunsaturated fat (fish oil) reduced the level of postprandial chylomicrons by 56% and 67%, and of chylomicron remnants by 38% and 53%, respectively, when compared with a saturated fat diet. Harris *et al.* [40] showed that adding fish oil to the background diet reduced postprandial lipemia regardless of the type of fat in the test meal. The mechanism for the reduced postprandial lipemia on a diet rich in n-3 or n-6 fatty acids is not currently clear. Postheparin lipoprotein lipase activity on a diet rich in n-3 fatty acids was not significantly different from that on a diet rich in saturated fat [39], but postprandial lipoproteins produced following an n-3 unsaturated fat load were more susceptible to *in vitro* lipolysis than those produced following a saturated fat load [39]. However, *in vivo*, test meals of n-3 and saturated fatty acids produced a similar lipemic response in individuals on the same background diet [40]. It seems most likely that chronic n-3 fatty acid intake reduces endogenous VLDL synthesis, thereby reducing competition between VLDL and gut-derived lipoproteins for lipolysis, and so increases the catabolism of postprandial lipoproteins.

A number of studies have shown that exercise can decrease the postprandial lipemic response [41,42]. These findings reflect the increase in adipose tissue and postheparin lipoprotein lipase activity brought about by endurance training.

In drug studies, several fibric acid derivatives (gemfibrozil, fenofibrate) have been shown to decrease the postprandial lipemic response. Gemfibrozil reduced the level of postprandial lipoproteins by 66% in Type IV hyperlipidemic patients without significantly increasing lipoprotein lipase activity [9]. Simpson *et al.* [43] showed that treatment of CHD patients with fenofibrate reduced triglycerides (d <1.006) by 50% with an associated 73% increase in postheparin lipoprotein lipase. Cholestyramine was shown to increase postprandial lipoproteins in patients with Type IIa hyperlipidemia even though there was no increase in fasting triglyceride level [9]. In Type I and Type II diabetics, improvement of glycemic control with a period of continuous subcutaneous insulin infusion resulted in a reduction in postprandial lipoproteins [44]. This is likely to be due to both reduced production of VLDL, increasing the rate of chylomicron lipolysis, and an increase in lipoprotein lipase activity.

Effect of postprandial lipemia on lipoprotein metabolism

Postprandial lipoproteins affect many facets of lipoprotein metabolism. Alimentary lipemia is associated with an acute rise in the concentration of phospholipids and proteins in HDL, particularly in the HDL_2 subfraction [7,10,34,45–47]. The increase of HDL_2 mass during the postprandial lipemic state was more pronounced in women than men and correlated positively with adipose tissue lipoprotein lipase [35]. Tall *et al.*

[46] have shown that postprandial lipemia caused a redistribution of HDL mass into larger, less dense HDL particles, and that these changes were mainly due to an increased concentration of phospholipids and apoprotein transfer within existing HDL species. *In vitro* lipolysis studies have shown that the lipoprotein lipase-mediated hydrolysis of triglycerides in the core of triglyceride-rich lipoproteins generated excess surface components which fused to existing HDL_3 particles, transforming them into HDL_2-like particles [48]. Groot and Scheek [49] have shown that the changes in the level, composition, and flotation rate of HDL which occurred during the postprandial lipemic state were mainly due to uptake of surface material from chylomicrons, not only by existing HDL_2 but also by HDL_3 particles. Redgrave *et al.* [50] reported that postprandial lipemia shifted the distribution of VLDL towards larger diameter particles, probably because of competition between chylomicrons and hepatic VLDL for lipoprotein lipase. This study showed that most chylomicron remnants were removed from the circulation without degradation to small VLDL or LDL.

A number of studies [51–53] have reported that postprandial lipemia stimulates cholesteryl ester transfer activity, thereby accelerating the redistribution of cholesteryl ester between lipoproteins. The cholesteryl ester transfer reaction in plasma involves a net transfer of cholesteryl ester from cholesterol-rich lipoproteins (HDL and/or LDL) to triglyceride rich lipoproteins, and of triglycerides from triglyceride-rich lipoproteins to cholesterol-rich lipoproteins [54]. Tall *et al.* [52] have shown that the cholesteryl ester transfer activity, as measured by the transfer of cholesteryl ester from HDL to apo B-containing lipoproteins, was two to three times greater during the postprandial lipemic state than the fasting state. Dullaart *et al.* [53] demonstrated that postprandial lipemia caused a significant shift in the lipoprotein cholesteryl ester distribution, from LDL and HDL to postprandial lipoproteins, without affecting total plasma cholesteryl ester. Thus, the levels of cholesteryl ester in LDL and HDL during the postprandial lipemic state were lower than during the fasting state. This alteration was more pronounced in normolipidemics and patients with combined hyperlipidemia than in hypercholesterolemic patients [53]. The HDL_2 in postprandial lipemic serum contained significantly more triglycerides, but less cholesteryl ester, and had a greater flotation rate than HDL_2 from fasting serum [55]. The extent of these changes correlated positively with the magnitude of postprandial lipemia [55]. The above changes in core lipid composition of HDL suggest that much of the compositional and physical change occurring during postprandial lipemia may be due to increased cholesteryl ester transfer activity. Tall *et al.* [56] found that an increase of cholesteryl ester transfer activity during the postprandial lipemic period was due to a modification of lipoproteins by lipolytic products which increased their binding to cholesteryl ester transfer proteins. It has been shown that triglyceride-rich lipoproteins having either a greater triglyceride:cholesteryl ester molar ratio or size were the preferential acceptor of cholesteryl ester from LDL [57,58]. Postprandial lipoproteins are therefore very efficient acceptors of cholesteryl ester from LDL or HDL.

Patsch *et al.* [55] suggested that postprandial lipemia may be a necessary step in converting HDL_2 to HDL_3, and that the magnitude of postprandial lipemia may determine the extent of conversion of HDL_2 to HDL_3 *in vivo*. These investigators demonstrated that triglyceride-rich HDL_2 particles from postprandial serum, but not HDL_2 from fasting serum, were converted into particles having a density, size, and apoprotein composition similar to that of native HDL_3 by *in vitro* incubation with hepatic lipase [55]. Deckelbaum *et al.* [59] found that triglyceride-rich HDL_2 which is similar to postprandial HDL_2 can be produced *in vitro* by incubating normal HDL_2 with triglyceride-rich lipoproteins in the presence of cholesteryl ester transfer proteins, and that this triglyceride-rich HDL_2 can be remodeled into more dense HDL_3 by the action of lipoprotein lipase.

An increase in plasma lecithin cholesterol acyltransferase (LCAT) activity is usually associated with postprandial lipemia [51,60,61]. The increase in LCAT activity was correlated with the increase in plasma triglyceride [60]. The LCAT reaction rate in plasma is determined not only by the concentration of catalytically active LCAT proteins, but also by the nature of the lipoprotein substrate. The increase in LCAT activity during the postprandial lipemic state may reflect the greater availability of substrate. Walletin *et al.* [61] showed that fat ingestion increases the plasma LCAT activity by increasing the level of phospholipids in plasma or HDL. Since chylomicrons do not interact with purified LCAT [62], an increase in the LCAT reaction rate during the postprandial state could occur through an increase in the affinity of the enzyme for HDL. It has been shown that product inhibition may be an important factor in determining the plasma LCAT rate [63], and that this inhibition may be decreased by the transfer of LCAT products to other lipoproteins [64]. It is possible that the increase in LCAT activity during the postprandial lipemic state may be related to an increase of cholesteryl ester transfer activity.

Postprandial lipoproteins and the relation to atherogenesis

It is generally considered that intact chylomicrons are not atherogenic because they consist mostly of triglycerides and are too large to filter into the arterial wall. Zilversmit [13] proposed that chylomicron remnants, formed at the endothelial surface by the action of lipoprotein lipase, may be atherogenic. Arterial lesions resembling the atherosclerosis of humans occur quickly after cholesterol feeding in rabbits, with the predominant cholesterol-containing particles in the lesions being chylomicron remnants [65]. Stender and Zilversmit [66,67] showed that in cholesterol-fed rabbits the cholesteryl esters of chylomicrons entered the aortic intima during the interaction between chylomicrons and lipoprotein lipase at the endothelial surface.

A number of *in vitro* studies have shown that chylomicron remnants may be taken up by various cells of the vessel wall, including monocyte-derived macrophages [68–72]. Floren *et al.* [70] reported that lipolytic remnants of chylomicrons, produced *in vitro*, bound to the LDL receptors of cultured skin fibroblasts, were internalized, and thus were able to downregulate LDL receptor activity; as the degree of chylomicron lipolysis increased, remnants were more efficiently taken up by these cells. Chylomicron remnants, produced following 70–80% hydrolysis of triglycerides in chylomicrons, were able to increase cellular cholesterol to the same extent as LDL when cultured cells were incubated at an equal cholesterol concentration [71]. When the culture dishes contained an equal number of particles of LDL or chylomicron remnants, the chylomicron remnants were two to three times more effective than LDL in delivering cholesterol to the fibroblasts [71]. Van Lenten *et al.* [72] have shown that thoracic duct chylomicrons obtained from fat-fed normolipidemic subjects can inhibit degradation of ^{125}I-labeled rabbit β-VLDL in human monocyte-derived macrophages, indicating that chylomicrons may bind to the β-VLDL receptor of macrophages. Incubation of human monocyte-derived macrophages with serum supplemented with chylomicron remnants resulted in an increase in cellular cholesteryl ester content which was four times greater than that caused by serum supplemented with LDL [72]

Bersot *et al.* [73] have shown that a subfraction of triglyceride-rich lipoproteins enriched with lipoprotein(a) (Lp(a)), which is only detectable in postprandial plasma, caused the accumulation of lipids in macrophages. Apo(a) has been found in postprandial chylomicrons and the triglyceride-rich lipoproteins of patients with various forms of endogenous hypertriglyceridemia [74]. An apo B_{100}–apo(a) complex, prepared in a lipid-free form, exhibited a marked avidity for chylomicrons [75]. Zioncheck *et al.* [76] reported that Lp(a) and pure recombinant apo(a) bound to macrophages through a specific high affinity receptor, which could lead to foam-cell formation. Gianturco and Bradley [77] have shown that a subfraction of triglyceride-rich lipoproteins (S_f100–400) from individuals with abnormal fasting lipid profiles (high VLDL and/or low HDL) produced an increase of cellular lipids in THP-1 monocyte-derived macrophages $10\times$ more than did the same fraction from normolipidemics. This response was maximal at 2–4 hours after the fat load and returned to baseline by 8 hours.

Although the above *in vitro* and *in vivo* studies suggest that post-prandial lipoproteins and their remnants are potentially atherogenic, they are usually cleared rapidly from the circulation. However, there are several situations in which the half-life of chylomicron remnants is prolonged, which may also increase their atherogenicity. The removal of chylomicron remnants from the circulation is a saturable process, so that a large fat load will substantially increase the plasma residence time of these lipoproteins [78]. In addition, during the postprandial phase, endogenous VLDL may increase due to either increased hepatic synthesis or decreased catabolism [79]. As described above, normolipidemic individuals with apo E phenotypes E-II/E-II or E-III/E-II have delayed clearance of chylomicron remnants [80]. This may help explain why apo E-II has been reported to be an independent CHD risk factor [80]. Groot *et al.* [16] found no significant difference in the postprandial lipemic response in normolipidemic individuals with and without CHD. However, CHD patients had a marked delay in clearance of chylomicron remnants.

The initiation of the atherogenic process involves injury to the arterial endothelium [81]. Zilversmit [82] proposed that lipolysis of postprandial lipoproteins in close proximity to the arterial surface may injure the vascular endothelium by exposing it to an excessive local concentration of lipolytic remnant products, especially fatty acid anions. This injury would then allow remnants and other cholesterol-rich lipoproteins to enter the arterial wall. In support of this hypothesis, in rabbits on an atherogenic diet, aortic lipoprotein lipase has been shown to increase in proportion to the aortic cholesterol content [83]. Dissection of the aorta revealed that increments of lipoprotein lipase activity were associated with raised fatty lesions [83]. Postprandial lipemia has also been shown to limit arterial oxygen diffusion and this is a further mechanism which may result in endothelial cell injury [84].

Lipolysis of hypertriglyceridemic serum *in vitro* by purified lipoprotein lipase or *in vivo* by heparinization caused whole serum to become cytotoxic and foam-cell inducing in both cultured macrophages and endothelial cells [85,86]. Lipolysis of serum from fasting normolipidemic subjects failed to produce cytotoxicity. However, postprandial serum from normolipidemic subjects with a brisk chylomicron response, when lipolyzed *in vitro*, was cytotoxic to cultured macrophages [84]. These data suggest that arterial endothelial injury could occur during the clearance phase of postprandial lipemia in hypertriglyceridemic subjects as well as normolipidemic individuals. Since lipolysis *in vivo* is a localized event, the concentration of fatty acids adjacent to the vascular endothelium would be expected to be high during the clearance phase of postprandial lipemia. It has been shown that serum containing an increased level of free fatty acids accelerated foam-cell formation [87] and altered the barrier function of endothelial cells [88].

Epidemiologic studies have established that high levels of plasma HDL are associated with reduced CHD risk [89]. The protective role of HDL has been attributed to its role in reverse cholesterol transport [90]. Castro and Fielding [51] suggested that postprandial lipoproteins may play an important role in stimulating reverse cholesterol transport. These investigators demonstrated that a high level of postprandial lipoproteins in serum increased the capacity of serum to promote net removal of cholesterol from cultured cells. The increased capacity of postprandial serum to promote reverse cholesterol transport was attributed to an increase in LCAT activity and cholesteryl ester transfer in postprandial serum [51]. The reverse cholesterol transport pathway involves (i) removal of cellular free cholesterol by HDL, (ii) esterification of free cholesterol into cholesteryl ester by LCAT, (iii) transfer of LCAT-generated cholesteryl esters into postprandial lipoproteins by cholesteryl ester transfer proteins, and (iv) the removal of the cholesteryl ester-enriched postprandial lipoproteins by the liver following their interaction with lipoprotein lipase. Although this may be an efficient way to deliver excess cellular cholesterol to the liver for excretion, the enrichment of postprandial lipoproteins with cholesteryl ester by the above pathway could also be atherogenic. Perfusion of cholesterol-enriched chylomicrons through the rat heart caused nonendocytic transfer of cholesteryl ester into the coronary artery tissue [91]. Cholesteryl ester-enriched β-VLDL, which are probably chylomicron remnants, are the most effective unmodified natural lipoproteins at promoting foam-cell formation in cultured macrophages [92]. Although it is uncertain whether an increase in cholesteryl ester transfer activity during postprandial lipemia increases the atherogenicity of postprandial and other lipoproteins, a number of studies have shown that an increase in plasma cholesteryl ester transfer activity may be associated with atherosclerosis [93,94].

The postprandial lipemic response is inversely related to the level of HDL [7,10,34], but the mechanism of this inverse relationship and the role of HDL in the atherogenicity of postprandial lipoproteins have not been clarified. It has been established that HDL is important in clearing the lipolytic surface remnants of triglyceride-rich lipoproteins [30]. The presence of an excess amount of surface remnant products (apo C-III) on lipolytic remnants has been shown to inhibit their apo E-mediated removal by the liver [31]. *In vitro* lipolysis studies have shown that lipolytic remnants of triglyceride-rich lipoproteins, produced in the presence of a low level of HDL, retained most of their surface remnant products. When the HDL was further increased to levels approximating normolipidemic serum, these surface remnant products could no longer be identified in the remnant particles [85]. It is possible that a low HDL and high postprandial lipoprotein level will result in circulating chylomicron remnants containing excess surface remnant products which may inhibit clearance and result in a longer plasma remnant residence time. It has been shown that the presence of HDL in lipolysis mixtures or in culture medium containing lipolytic remnants could inhibit the cytotoxicity produced by lipolytic remnants of triglyceride-rich lipoproteins to both cultured macrophages and endothelial cells [85,86]. These results suggest that HDL may prevent atherogenesis by inhibiting the cytotoxicity produced by remnants of postprandial lipoproteins and/or by promoting rapid hepatic clearance of remnants of postprandial lipoproteins by accepting their excess surface remnant products.

Summary

Postprandial lipoproteins are the principal carriers of dietary cholesterol and fat in the bloodstream. The current approach to assessment of CHD risk has been based on measurement of serum total cholesterol, triglycerides, and cholesterol associated with various lipoproteins in fasting blood. There is considerable evidence, of a diverse nature, which supports the hypothesis that postprandial lipoproteins and their remnants are a major atherogenic factor. However, until the development of more widely applicable assays for chylomicrons and their remnants, clinicians must rely on the correlations which exist between the postprandial lipemic response and fasting triglyceride and HDL cholesterol. The postprandial lipemic phase is also associated with important changes in the level and composition of other lipoproteins. Postprandial lipoproteins may be involved directly in atherogenesis by causing endothelial injury and subsequently by transporting cholesterol into the arterial wall, or indirectly by altering the metabolic and functional properties of other plasma lipoproteins.

References

1 Stamler J. Life style, major risk factors, proof and public policy. *Circulation* 1978;58: 3–19.
2 Scott RF, Daoud AS, Florentin RA. Animal models in atherosclerosis. In *The Pathogenesis of Atherosclerosis* (eds RW Wissler, JC Geer). Baltimore: Williams and Wilkins, 1972: 120–54.
3 Kannel WB, Castelli WP, Gordon T. Serum cholesterol, lipoproteins, and the risk of coronary heart disease. *Ann Intern Med* 1971;74:1–12.
4 Nestel PJ. Relationship between plasma triglycerides and removal of chylomicrons. *J Clin Invest* 1964;43:943–9.
5 Grundy SM, Mok HYI. Chylomicron clearance in normal and hyperlipidemic man. *Metabolism* 1976;25:1225–39.
6 Redgrave TG, Carlson LA. Change in plasma very low density and low density lipoprotein content, composition and size after a fatty meal in normo- and hyperlipidemic man. *J Lipid Res* 1979;20:217–29.
7 Patsch JR, Karlin JB, Scott LW, Smith LC, Gotto AM. Inverse relationship between blood levels of high density lipoprotein subfraction 2 and magnitude of postprandial lipemia. *Proc Natl Acad Sci USA* 1983;80:1449–53.
8 Cortner JA, Coates PM, Le NA *et al*. Kinetics of chylomicron remnant clearance in normal and hyperlipoproteinemic subjects. *J Lipid Res* 1987;28:195–206.
9 Weintraub MS, Eisenberg S, Breslow JL. Different patterns of postprandial lipoprotein metabolism in normal, type IIa, type III and type IV hyperlipoproteinemic individuals. Effect of treatment with cholestyramine and gemfibrozil. *J Clin Invest* 1987;79: 1110–19.
10 Kashyap ML, Barnhart RL, Srivastava LS *et al*. Alimentary lipemia: Plasma high density lipoproteins and apolipoproteins C-II and C-III in healthy subjects. *Am J Clin Nutr* 1983;37:233–43.
11 Dullaart RPF, Groener JEM, Wijk HV, Sluiter WJ, Erkelens DW. Alimentary lipemia-induced redistribution of cholesteryl ester between lipoproteins. Studies in normolipidemic, combined hyperlipidemic, and hypercholesterolemic men. *Arteriosclerosis* 1988;9:614–22.
12 Cohn JS, McNamara JR, Cohn SD, Ordovas JM, Schaefer EJ. Postprandial plasma lipoprotein changes in human subjects of different ages. *J Lipid Res* 1988;29:469–79.
13 Zilversmit DB. Atherogenesis: A postprandial phenomenon. *Circulation* 1979;60: 473–85.
14 Shekelle RB, Stamler J. Dietary cholesterol and ischemic heart disease. *Lancet* 1989;i: 1177–8.
15 Simons LA, Dwyer D, Simons J *et al*. Chylomicrons and chylomicron remnants in coronary artery disease: a case-control study. *Atherosclerosis* 1987;65:181–9.
16 Groot PHE, Van Stipout WAHJ, Krauss XH *et al*. Postprandial lipoprotein metabolism in normolipidemic men with and without coronary artery disease. *Arteriosclerosis* 1991; 11:653–62.
17 Green PH, Glickman RM. Intestinal lipoprotein metabolism. *J Lipid Res* 1981;22: 1153–72.
18 Fraser R. Size and lipid composition of chylomicrons of different svedberg units of flotation. *J Lipid Res* 1970;11:60–5.

19 Skipski VP. Lipid composition of lipoproteins in normal and disease states. In *Blood Lipids and Lipoproteins: Quantitation, Composition, and Metabolism* (ed GL Nelson). New York: Wiley-Interscience, 1972:471–583.
20 Haberbough W, Doli A, Augstin J. Characterization of human chylomicrons. *Biochim Biophys Acta* 1982;713:390–409.
21 Kane JP, Hardman DA, Paulus HE. Heterogeneity of apolipoprotein B: isolation of a new species from human chylomicrons. *Proc Natl Acad Sci USA* 1981;77:2465–9.
22 Dullaart RPF, Speelberg B, Schuurman HJ *et al*. Epitopes of apolipoprotein B-100 and B-48 in both liver and intestine. *J Clin Invest* 1986;78:1397–404.
23 Imaizumi K, Fainaru M, Havel RJ. Composition of proteins of mesenteric lymph chylomicrons in the rat and alterations produced upon exposure of chylomicrons to blood serum and serum proteins. *J Lipid Res* 1978;19:712–22.
24 LaRosa JC, Levy RI, Herbert P, Lux SE, Fredrickson DS. A specific apoprotein activator for lipoprotein lipase. *Biochim Biophys Res Commun* 1970;41:57–62.
25 Havel RJ, Shore VG, Shore B, Bier DM. Role of specific glycopeptides of human serum lipoproteins in activation of lipoprotein lipase. *Circ Res* 1970;27:595–600.
26 Windler E, Chao Y, Havel RJ. Determinants of hepatic uptake of triglyceride-rich lipoproteins and their remnants in the rat. *J Biol Chem* 1980;255:5475–80.
27 Shelburne E, Hanks J, Meyers W, Quarfordt S. Effect of apoproteins on hepatic uptake of triglyceride emulsions in the rat. *J Clin Invest* 1980;65:652–8.
28 Fielding CJ, Havel RJ. Lipoprotein lipase: properties of the enzyme in solution. *Arch Pathol Lab Med* 1977;101:225–9.
29 Smith LC, Scow RO. Chylomicrons: Mechanism of transfer of lipolytic products to cells. *Prog Biochem Pharmacol* 1979;15:109–38.
30 Havel RJ. Origin of HDL. In *High Density Lipoproteins and Atherosclerosis* (eds AM Gotto Jr, NE Miller, MF Oliver). Amsterdam: Elsevier/North Holland Biomedical Press, 1978:21.
31 Havel RJ. Functional activities of hepatic lipoprotein lipase. *Annu Rev Physiol* 1986;48:119–34.
32 Craig WY, Nutik R, Cooper BAD. Regulation of apoprotein synthesis and secretion in the human hepatoma Hep G2. *J Biol Chem* 1988;263:13880–90.
33 Olefsky JM, Crapo P, Reaven GM. Postprandial plasma triglyceride and cholesterol response to a low fat meal. *Am J Clin Nutr* 1976;29:535–9.
34 Patsch JR, Prasad S, Gotto AM, Patsch W. High density lipoprotein-2. Relationship of the plasma levels of this lipoprotein species to its composition, to the magnitude of postprandial lipemia, and to the activities of lipoprotein lipase and hepatic lipase. *J Clin Invest* 1987;80:341–7.
35 Taskinen MR, Kuusi T. High density lipoproteins in postprandial lipemia. Relation to sex and lipoprotein lipase activity. *Atherosclerosis* 1986;59:121–30.
36 Krasinski SD, Cohn JS, Schaefer EJ, Russell RM. Postprandial plasma retinyl ester response is greater in older subjects compared with young subjects. Evidence for delayed plasma clearance of intestinal lipoproteins. *J Clin Invest* 1990;85:883–92.
37 Weintraub MS, Eisenberg S, Breslow JL. Dietary fat clearance in normal subjects is regulated by genetic variation in apolipoprotein E. *J Clin Invest* 1987;80:1571–7.
38 Rubinsztein DC, Cohen JC, Berger GM *et al*. Chylomicron remnant clearance from the plasma is normal in familial hypercholesterolemic homozygotes with defined receptor defects. *J Clin Invest* 1990;86:1306–12.
39 Weintraub MS, Zechner R, Brown A, Eisenberg S, Breslow JL. Dietary polyunsaturated fats of the w-6 and w-3 series reduce postprandial lipoprotein levels. Chronic and acute effects of fat saturation on postprandial lipoprotein metabolism. *J Clin Invest* 1988;82:1884–93.
40 Harris WS, Connor WE, Alam N, Illingworth DR. Reduction of postprandial triglyceridemia in humans by dietary n-3 fatty acids. *J Lipid Res* 1988;29:1451–60.
41 Merrill JR, Holly RG, Anderson RL *et al*. Hyperlipidemic response of young trained and untrained men after a high fat meal. *Arteriosclerosis* 1989;9:217–23.

42 Weintraub MS, Rosen Y, Otto R, Eisenberg S, Breslow JL. Physical exercise conditioning in the absence of weight loss reduces fasting and postprandial triglyceride-rich lipoprotein levels. *Circulation* 1989;79:1007−14.

43 Simpson HS, Williamson CM, Olivecrona T *et al.* Postprandial lipemia, fenofibrate and coronary artery disease. *Atherosclerosis* 1990;85:193−202.

44 Georgopoulos A, Margolis S, Bachorik P, Kwiterovich PO. Effect of improved glycemic control on the response of plasma triglycerides to ingestion of a saturated fat load in normotriglyceridemic and hypertriglyceridemic diabetic subjects. *Metabolism* 1988; 37:866−71.

45 Kay RM, Rao S, Arnott C, Miller NE, Lewis B. Acute effects of the pattern of fat ingestion on plasma high density lipoprotein components in man. *Atherosclerosis* 1980; 36:567−73.

46 Tall AR, Blum CB, Forester GP, Nelson CA. Change in the distribution and composition of plasma high density lipoproteins after ingestion of fat. *J Biol Chem* 1982;257: 198−207.

47 Havel RJ. Early effect of fat ingestion on lipids and lipoproteins of serum in man. *J Clin Invest* 1957;36:848−54.

48 Patsch JR, Gotto AM, Olivecrona T, Eisenberg S. Formation of high density lipoprotein-2 like particles during lipolysis of very low density lipoproteins *in vitro. Proc Natl Acad Sci USA* 1978;75:4519−23.

49 Groot PHE, Scheek LM. Effect of fat ingestion on high density lipoprotein profiles in human sera. *J Lipid Res* 1984;25:684−92.

50 Redgrave TG, Carlson LA. Change in plasma very low density and low density lipoprotein content, composition, and size after a fatty meal in normo- and hypertriglyceridemic man. *J Lipid Res* 1979;20:217−29.

51 Castro GR, Fielding CJ. Effect of postprandial lipemia on plasma cholesterol metabolism. *J Clin Invest* 1985;75:874−82.

52 Tall A, Sammett D, Granot E. Mechanisms of enhanced cholesteryl ester transfer from high density lipoproteins to apolipoprotein B-containing lipoproteins during alimentary lipemia. *J Clin Invest* 1986;77:1163−72.

53 Dullaart RPF, Groener JEM, Wijk IIV, Sluiter WJ, Erkelens DW. Alimentary lipemia-induced redistribution of cholesteryl ester between lipoproteins. Studies in normolipidemic, combined hyperlipemic, and hypercholesteremic men. *Arteriosclerosis* 1989;9:614−22.

54 Nichols AV, Smith L. Effect of very low density lipoproteins on lipid transfer in incubated serum. *J Lipid Res* 1965;6:206−10.

55 Patsch JR, Prasad S, Gotto AM, Bengtsson-Olivecrona G. Postprandial lipemia. A key for the conversion of high density lipoprotein-2 into high density lipoprotein-3 by hepatic lipase. *J Clin Invest* 1984;74:2017−23.

56 Tall AR, Sammett D, Vita G, Deckelbaum RJ, Olivecrona T. Lipoprotein lipase enhances the cholesteryl ester transfer protein-mediated transfer of cholesteryl ester from high density lipoproteins to very low density lipoproteins. *J Biol Chem* 1984;259:9589−94.

57 Dullaart RPF, Goerner JEM, Erkelens DW. Effect of the composition of very low density lipoproteins on the rate of cholesteryl ester transfer from high density lipoproteins in man, studied *in vitro. Eur J Clin Invest* 1987;17:241−8.

58 Eisenberg S. Preferential enrichment of large sized very low density lipoprotein population with transferred cholesteryl ester. *J Lipid Res* 1984;25:684−92.

59 Deckelbaum RJ, Eisenberg S, Oschry Y *et al.* Conversion of human plasma high density lipoprotein-2 to high density lipoprotein-3. *J Biol Chem* 1986;261:5201−8.

60 Rose HG, Juliano J. Regulation of plasma lecithin cholesterol acyltransferase in man. Activation during alimentary lipemia. *J Lab Clin Med* 1977;89:524−32.

61 Walletin L, Vikrot O. Influence of fat ingestion on lecithin cholesterol acyltransferase in plasma of normal persons. *Scand J Clin Lab Invest* 1976;36:473−9.

62 Chung BH, Nishida T, Segrest JP. Reactivity of lecithin cholesterol acyltransferase with the lipolytic surface remnants of triglyceride-rich lipoproteins. *Circulation* 1983; 68:928.

63 Fielding CJ, Shore VG, Fielding PE. Lecithin cholesterol acyltransferase. Effect of substrate composition upon enzyme activity. *Biochim Biophys Acta* 1972;270:513–19.

64 Hopkins GJ, Barter PJ. Role of esterified cholesterol transfers in regulation of plasma cholesterol esterification. *Atherosclerosis* 1983;49:177–85.

65 Ross AL, Zilversmit DB. Chylomicron remnant cholesteryl ester as the major constituent of very low density lipoproteins in plasma of cholesterol fed rabbits. *J Lipid Res* 1977;18:169–81.

66 Stender S, Zilversmit DB. Comparison of cholesteryl ester transfer from chylomicrons and other lipoproteins to aortic intima media of cholesterol fed rabbits. *Arteriosclerosis* 1982;2:493–9.

67 Stender S, Zilversmit DB. Arterial influx of esterified cholesterol from two plasma lipoprotein fractions and its hydrolysis *in vivo* in hypercholesterolemic rabbits. *Atherosclerosis* 1981;39:97–109.

68 Ellsworth JL, Fong LG, Kramer FB, Cooper AD. Difference in processing chylomicron remnants and β-VLDL by macrophages. *J Lipid Res* 1990;31:1399–419.

69 Redgrave TG, Fidge NH, Yin J. Specific saturable binding, and uptake of rat chylomicron remnants by rat skin fibroblasts. *J Lipid Res* 1982;23:638–44.

70 Floren CJ, Alber JJ, Kudchodkar BJ, Bierman EL. Receptor dependent uptake of chylomicron remnants by cultured skin fibroblasts. *J Biol Chem* 1981;256:424–35.

71 Floren CJ, Alber JJ, Bierman EL. Uptake of chylomicron remnants causes cholesterol accumulation in cultured human arterial smooth muscle cells. *Biochim Biophys Acta* 1981;663:336–49.

72 Van Lenten BJ, Fogelman AM, Jackson RL et al. Receptor mediated uptake of remnant lipoproteins by cholesterol loaded human monocyte–macrophages. *J Biol Chem* 1985; 260:8783–8.

73 Bersot TP, Innerarity RW, Pitas RE et al. Fat feeding in humans induces lipoproteins of density less than 1.006 that are enriched in apoprotein(a) and that cause lipid accumulation in macrophages. *J Clin Invest* 1986;77:622–30.

74 Fless GM. Heterogeneity of particles containing the apo B–apo(a) complex. In *Lipoprotein(a): 25 Years of Progress* (ed. AM Scanu). New York: Academic Press, 1990:41–51.

75 Bersot TP, Innerarity RW, Mahley RW. Apo Lp(a)-enriched chylomicrons induced by fat feeding bind to the macrophage β-VLDL receptor. *Arteriosclerosis* 1984;4:536a.

76 Zioncheck TF, Powell LM, Rice GC, Eaton DL, Lawn RM. Interaction of recombinant apolipoprotein(a) and lipoprotein(a) with macrophages. *J Clin Invest* 1991;87:767–71.

77 Gianturco SH, Bradley WA. A cellular basis for the atherogenicity of triglyceride-rich lipoproteins. In *Atherosclerosis Reviews*, Vol. 22 (eds AM Gotto, R Paoletti). New York: Raven Press, 1990:9–14.

78 Berr K, Kern F. Characteristics of removal of labelled chylomicron remnants from plasma in normal men. *Hepatology* 1985;5:1022.

79 Brunzell JP, Hazzard WR, Porte D, Bierman EL. Evidence for common saturable triglyceride removal mechanism for chylomicron and very low density lipoproteins in man. *J Clin Invest* 1973;52:1578–86.

80 Eichner J, Kuller L, McCallum L, Grandits G, Neaton J. Apolipoprotein E: an inherited metabolic risk factor. Abstracts of the 31st Annual Conference on Cardiovascular Disease Epidemiology. *Circulation* 1991;83:6.

81 Ross R. The pathogenesis of atherosclerosis—an update. *N Engl J Med* 1986;314: 488–500.

82 Zilversmit DB. A proposal linking atherogenesis to the interaction of endothelial lipoprotein lipase with triglyceride-rich lipoproteins. *Circ Res* 1973;33:633–8.

83 Corby JE, Zilversmit DB. Effect of cholesterol feeding on arterial lipolytic activity in the rabbit. *Atherosclerosis* 1977;27:201–6.

84 Engelberg H. Serum lipemia: an overlooked cause of tissue hypoxia. *Cardiology* 1983; 70:273–9.

85 Chung BH, Segrest JP, Smith K, Griffin FM, Brouillette CG. Surface remnants of triglyceride-rich lipoproteins are cytotoxic to cultured macrophages but not in the

presence of high density lipoproteins. A possible mechanism of atherogenesis. *J Clin Invest* 1989;83:1363−74.

86 Speidel MT, Booyse FM, Abrams A, Moore MA, Chung BH. Lipolyzed hypertriglyceridemic serum and triglyceride-rich lipoproteins are cytotoxic to cultured human endothelial cells. High density lipoproteins inhibit this cytotoxicity. *Thromb Res* 1990; 58:251−64.

87 Lindqvist P, Ostlund Lindqvist AM, Witztum JL, Steinberg D. The role of lipoprotein lipase in metabolism of triglyceride-rich lipoproteins by macrophages. *J Biol Chem* 1984;258:9086−92.

88 Hennig B, Shasby DM, Fulton AB, Spector AA. Exposure to free fatty acid increases the transfer of albumin across cultured endothelial monolayers. *Arteriosclerosis* 1984; 4:489−97.

89 Castelli WP, Doyle JT, Gordon T *et al.* HDL cholesterol and other lipids in coronary heart disease. The co-operative lipoprotein phenotyping study. *Circulation* 1977;55: 767−72.

90 Miller GJ, Miller NE. Plasma high density lipoprotein concentration and development of ischemic heart disease. Lancet 1975;i:16−17.

91 Fielding CJ. Metabolism of cholesterol-rich chylomicrons. Mechanism of binding and uptake of cholesteryl ester by the vascular bed of the perfused rat heart. *J Clin Invest* 1978;62:141−51.

92 Bersot TP, Innerarity TL, Mahley RW. Stimulation of macrophage cholesteryl ester formation by β-VLDL from cholesterol-fed and hyperlipidemic subjects. *Clin Res* 1981; 29:536a.

93 Quig DW, Zilversmit DB. Plasma lipid transfer activity in rabbits. Effects of dietary hyperlipidemia. *Atherosclerosis* 1988;70:263−71.

94 Tall A, Granot E, Borcia B *et al.* Accelerated transfer of cholesteryl ester in dyslipidemic plasma. Role of cholesteryl ester transfer proteins. *J Clin Invest* 1987;79:1217−25.

95 Shen BW, Scanu AM, Kezdy FJ. Structure of human serum lipoproteins inferred from compositional analysis. *Proc Natl Acad Sci USA* 1977;74:837−41.

96 Redgrave TG. Postprandial remnants and their relation to atherosclerosis. In *Latent Dyslipoproteinemia and Atherosclerosis* (ed. H. De Gennes) New York: Raven Press, 1984:9−15.

Chapter 9
Oxidized Lipoproteins

GUY M. CHISOLM

Introduction

Although the plasma lipoproteins carry endogenous lipophilic anti-oxidants, vitamin E, vitamin A, and ubiquinols, among others, free radical-mediated oxidation can occur at a level sufficient to consume these protective agents and, as they are consumed, attack the particularly vulnerable unsaturated sites on the fatty acid moieties of cholesteryl esters, triglycerides, and phospholipids, and as well, attack cholesterol and other components of the lipoprotein complex [1,2]. Exposure to an oxidizing milieu can markedly change a lipoprotein. The chemical nature of the lipoprotein is altered as the dozens of distinct lipids present in normalcy are transformed into a multitude of new products, some of which are sufficiently hydrophilic to leave the lipoprotein complex. Physical changes take place as a result: the density of the particles increases, their surface charge is changed, and if the lipoprotein concentration and its degree of oxidation is sufficient the lipoprotein particles can aggregate.

With such far-reaching changes, it is perhaps not surprising that the biologic properties of oxidized lipoproteins are different from their unaltered, "native" counterparts. Recognition of the lipoprotein by receptors, intracellular hydrolysis, and intracellular distribution are all changed, as is the catalog of cellular functions that can be induced or inhibited by the lipoprotein.

To date most of the studies of oxidized lipoproteins have been performed *in vitro*, i.e., as experiments which compare the interactions between cells and oxidized or native lipoproteins. Enthusiasm for such studies has steadily grown because functions observed in cells incubated with oxidized lipoproteins parallel cellular phenomena that have been observed *in vivo* for decades in both early and developing atherosclerotic lesions. In addition to these observations, it has been demonstrated in cell culture that the cells present in early lesions, endothelial cells, vascular smooth-muscle cells, and monocyte-derived macrophages, are capable of oxidizing low-density lipoprotein (LDL).

Theories based on these results which propose a role for lipoprotein oxidation in atherosclerosis have gained momentum with increasing evidence that oxidized LDL exists in atherosclerotic lesions of human and experimental animals; however, whether or not lipoprotein oxidation actually causes atherosclerosis is still unknown. There are reported instances of retarded progression of atherosclerosis in experimental animals treated with antioxidants which offer circumstantial evidence for such theories, but currently such a causal role should be regarded as theory worthy of further study.

The strong and nearly universally accepted correlation between high plasma concentrations of LDL and increased risk of atherosclerosis has focused the attention of physicians and researchers on LDL as a probable causative factor in arterial lesion formation. While it is clear that other lipoprotein patterns (e.g., high very low-density lipoproteins (VLDL) with low high-density lipoproteins (HDL)) and nonlipid factors (hypertension, diabetes, cigarette smoking) contribute significantly to risk profiles, and while it is clear that some patients with high LDL do not have severe atherosclerosis and some with low LDL do, the connection between plasma LDL and atherosclerosis is sufficiently strong that its study has played a prominent role in atherosclerosis research. The study of oxidized lipoproteins has likewise been dominated by experiments with LDL. Studies of oxidized HDL, VLDL, and β-VLDL have been reported, and such will no doubt ultimately lead to novel concepts, but the present chapter deals with available data, most of which pertains to oxidized LDL.

The purpose of this chapter is to discuss the possible implications of the experimental work related to lipoproteins which have been altered by free radical oxidation. In addition, a current version of the evolving theory of how lipoprotein oxidation could play a role in the initiation and development of an atherosclerotic lesion will be presented. There are a number of review articles related to oxidized lipoproteins on which the reader should rely for further sources of primary experimental studies and for alternate perspectives on the results of these [3–5].

Heterogeneity of oxidized lipoproteins

Unfortunately, the concept of oxidized lipoproteins is ill-defined. Each of the lipoprotein categories, VLDL, LDL, and HDL, is well known to be heterogeneous, both with respect to apolipoprotein composition and to the make-up of the lipid moieties. Fatty acid variations among triglycerides, cholesteryl esters, and the several classes of phospholipids present on lipoproteins amplify further the heterogeneity within each category. Upon free radical attack, the products produced vary widely, depending in large part upon the composition of the available substrate. For example, polyunsaturated fatty acids can be oxidized to form a number of different aldehydes, some of which, e.g., malondialdehyde and 4-hydroxynonenal, have been studied extensively for their biologic effects [3]. Thus, the concentrations of the various polyunsaturated fatty acids, which can be altered by diet, can influence the amount of such products produced upon oxidation [6]. In addition, unesterified cholesterol and the various cholesteryl esters can be transformed into numerous compounds. Several hydroxycholesterols, cholesterol epoxides, and 7-ketocholesterol are produced from free cholesterol when LDL is oxidized [7].

Other major sources of variability are in the ways in which the lipoprotein is oxidized and in the degree of oxidation. *In vitro*, LDL can be oxidized in a cell-free environment by exposure to oxygen, cupric ion, ferrous or ferric ion, ultraviolet irradiation, gamma irradiation, azo-initiators and, no doubt, numerous other agents [8–13]. Cultured cells can also mediate the oxidation. Vascular endothelial cells [10,14], vascular smooth-muscle cells [12,14], and a variety of leukocytes [15,16] have been shown capable of facilitating LDL oxidation. Some of the instances of cell-mediated oxidation have been found to be dependent on the presence of metal ions in the culture media; however, even in culture media with low metal ion levels, human monocytes can oxidize LDL after treatment with certain phagocytic stimuli [15,17].

As would be expected, the lipoprotein concentration, the concentration of the free radical generator (or number of free radical-producing cells), and the time and temperature of incubation can each influence the degree of oxidation and the degree of particle interactions, including aggregation. With increasing oxidation new products are formed; "intermediate" products formed by mild oxidation can disappear with more extensive oxidation.

The mechanism for these changes likely includes initiating oxidative events, in which free radicals abstract hydrogen atoms from poly-unsaturated fatty acids. The subsequent cascade of events results in the formation of lipid radicals which can propagate the oxidative reaction further in the lipid core of the lipoprotein complex. Uniformity in this propagation itself may be responsible for the fact that many of the biologic properties of oxidized LDL can be observed regardless of the mode of oxidation. For example, oxidized LDL is cytotoxic whether the oxidation is mediated by metal ions, cells, or ultraviolet irradiation [8,9,14,15,18]. Much of the reported variations in biologic functions can be attributed to the degree of oxidation rather than the mode of oxidation, although this topic is still under investigation.

Defining oxidized lipoproteins *in vivo* adds yet another layer of complexity to the definitions. For example, LDL, which is perceived to be oxidized *in vivo*, may have been exposed to free radical attack directly, as occurs in the *in vitro* systems, but could also result from the incorporation into the lipoprotein of lipid peroxidation products derived from cellular lipids or other sources. Due to the potential for exchange of oxidized lipids with cell membranes and other lipoproteins, it is possible that the composition of lipoproteins oxidized *in vivo* is highly variable and distinct from the isolated lipoproteins which are oxidized *in vitro*.

In addition to the far-reaching changes in lipoprotein lipids resulting from oxidation there are important reactions involving the apolipoproteins. In LDL, the apolipoprotein expresses a phospholipase A_2 activity for which the preferred substrates are oxidized phospholipids [10,19,20]. Thus, upon oxidation, lysophosphatidylcholine is produced in the LDL particle. This enzymatic activity is believed to be intrinsic to apolipoprotein (apo) B_{100} [20]. The apolipoprotein also reacts with the aldehyde products of fatty acid; 4-hydroxynonenal for example can react with lysyl, histidyl, and other amino acid residues [3]. In addition, the apolipoprotein is fragmented via nonenzymatic processes [21]. The change in surface charge and the aggregation of oxidized LDL are two of the functionally important manifestations of these protein changes.

The evidence for oxidized LDL *in vivo*

There are several lines of evidence suggesting that, under certain conditions, LDL existing *in vivo* is oxidatively modified. Perhaps most convincing are the data from several laboratories showing that antibodies which recognize epitopes on oxidized LDL but not native LDL also recognize epitopes in the atherosclerotic lesions of experimental animals and humans [22–26]. These include polyclonal and monoclonal antibodies produced against malondialdehyde or 4-hydroxynonenal-treated LDL which recognize these adducts linked to the lysyl residues of any protein, as well as antibodies produced against oxidized LDL which recognize unknown epitopes. These antibodies indicate the presence of their antigens at both intracellular and extracellular sites in lesions [24]. While these antibodies may all recognize particular lipid peroxidation products linked to any protein, LDL oxidation is strongly suggested by the finding that antibodies recognizing apo B_{100} at least in part colocalize with those recognizing oxidized LDL [22]. It is this colocalization that has led researchers to conclude that a portion of the high levels of LDL accumulating in lesions has been modified by oxidation.

Several studies have examined the characteristics of LDL-like particles extracted from atherosclerotic lesions. Early studies performed prior to suggestions that LDL might be oxidized revealed increases in the electrophoretic mobility and a variety of changes in composition [27]. More recently these LDL-like preparations from lesions have been shown to react with thiobarbituric acid [28], to be taken up by macrophages [29–31], and to react with antibodies which recognize oxidized LDL but not native LDL [29].

There are, in addition, studies which reveal that oxidized LDL may exist in plasma. A small chromatographically separable fraction of human plasma LDL has been identified which has characteristics resembling oxidized LDL [32]. Oxidized lipoproteins have been reported in the plasma of diabetic rats [33]. Earlier, it was demonstrated that LDL modified by endothelial cells (later shown to be oxidized) was cleared very rapidly from plasma [34]. Subsequent studies showed that removal of oxidized LDL from plasma was dependent on the degree of oxidation and that mildly oxidized LDL circulated with a half-life close to that of native LDL [35]. Recent studies have further shown that antibodies circulate in human plasma which can recognize oxidized LDL (and other malondialdehyde-modified protein) but not native LDL [23]. Thus, oxidation of LDL or modification of LDL by lipid peroxidation products may occur to variable extents even in normal humans. Further study will determine whether quantifying the fraction of plasma LDL-resembling oxidized forms of the lipoprotein will correlate with vascular disease.

The interactions of cells with oxidized lipoproteins *in vitro*

Recognition and metabolism of oxidized lipoproteins

The binding of native LDL to its receptor in general results in hydrolysis by lysosomes, contributes free cholesterol to cellular pools, decreases *de novo* cellular cholesterol synthesis, and downregulates LDL receptor synthesis [36]. Upon oxidation, multiple changes take place to the apolipoprotein, such as reaction of lipid peroxidation products with lysyl residues [3,37]. With progressive modification, the changes result in diminished LDL receptor recognition [38,39]. One would speculate that as a consequence the removal of oxidized LDL via this pathway would be decreased and the control of cellular cholesterol synthesis would be compromised. However, upon further oxidation oxidized LDL becomes recognizable by scavenger receptors expressed on macrophages and on confluent endothelial cells [10,40]. Scavenger receptors were characterized earlier in terms of their capacity to bind LDL after certain chemical modifications of the lipoprotein, including acetylation and treatment with malondialdehyde [41]. In macrophages, acetylated LDL and malondialdehyde-modified LDL cause scavenger receptor-mediated uptake and metabolism [38,41]. The uptake of modified LDL by this mechanism leads to a stimulation of reesterification of the cholesterol liberated from hydrolysis of the lipoprotein-borne cholesteryl ester. The receptor is not downregulated by the accumulation of lipoprotein products; unregulated incorporation and cellular storage of cholesteryl ester can occur. The resulting lipid-laden macrophage resembles the foam cells observed in the early fatty streak lesions of atherosclerosis.

Oxidized LDL does not appear to be as efficiently metabolized as the chemically modified forms of (unoxidized) LDL that are ligands of scavenger receptors [7,42]. However, it has been proposed that oxidized LDL may be an *in vivo* ligand for these receptors since the existence of acetylated LDL *in vivo* is doubted. Macrophages in atherosclerotic lesions of animals have been shown to express the scavenger receptor and to contain material reactive with antibodies recognizing oxidized LDL [30].

There are alternate mechanisms for the uptake of oxidized LDL by macrophages. *In vitro* incubations of oxidized LDL with macrophages have demonstrated a number of pathways by which the lipoprotein-borne lipid can enter these cells. The LDL receptor allows the entry of mildly oxidized LDL and the scavenger receptors facilitate entry of more severely oxidized LDL. In addition, Fc receptors can internalize large immune complexes via recognition of the Fc region of immunoglobulin molecules. Complexes of oxidized LDL recognized by and associated with endogenous antibodies, such as those found to occur in human plasma [23], could theoretically serve as a means of entry into macrophages.

Animals fed cholesterol-supplemented diets to induce atherosclerosis develop an aberrant lipoprotein, called β-VLDL, which is enriched with apo E. As the name implies, this is a lipoprotein particle with buoyancy properties in the ultracentrifuge similar to VLDL, but which upon electrophoresis migrates with LDL in the "beta" band. These β-VLDL particles are also taken up by macrophages in a process that involves the LDL receptor. Upon oxidation, β-VLDL is internalized to an even greater extent [43]. A β-VLDL-like particle is also formed in humans with the Type III form of hyperlipemia. Thus, β-VLDL and its oxidized counterpart offer additional pathways for enhanced lipid accumulation by macrophages.

It has been observed that when LDL is oxidized at concentrations close to those that exist in normal plasma or those that have been observed in human atherosclerotic lesions, aggregation can occur. Such aggregates suggest another, distinct mode of entry into macrophages, i.e., by phagocytosis. Aggregates of LDL induced by treatment with lipid peroxidation products were shown to enter cultured macrophages by this mechanism [44].

Which, if any, of these mechanisms is operable *in vivo* is unknown but these *in vitro* findings strongly suggest the possibility that the oxidation of LDL contributes to the foam-cell formation characteristic of fatty streak lesions. Supporting the speculation is the observation that incubation of macrophages with oxidized LDL, but not with native or acetylated LDL, leads to "ceroid" deposition in these cells [45]. Ceroid is an insoluble mix of protein and lipid oxidation material that has for decades been known to accumulate in the developed lesions of atherosclerosis.

Effects of oxidized LDL on cellular lipid metabolism

LDL internalization generally affects cellular metabolism; cholesterol esterification is stimulated and *de novo* cellular cholesterol synthesis is inhibited, for example [36]. Oxidized LDL affects lipid metabolism in ways distinct from those of native LDL. This is particularly true for pathways of arachidonic acid metabolism as well as metabolism of cholesterol

In smooth-muscle cell cultures, moderately oxidized LDL was reported to stimulate cyclooxygenase, but at higher oxidation levels the enzyme was inhibited. This inhibition was separable from the injurious effects of the oxidized lipoprotein [46]. Stimulation of certain arachidonic acid metabolites by oxidized LDL has also been observed *in vitro* in macrophages and endothelial cells [47,48].

In cultured macrophages it has been shown that oxidized LDL and the oxidized sterols present in the particle have various effects on cholesterol metabolism. Upon oxidation of LDL *in vitro*, both free and esterified cholesterol are decreased as oxidized versions of both are formed. Major oxysterol products include 7-ketocholesterol, 5,6-epoxycholesterol, and 7-hydroxycholesterol [7]. While some oxysterols enhance and others inhibit cholesterol esterification, the oxysterol extract of oxidized LDL was shown to inhibit the cholesterol esterification in macrophages that was stimulated by acetylated LDL [7]. Despite the fact that acetylated LDL and oxidized LDL are both recognized by scavenger receptors [40], the macrophage degradation of oxidized LDL is slower than that of acetylated LDL [7]. Thus, with its reduced quantity of cholesterol per particle and its slower cellular processing, the ability of oxidized LDL to stimulate cholesterol ester accumulation in macrophages can be considered greater than that of native LDL, but less than that of unoxidized acetylated LDL. Similar observations in the intracellular processing of oxidized LDL have been made in endothelial cells [42].

Effects of oxidized LDL on monocyte and macrophage motility

Recent research has suggested that oxidized LDL could be responsible for the observed involvement of macrophages in atherosclerotic lesions. There are several findings which indicate that oxidized LDL at least has the capacity to play a role in the process. Oxidized LDL could mediate the chemoattraction of monocytes to a particular tissue site by two distinct pathways. LDL that is moderately oxidized (such that the modified lipoprotein is still recognized by the LDL receptor) induces endothelial cells in culture to produce monocyte chemotactic protein-1 (MCP-1) [49,50]. More severely oxidized LDL is itself chemotactic for monocytes [51,52]. This is at least in part via the presence of lysophosphatidylcholine produced by the intrinsic phospholipase A_2 activity of oxidized LDL acting on oxidized phosphatidylcholine substrate [52]. Studies in culture have also shown that oxidized LDL reduces the motility of murine macrophages [51]. These observations have led to the speculation that oxidized LDL accumulating at a tissue site could draw monocytes to the site and upon transformation of the monocyte to a macrophage could immobilize the macrophage locally. Possibly contributing further to this process is the finding that oxidized LDL induces endothelial cells to express a specific monocyte-binding protein on the cell surface [49]. This observation may indicate another important avenue through which lipid oxidation may facilitate the invasion of a tissue site with monocyte-derived macrophages.

Cholesterol feeding in animals susceptible to atherosclerosis leads to a significant increase in binding of monocytes to endothelium, followed by their diapedesis into the intima and subsequent lipid engorgement [53,54]. It is tempting to speculate that these early events in experimental atherosclerosis are manifestations of lipoprotein oxidation.

It is unproved whether the *in vitro* processes described above are active *in vivo*, but aspects of these observations are now being tested. For example, injection of oxidized LDL into mice results in an increase in tissue expression of the gene *JE*, the murine equivalent of MCP-1 [55].

Oxidized lipoproteins and cell injury

Among the earliest studies of the properties of oxidized VLDL and LDL were those describing its capacity to injure vascular cells *in vitro*. LDL is cytotoxic when oxidized whether it is oxidized in a cell-free system enhanced by oxygen, iron or copper ion [8,9,11], or ultraviolet irradiation [18], or whether it is modified by endothelial cells [14], vascular smooth-muscle cells [14], or stimulated monocyte-derived macrophages [15]. Furthermore, the VLDL plus LDL fraction of plasma oxidized *in vivo* and circulating in streptozotocin-treated (diabetic) rats is also cytotoxic [33].

The injurious effects are not specific to cell type, since endothelial cells, vascular smooth-muscle cells, fibroblasts, and lymphocytes are all susceptible [8,18,56–58]. LDL receptors are not required for oxidized LDL to kill cells [57,59], but if LDL is oxidized mildly such that it is a recognizable ligand for the LDL receptor, receptor interactions enhance the rate of cell killing [18]. The toxins are known to be associated with the lipid moiety of the lipoprotein particle [56]. The primary cytotoxins have not been identified; however, among the collection of oxidized lipids that have been identified following LDL oxidation *in vitro* are a number of substances known from previous studies to be cytotoxic. Numerous cholesterol oxidation products, for example, are potent cytotoxins. Cholesterol epoxides, various triol derivatives of cholesterol, and certain hydroxycholesterols have been demonstrated by some to be formed on oxidized LDL [7,60] and by others to be cytotoxic to vascular cells [60,61]. Lysophosphatidylcholine, various aldehyde derivatives of polyunsaturated fatty acid oxidation (including 4-hydroxynonenal), and hydroperoxy derivatives of polyunsaturated fatty acids have also been identified as products of LDL oxidation which are known to injure cells. Given the number of toxic agents produced, it is possible that different injurious substances may predominate in the different preparations of oxidized lipoproteins.

By the same reasoning, there may be multiple mechanisms by which cell injury is induced by oxidized LDL. A potent toxicity observed on endothelial cells with certain preparations of oxidized LDL was found to be dependent upon metal ions bound to LDL that were not removed after copper- or iron-mediated oxidation [62]. However, oxidized LDL is cytotoxic even if oxidized in the absence of added metal ion [8,9] or if the metal ion is stripped away by chelation after metal ion-mediated oxidation [11]. The mechanisms of cell death may be distinct in the two cases [63].

It has been shown that HDL [8,56] and various antioxidants [64] can inhibit the cytotoxic effects of oxidized LDL, and that proliferating cells exposed to oxidized LDL during the DNA-synthesis (S) phase of the cell cycle are more vulnerable then their quiescent counterparts [11]. It has been speculated that the cell-injuring capabilities of oxidized LDL may also play a role in atherosclerosis [3−5,63], either in the subtle endothelial injury believed to facilitate the initiation of lesions or in the accumulation of dead cell debris present in advanced plaque.

The influence of oxidized LDL on cytokine and growth factor production

There have been a number of observations made *in vitro* that can loosely be grouped as positive or negative influences on cellular gene expression and production of factors influencing cell behavior, including cell growth. The production of MCP-1 [50], noted above, is an example. The diversity of these likely reflects that a number of different oxidized lipids are separately exerting distinct cellular effects.

Relatively low concentrations of moderately oxidized LDL can stimulate the production by vascular endothelial cells of colony stimulating factors (CSFs) [65]. Granulocyte-CSF (G-CSF), monocyte-CSF (M-CSF), and GM-CSF are all expressed in endothelial cells exposed to relatively low concentrations of oxidized LDL [65]. If injected intravenously into mice, a single dose of oxidized LDL results in increased levels of M-CSF in plasma [55].

In other contexts oxidized LDL exerts marked inhibitory effects. Pretreatment of murine macrophages for 6−24 hours with 50−100 µg LDL/ml suppresses the expression of genes for tumor necrosis factor-α (TNF-α) and interleukin-1α (IL-1α) upon macrophage simulation [66]. The potent inhibition is independent of a cytotoxic effect, a reduction in total protein synthesis, or the effects of contaminating endotoxin. The inhibitory activity resides in the organic solvent-extractable (lipid) moiety of the LDL. It appears that these suppressive effects of oxidized LDL can be generalized to other cytokines, including IL-1β [67].

Oxidized LDL is a potent suppressor of platelet-derived growth factor (PDGF) constitutively produced by vascular endothelial cells in culture [68]. This activity also resides in the lipid fraction of the oxidized LDL complex. Acetylated LDL, which is efficiently internalized in confluent endothelium via scavenger receptors, is also a potent suppressor of PDGF production but only when oxidized [68]. The degree of oxidation of acetylated LDL required to suppress PDGF is much less than that required for LDL that is not chemically modified. This is likely related to the fact that extensive oxidation of LDL is required to transform it into a ligand for scavenger receptors, whereas acetylation would lead to a very efficient delivery of even mildly oxidized LDL.

It is currently unknown how or whether these diverse effects fit into a pattern of relevance to atherosclerosis or to other *in vivo* examples of tissue injury or inflammation. These are obvious avenues of continuing study.

Lipoprotein oxidation and vasoreactivity

There are data which show that oxidized LDL alters vascular relaxation and constriction. In preparations of vascular tissue *in vitro*, oxidized LDL, but not native LDL, induces moderate vasoconstriction [69,70]; these vasoconstrictive effects are enhanced in the absence of endothelium. A more dramatic effect occurs in agonist-induced vasoconstriction in which a marked increase in constriction is observed in the presence of oxidized but not native LDL [69]. The enhancement is dependent on the degree of LDL oxidation. Pretreatment of the tissue with calcium blocking agents blunts the vasoconstrictive effects of oxidized LDL [69].

Oxidized LDL has also been shown to inhibit endothelium-dependent relaxation [70−74]. The lipid phase of the oxidized lipoprotein contains the inhibitory activity and lysophophatidylcholine, which is produced in and carried by oxidized LDL, has been shown to be capable of this inhibitory effect. This effect is not secondary to oxidized LDL-mediated endothelial cell toxicity or desquamation.

The mechanism by which oxidized LDL mediates these effects is unknown but may be related to the fact that the stimulation of guanylate cyclase by a number of agents is inhibited by oxidized LDL [75].

This phenomenon, too, may ultimately be shown to contribute to atherosclerosis and its complications. Potentiation of vasoconstrictive effects and inhibition of vascular relaxation mediated by oxidized LDL could theoretically contribute to angina pectoris or to occlusive effects in a vessel already comprised by lesions.

A theory for a causal role for oxidized lipoproteins in atherosclerosis

With due respect for the caveats inherent in extrapolating from *in vitro* data to *in vivo* situations, one can construct a plausible sequence of events that applies to the formation and development of atherosclerotic lesions which is based on published observations *in vitro*. There are no doubt variations on this theme, so what follows should be regarded as an example of such a theory.

It is known that elevated levels of LDL in plasma will increase the interstitial concentration of LDL in the artery wall. Even acutely raising LDL in the plasma of a normal animal proportionately raises the arterial wall concentration [76]. Increased levels of LDL increase the residence time of the lipoprotein in the interstitium [77], inviting the possibility for opportunistic oxidation—perhaps mediated by adjacent endothelial cells or smooth-muscle cells following the depletion of lipoprotein-borne antioxidants (Fig. 9.1a). With even moderate oxidation the LDL can interact with the endothelium, stimulating the production of MCP-1 [50], inducing the expression of a monocyte-specific binding protein on the cell surface [49], and injuring those few endothelial cells in the DNA-synthesis phase of the cell cycle [11]. These events could facilitate the attraction and binding of monocytes to the endothelium focally, which is known to occur early in diet-induced experimental athero-sclerosis [53,54]. The increased turnover of endothelial cells could allow enhanced entry of lipoproteins and other plasma-derived macro-molecules (Fig. 9.1b). Accelerated endothelial cell turnover itself can promote monocyte adhesion [78].

The entry of monocytes into the intima introduces further oppor-tunity for the oxidation of the accumulating lipoprotein, since it has been shown that LDL is oxidized when exposed to monocyte-derived macrophages which have been given a phagocytic stimulus [15]. At this point we can presume that the interstitial space would contain LDL molecules oxidized to varying extents. Those which are highly oxidized may be taken up by macrophage scavenger receptors [10,40] or other receptors recognizing oxidized forms of LDL [79,80]. Where LDL is present in tissue in relatively high concentrations, e.g., above about 50% that in plasma, oxidized LDL can aggregate and be taken up by macrophages via a phagocytic pathway [44]. Oxidized LDL may also retard movement of the established macrophages [51] and may act as a chemoattractant to smooth-muscle cells [81]. Thus, migration of medial cells into the intima may be in response to lipoprotein modification (Fig. 9.1c). The variety of cytokines and growth factors either inhibited or induced by oxidized LDL in the various cells present, particularly the endothelial cells and macrophages, may also variably influence smooth-muscle cell proliferation and injury. High levels of HDL infiltrating the intima from plasma could potentially provide antioxidant capacity [82] as well as protect cells from oxidized LDL-induced injury [56].

Whether such a theory pertains to the *in vivo* situation is as yet unknown. Other mysteries of the disease process—the hemodynamic

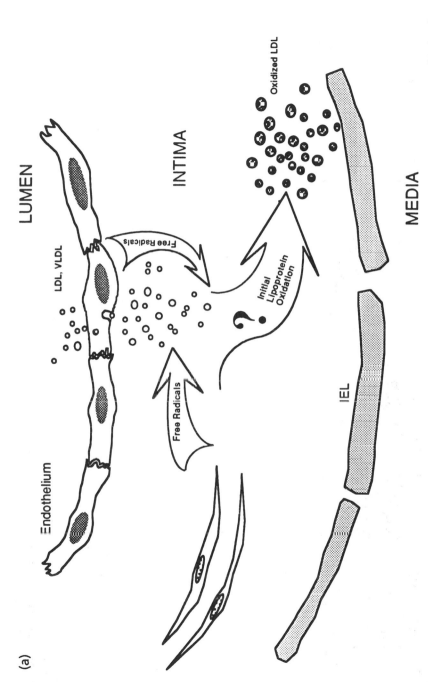

Fig. 9.1 Hypothetical role of oxidized lipoproteins in the development of atherosclerotic lesions. (a) VLDL and LDL can enter the arterial intima from plasma by crossing endothelium through pinocytotic vesicles or vesicular channels. With increases in plasma lipoprotein concentration, the resulting increase in intimal concentration extends the residence time of the molecules in the tissue and may afford an increased opportunity for oxidation. This could be mediated by free radicals emanating from endothelial cells or the occasional smooth-muscle cell residing in the intima.

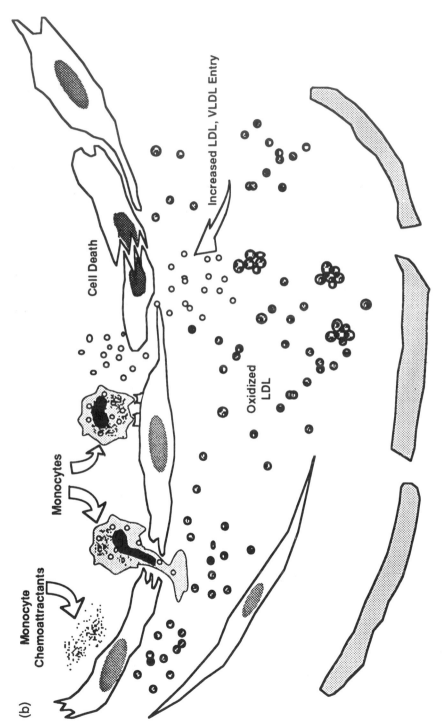

Fig. 9.1 *(cont.)* (b) Oxidation of LDL changes its properties and the way it interacts with cells. It can injure or kill cells, particularly those going through the cell cycle. It may recruit monocytes by acting as a chemoattractant itself, by inducing endothelial cells to produce monocyte chemoattractants, and by causing the expression of a monocyte-binding protein on the endothelial cell surface.

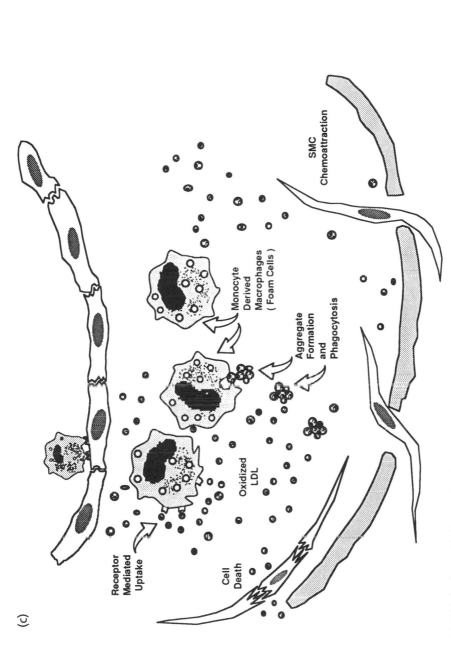

Fig. 9.1 (*cont.*) (c) With further oxidation, oxidized LDL can become a ligand for scavenger receptors on monocyte-derived macrophages. Aggregated oxidized LDL may be taken up by phagocytotic processes. Oxidized LDL may also be a chemoattractant for smooth-muscle cells from the media, a process which may set the stage for the smooth-muscle cell proliferative phase of atherosclerotic lesion development.

influences which govern why lesions begin at arterial branches, the ambiguities surrounding an initial unchecked oxidative event, the role of lipoprotein(a) in the disease process, etc.—complicate the adoption of an oxidative theory and emphasize the complexity and variability of the vascular events.

Antioxidants and atherosclerosis

Interest in a theory such as that outlined above has prompted vigorous recent activity in examining the effects of antioxidants on atherosclerosis development in humans and experimental animals. A number of studies are underway using a variety of antioxidants which may help to settle the impact of oxidation on atherosclerosis risk. The existing data have recently been evaluated [83,84] and can briefly be summarized. There are several studies in which a beneficial effect on atherosclerosis progression has been reported using the potent lipophilic antioxidant probucol in cholesterol-fed rabbits [85], in the Watanabe heritable hyperlipemic (WHHL) rabbit [86,87] which has a defective LDL receptor pathway, and in atherosclerotic rats [88] and primates [89]. In some of these studies, it could be argued that the decreased atherosclerosis may be secondary to the cholesterol-lowering effects of the drug; however, in one study using the WHHL rabbit, cholesterol-lowering agents were given so as to match the probucol-mediated decrease [87], and in another study using cholesterol-fed rabbits cholesterol levels were not significantly changed by probucol [85]. In both of these latter cases, atherosclerosis development was significantly reduced by the drug. In another study using cholesterol-fed rabbits, cholesterol was fed intermittently to a control group to inhibit the rise in cholesterol above a parallel group continuously fed cholesterol plus probucol [90]. In this study atherosclerosis was *not* significantly different between the groups. An analog of probucol, having antioxidant capabilities, but without lipid-lowering effects, was also shown to retard atherosclerosis in a variant strain of the WHHL rabbit [91]. Probucol is known to have numerous other biologic effects that may be unrelated to its antioxidant properties and that may or may not be shared by analogs. It is important therefore to assess whether other antioxidants retard atherosclerosis. Vitamin E and/or vitamin A have been reported to lessen atherosclerosis development in chickens, rabbits, and primates, but in the hands of others with various experimental models, these vitamins have failed [63]. In one report in humans, β-carotene, considered to have anti-oxidant properties in certain circumstances, was observed to reduce adverse myocardial events [92]. In another recent study butylated hydroxytoluene, a potent radical scavenger, was observed to lessen atherosclerosis development in cholesterol-fed rabbits in the absence of any lipid-lowering effect [93]. With such equivocal data, the theory of a causal role for oxidized lipoproteins in atherosclerosis, and the concept that antioxidants can safely impede lesion development, should be regarded as of interest and worthy of study, but as yet unproved.

Summary and perspective

It is currently appropriate to consider oxidatively modified lipoproteins as entities that exist *in vivo* in certain pathologic circumstances that are still being identified and further characterized. It is possible that their existence is a manifestation of appropriate inflammatory responses or injury- and disease-fighting processes. After all, lipoproteins resembling oxidized LDL have been found in "normal" human plasma and antibodies recognizing oxidized but not native LDL have been shown to exist in "normal" human plasma. The proposition that oxidized lipoproteins cause atherosclerosis has not been demonstrated, nor has the corollary that antioxidants can prevent the disease. Because of the promising results from *in vitro* studies demonstrating interactions with cells that are distinct from those of native LDL and that are consistent with features of lesion development, and because of success with some antioxidants in the inhibition of lesion development in certain animal models, the theory will continue to stimulate further research.

Many of the cell biologic effects of oxidized LDL are the result of a particular lipid derivative or a group of lipids created by the oxidation of the normal lipid constituency of the parent lipoprotein. The study of these lipid derivatives and their cellular effects are of interest *per se*. Research is being directed in each of these biologic effects of oxidized LDL to isolate and identify the responsible lipid(s) and study the mechanisms by which cell functions are altered. Certainly, it would be of interest beyond understanding atherosclerosis to know which agents on oxidized LDL inhibit PDGF production, or alter the production of various other growth factors and cytokines.

References

1 Frei B, Kim MC, Ames BN. Ubiquinol-10 is an effective lipid-soluble antioxidant at physiological concentrations. *Proc Natl Acad Sci USA* 1990;87:4879–83.
2 Esterbauer H, Jurgens G, Quehenberger O, Koller E. Autoxidation of human low density lipoprotein: loss of polyunsaturated fatty acids and vitamin E and generation of aldehydes. *J Lipid Res* 1987;28:495–509.

3 Jurgens G, Hoff HF, Chisolm GM, Esterbauer H. Modification of human serum low density lipoprotein by oxidation—characterization and pathophysiologic implications. *Chem Phys Lipids* 1987;45:315−36.

4 Steinberg D, Parthasarathy S, Carew TE, Khoo JC, Witztum JL. Beyond cholesterol: modifications of low-density lipoprotein that increase its atherogenicity. *N Engl J Med* 1989;320:915−24.

5 Steinbrecher UP, Zhang H, Lougheed M. Role of oxidatively modified LDL in atherosclerosis. *Free Radic Biol Med* 1990;9:155−68.

6 Parathasarathy S, Khoo JC, Miller E, et al. Low density lipoprotein rich in oleic acid is protected against oxidative modification: implications for dietary prevention of atherosclerosis. *Proc Natl Acad Sci USA* 1990;87:3894−38.

7 Zhang H, Harkamal JKB, Steinbrecher UP. Effects of oxidatively modified LDL on cholesterol esterification in cultured macrophages. *J Lipid Res* 1990;31:1361−9.

8 Hessler JR, Morel DW, Lewis LJ, Chisolm GM. Lipoprotein oxidation and lipoprotein-induced cytotoxicity. *Arteriosclerosis* 1983;3:215−22.

9 Morel DW, Hessler JR, Chisolm GM. Low density lipoprotein cytotoxicity induced by free radical peroxidation of lipid. *J Lipid Res* 1983;24:1070−6.

10 Steinbrecher UP, Parthasarathy S, Leake DS, Witztum JL, Steinberg D. Modification of low density lipoprotein by endothelial cells involves lipid peroxidation and degradation of low density lipoprotein phospholipids. *Proc Natl Acad Sci USA* 1984;81:3883−7.

11 Kosugi K, Morel DW, DiCorleto PE, Chisolm GM. Toxicity of oxidized low density lipoprotein to cultured fibroblasts is selective for the S phase of the cell cycle. *J Cell Physiol* 1987;102:119−27.

12 Heinecke JW, Rosen H, Chait A. Iron and copper promote modification of low density lipoprotein by human arterial smooth muscle cells in culture. *J Clin Invest* 1984;74:1890−4.

13 Dousset N, Negre-Salvayre A, Lopez M, Salvayre R, Dousteblazy L. Ultraviolet-treated lipoproteins as a model system for the study of the biological effects of lipid peroxides on cultured cell. I. Chemical modifications of ultraviolet-treated low-density lipoproteins. *Biochim Biophys Acta* 1990;1045:219−23.

14 Morel DW, DiCorleto PE, Chisolm GM. Endothelial and smooth muscle cells alter low density lipoprotein *in vitro* by free radical oxidation. *Arteriosclerosis* 1984;4:357−64.

15 Cathcart MK, Morel DW, Chisolm GM III. Monocytes and neutrophils oxidize low density lipoproteins making it cytotoxic. *J Leukoc Biol* 1985;38:341−50.

16 Parthasarathy S, Printz DJ, Boyd D, Joy L, Steinberg D. Macrophage oxidation of low density lipoprotein generates a form recognized by the scavenger receptor. *Arteriosclerosis* 1986;6:505−10.

17 Cathcart MK, McNally AK, Morel DW, Chisolm GM III. Superoxide anion participation in human monocyte-mediated oxidation of low density lipoprotein and conversion of low-density lipoprotein to a cytotoxin. *J Immunol* 1989;142:1963−9.

18 Negre-Salvayre A, Lopes M, Levade T et al. Ultraviolet-treated lipoproteins as a model system for the study of the biological effects of lipid peroxides on cultured cells. II. Uptake and cytotoxicity of ultraviolet-treated LDL on lymphoid cell lines. *Biochim Biophys Acta* 1990;1045:224−32.

19 Parthasarathy S, Steinbrecher UP, Barnett J, Witztum JL, Steinberg D. Essential role of phospholipase A_2 activity in endothelial cell-induced modification of low density lipoprotein. *Proc Natl Acad Sci USA* 1985;82:3000−4.

20 Parthasarathy S, Barnett J. Phospholipase A_2 activity of low density lipoprotein: evidence for an intrinsic phospholipase A_2 activity of apoprotein B-100. *Proc Natl Acad Sci USA* 1990;87:9741−5.

21 Fong LG, Parthasarathy S, Witztum JL, Steinberg D. Nonenzymatic oxidative cleavage of peptide bonds in apoprotein B100. *J Lipid Res* 1987;28:1466−77.

22 Haberland M, Fong D, Cheng L. Malondialdehyde-altered protein occurs in atheroma of Watanabe heritable hyperlipidemic rabbits. *Science* 1988;241:215−18.

23 Palinski W, Rosenfeld ME, Ylä-Herttuala S *et al*. Low density lipoprotein undergoes oxidative modification *in vivo*. *Proc Natl Acad Sci USA* 1989;86:1372−6.

24 Palinski W, Ylä-Herttuala S, Rosenfeld ME *et al*. Antisera and monoclonal antibodies specific for epitopes generated during oxidative modification of low density lipoprotein. *Arteriosclerosis* 1990;10:325−35.

25 Mowri H, Ohkuma S, Takano T. Monoclonal DLR1a/104G antibody recognizing peroxidized lipoproteins in atherosclerotic lesions. *Biochim Biophys Acta* 1988;963:208−14.

26 Boyd HC, Gown AM, Wolfbauer G, Chait A. Direct evidence for a protein recognized by a monoclonal antibody against oxidatively modified LDL in atherosclerotic lesions from a Watanabe heritable hyperlipidemic rabbit. *Am J Pathol* 1989;135:815−25.

27 Hoff HF, Gaubatz JW. Isolation, purification and characterization of a lipoprotein containing apo B from the human aorta. *Atherosclerosis* 1982;42:273−97.

28 Daugherty A, Zwiefel BS, Sobel BE, Schonfeld G. Isolation of low density lipoprotein from atherosclerotic vascular tissue of Watanabe heritable hyperlipidemic rabbits. *Arteriosclerosis* 1988;8:768−77.

29 Ylä-Herttuala S, Palinski W, Rosenfeld ME *et al*. Evidence for the presence of oxidatively modified LDL in atherosclerotic lesions of rabbit and man. *J Clin Invest* 1989;84:1086−95.

30 Rosenfeld ME, Khoo JC, Miller E *et al*. Macrophage-derived foam cells freshly isolated from rabbit atherosclerotic lesions degrade modified lipoproteins, promote oxidation of low-density lipoproteins, and contain oxidation-specific lipid-protein adducts. *J Clin Invest* 1991;87:90−9.

31 Morton EE, West GE, Hoff HF. A low density lipoprotein-sized particle isolated from human atherosclerotic lesions is internalized by macrophages via a non-scavenger-receptor mechanism. *J Lipid Res* 1986;27:1124−34.

32 Avogaro P, Bon GB, Cazzolato G. Presence of a modified low density lipoprotein in humans. *Arteriosclerosis* 1988;8:79−87.

33 Morel DW, Chisolm GM. Antioxidant treatment of diabetic rats inhibits lipoprotein oxidation and cytotoxicity. *J Lipid Res* 1989;30:1827−34.

34 Nagelkerke JF, Havekes L, van Hinsbergh VW, van Berkel TJ. *In vivo* catabolism of biologically modified LDL. *Arteriosclerosis* 1984;4:256−94.

35 Steinbrecher UP, Witztum JL, Parthasarathy S, Steinberg D. Decrease in reactive amino groups during oxidation or endothelial cell modification of LDL. Correlation with changes in receptor-mediated catabolism. *Arteriosclerosis* 1987;7:135−43.

36 Goldstein JL, Brown MS. The low-density lipoprotein pathway and its relation to atherosclerosis. *Annu Rev Biochem* 1977;46:897−930.

37 Steinbrecher UP. Oxidation of human low density lipoproteins results in derivatization of lysine residues of apolipoprotein B by lipid peroxide decomposition products. *J Biol Chem* 1987;262:3603−8.

38 Haberland ME, Fogelman AM, Edwards PA. Specificity of receptor mediated recognition of malondialdehyde modified low density lipoproteins. *Proc Natl Acad Sci USA* 1982;79:1712−16.

39 Jessup W, Jurgens G, Lang J, Esterbauer H, Dean RT. Interaction of 4-hydroxynonenal-modified low-density lipoproteins with the fibroblast apolipoprotein B/E receptor. *Biochem J* 1986;234:245−8.

40 Freeman M, Ekkel Y, Rohrer L *et al*. Expression of type I and type II bovine scavenger receptors in Chinese hamster ovary cells: lipid droplet accumulation and nonreciprocal cross competition by acetylated and oxidized low density lipoprotein. *Proc Natl Acad Sci USA* 1991;88:4931−5.

41 Brown MS, Goldstein JL. Lipoprotein metabolism in the macrophage implications for cholesterol deposition in atherosclerosis. *Annu Rev Biochem* 1983;52:223−61.

42 Jialal I, Vega GL, Grundy SM. Physiologic levels of ascorbate inhibit the oxidative modification of low density lipoprotein. *Atherosclerosis* 1990;82:185−91.

43 Parthasarathy S, Quinn MT, Schwenke DC, Carew TE, Steinberg D. Oxidative modification of beta-very low density lipoprotein. *Arteriosclerosis* 1989;9:398–404.
44 Hoff HF, O'Neil J, Chisolm GM III *et al*. Modification of low density lipoprotein with 4-hydroxynonenal induces uptake by macrophages. *Arteriosclerosis* 1989;9:538–49.
45 Ball RY, Bindman JP, Carpenter KLH, Mitchinson MJ. Oxidized low density lipoprotein induces ceroid accumulation by murine peritoneal macrophages *in vivo*. *Atherosclerosis* 1986;60:173–81.
46 Zhang H, Davis WB, Chen X *et al*. The effects of oxidized low density lipoproteins on arachidonic acid metabolism in smooth muscle cells. *J Lipid Res* 1990;31:551–65.
47 Triau JE, Meydani SM, Schaefer EJ. Oxidized low density lipoprotein stimulates prostacyclin production by adult vascular endothelial cells. *Arteriosclerosis* 1988;8: 810–18.
48 Yokode M, Kita T, Kikawa Y *et al*. Stimulated arachidonate metabolism during foam cell transformation of mouse peritoneal macrophages with oxidized low density lipoprotein. *J Clin Invest* 1988;81:720–9.
49 Berliner JA, Territo MC, Sevanian A *et al* Minimally modified LDL stimulates monocyte endothelial interactions. *J Clin Invest* 1990;85:1260–6.
50 Cushing SD, Berliner JA, Valente AJ *et al*. Minimally modified low density lipoprotein induces monocyte chemotactic protein (MCTP-1) in human endothelial smooth muscle cells. *Proc Natl Acad Sci USA* 1990;87:5134–8.
51 Quinn MT, Parthasarathy S, Fong LG, Steinberg D. Oxidatively modified low density lipoproteins: a potential role in recruitment and retention of monocyte/macrophages during atherogenesis. *Proc Natl Acad Sci USA* 1987;84:2995–8.
52 Quinn MT, Parthasarathy S, Steinberg D. Lysophosphatidylcholine: a chemotactic factor for human monocytes and its potential role in atherogenesis. *Proc Natl Acad Sci USA* 1988;85:2805–9.
53 Faggiotto A, Ross R, Harker L. Studies of hypercholesterolemia in the nonhuman primate. I. Changes that lead to fatty streak formation. *Arteriosclerosis* 1984;4:323–40.
54 Gerrity RG. The role of the monocyte in atherogenesis. I. Transition of blood-borne monocytes into foam cells in fatty lesions. *Am J Pathol* 1981;103:181–90.
55 Liao F, Berliner JA, Mehrabian M *et al*. Minimally modified low density lipoprotein is biologically active *in vivo* in mice. *J Clin Invest* 1991;87:2253–7.
56 Hessler JR, Robertson AL Jr, Chisolm GM. LDL-induced cytotoxicity and its inhibition by HDL in human vascular smooth muscle and endothelial cells in culture. *Atherosclerosis* 1979;32:213–29.
57 Henriksen T, Evensen SA, Carlander B. Injury to human endothelial cells in culture induced by low density lipoproteins. *Scand J Clin Lab Invest* 1979;39:361–8.
58 Schuh J, Novogrodsky A, Haschemeyer RH. Inhibition of lymphocyte mitogenesis by autoxidized low-density lipoprotein. *Biochem Biophys Res Commun* 1978;84:763–8.
59 Børsum T, Henriksen T, Carlander B, Reisvaag A. Injury to human cells in culture induced by low-density lipoprotein—An effect independent of receptor binding and endocytotic uptake of low density lipoprotein. *Scand J Clin Lab Invest* 1982;42:75–81.
60 Sevanian A, Berliner J, Peterson H. Uptake, metabolism, and cytotoxicity of isomeric cholesterol-5,6-epoxides in rabbit aortic endothelial cells. *J Lipid Res* 1991;32:147–55.
61 Peng S-K, Hu B, Morin RJ. Angiotoxicity and atherogenicity of cholesterol oxides. *J Clin Lab Anal* 1991;5:144–52.
62 Kuzuya M, Naito M, Funaki C *et al*. Lipid peroxide and transition metals are required for the toxicity of oxidized low density lipoprotein to cultured endothelial cells. *Biochim Biophys Acta* 1991;1096:155–61.
63 Chisolm GM. Cytotoxicity of oxidized lipoproteins. *Curr Opin Lipidol* 1991;2:311–16.
64 Negre-Salvayre A, Alomar Y, Troly M, Salvayre R. Ultraviolet-treated lipoproteins as a model system for the study of the biological effects of lipid peroxides on cultured cells. III. The protective effect of antioxidants (probucol, catechin, vitamin E) against the cytotoxicity of oxidized LDL occurs in two different ways. *Biochim Biophys Acta* 1991; 1096:291–300.

65 Rajavashisth TB, Andalibi A, Territo MC *et al.* Induction of endothelial cell expression of granulocyte and monocyte–macrophage chemotactic factors by modified low density lipoproteins. *Nature* 1990;344:254–7.

66 Hamilton TA, Ma G, Chisolm GM. Oxidized low density lipoprotein suppresses the expression of tumor necrosis factor-alpha mRNA in stimulated murine peritoneal macrophages. *J Immunol* 1990;144:2343–50.

67 Fong LG, Fong TAT, Cooper AD. Inhibition of macrophage interleukin-1-β mRNA expression by oxidized-LDL (abstract). *Circulation* 1990;82:III-207.

68 Fox PL, Chisolm GM, DiCorleto PE. Lipoprotein-mediated inhibition of endothelial cell production of platelet-derived growth factor-like protein depends on free radical lipid peroxidation. *J Biol Chem* 1987;262:6046–54.

69 Galle J, Bassenge E, Busse R. Oxidized low density lipoproteins potentiate vasoconstrictions to various agonists by direct interaction with vascular smooth muscle. *Circ Res* 1990;66:1287–93.

70 Simon BC, Cunningham LD, Cohen RA. Oxidized low density lipoproteins cause contraction and inhibit endothelium-dependent relaxation in the pig coronary artery. *J Clin Invest* 1990;86:75–9.

71 Tanner FC, Noll G, Boulanger CM, Lüscher TF. Oxidized low density lipoproteins inhibit relaxations of porcine coronary arteries. Role of scavenger receptor and endothelium-derived nitric oxide. *Circulation* 1991;83:2012–20.

72 Jacobs M, Plane F, Bruckdorfer KR. Native and oxidized low-density lipoproteins have different inhibitory effects on endothelium-derived relaxing factor in the rabbit aorta. *Br J Pharmacol* 1990;100:21–6.

73 Yokoyama M, Hirata K, Miyake R *et al.* Lysophosphatidylcholine: essential role in the inhibition of endothelium-dependent vasorelaxation by oxidized low density lipoprotein. *Biochem Biophys Res Commun* 1990;168:301–8.

74 Kugiyama K, Kerns SA, Morrisett JD, Roberts R, Henry PD. Impairment of endothelium-dependent arterial relaxation by lysolecithin in modified low-density lipoproteins. *Nature* 1990;344:160–2.

75 Schmidt K, Graier WF, Kostner GM, Mayer B, Kukovetz WF. Activation of soluble guanylate cyclase by nitrovasodilators is inhibited by oxidized low density lipoprotein. *Biochem Biophys Res Commun* 1990;172:614–19.

76 Bratzler RL, Chisolm GM, Colton CK, Smith KA, Lees RS. The distribution of labeled low-density lipoproteins across the rabbit thoracic aorta *in vivo. Atherosclerosis* 1977;28:289–307.

77 Schwenke DC, Carew TE. Initiation of atherosclerotic lesions in cholesterol-fed rabbits. I. Focal increases in arterial LDL concentration precede development of fatty streak lesions. *Arteriosclerosis* 1989;9:895–907.

78 DiCorleto PE, de la Motte CA. Characterization of the adhesion of the human monocytic cell line U937 to cultured endothelial cells. *J Clin Invest* 1985;75:1153–61.

79 Sparrow CP, Parthasarathy S, Steinberg D. A macrophage receptor that recognizes oxidized low density lipoprotein but not acetylated low density lipoprotein. *J Biol Chem* 1989;264:2599–604.

80 Arai H, Kita T, Yokode M, Narumiya S, Kawai C. Multiple receptors for modified low density lipoproteins in mouse peritoneal macrophages: different uptake mechanisms for acetylated and oxidized low density lipoproteins. *Biochem Biophys Res Commun* 1989;159:1375–82.

81 Autio I, Jaakkola O, Solakivi T, Nikkari T. Oxidized low-density lipoprotein is chemotactic for arterial smooth muscle cells in culture. *FEBS Lett* 1990;277:247–9.

82 Parthasarathy S, Barnett J, Fong LG. High-density lipoprotein inhibits the oxidative modification of low-density lipoprotein. *Biochim Biophys Acta* 1990;1044:275–83.

83 Chisolm GM. Antioxidants and atherosclerosis: a current assessment. *Clin Cardiol* 1991;14:25–30.

84 Steinberg D. Antioxidants and atherosclerosis: a current assessment. *Circulation* 1991;84:1420–4.

85 Daugherty A, Zweifel BS, Schonfeld G. Probucol attenuates the development of aortic atherosclerosis in cholesterol-fed rabbits. *Br J Pharmacol* 1989;98:612−18.

86 Kita T, Nagano Y, Yokode M *et al.* Probucol prevents the progression of atherosclerosis in Watanabe heritable hyperlipidemic rabbit, an animal model for familial hypercholesterolemia. *Proc Natl Acad Sci USA* 1987;84:5928−31.

87 Carew TE, Schwenke DC, Steinberg D. Antiatherogenic effect of probucol unrelated to its hypocholesterolemic effect: evidence that antioxidants *in vivo* can selectively inhibit low density lipoprotein degradation in macrophage-rich fatty streaks and slow the progession of atherosclerosis in the Watanabe heritable hyperlipidemic rabbit. *Proc Natl Acad Sci USA* 1987;84:7725−9.

88 Shankar R, Sallis JD, Stanton H, Thomson R, Influence of probucol on early experimental atherogenesis in hypercholesterolemic rats. *Atherosclerosis* 1989;78:91−7.

89 Wissler RW, Vesselinovitch D. Combined effects of cholestyramine and probucol on regression of atherosclerosis in rhesus monkey aortas. *Appl Pathol* 1983;1:89−96.

90 Stein Y, Stein O, Delplanque B *et al.* Lack of effect of probucol on atheroma formation in cholesterol-fed rabbits kept at comparable plasma cholesterol levels. *Atherosclerosis* 1989;75:145−55.

91 Mao SJT, Yates MT, Rechtin AE, Jackson RL, Van Sickel WA. Antioxidant activity of probucol and its analogues in hypercholesterolemic Watanabe rabbits. *J Med Chem* 1991;34:298−302.

92 Gaziano JM, Manson JE, Ridker PM, Buring JE, Hennekens CH. Beta carotene therapy for chronic stable angina (abstract). *Circulation* 1990;82:III-201.

93 Björkhem I, Henriksson-Freyschuss A, Breuer O *et al.* The antioxidant butylated hydroxytoluene protects against atherosclerosis. *Arterioscler Thromb* 1991;11:15−22.

Chapter 10
Lipoprotein Receptors

JOHN F. ORAM

Plasma membrane receptors are macromolecules that mediate biologic responses upon binding specific extracellular molecules called ligands. Receptors can be grouped into two major classes based on their biologic functions [1]. Binding of ligands to class I receptors directly alters the behavior of the target cells. This action, which does not necessarily require internalization of bound ligands, is usually elicited by intracellular signals that influence specific metabolic processes. Well known examples of class I receptors are ligand-gated ion channels and receptors for hormones, growth factors, and cytokines. Of the lipoprotein receptors, only the high-density lipoprotein (HDL) receptor that facilitates removal of cholesterol from cells has been postulated to be a class I receptor. Class II receptors function to mediate selective uptake of ligands by the target cells, either to deliver nutrients or metabolic factors into cells or to promote clearance (scavenging) of extracellular molecules. For class II receptors, ligand binding *per se* does not necessarily elicit a metabolic response. Any response that occurs is usually secondary to cellular uptake and processing of the ligand. Most lipoprotein receptors function as class II receptors. The most thoroughly studied and best understood of these is the low-density lipoprotein (LDL) receptor.

The LDL receptor

The LDL receptor is a cell-surface glycoprotein that binds apolipoprotein (apo) B_{100}, the single protein component of LDL, and apo E, a protein associated with intermediate-density lipoproteins (IDL) and a minor subclass of HDL. It is a class II receptor that functions both to deliver a vital nutrient into cells and to remove LDL particles from the extracellular environment. In extrahepatic tissues, the LDL receptor functions to deliver cholesterol into cells to be utilized as a structural component of membranes. LDL-derived cholesterol is also used as a precursor for production of steroid hormones, thus accounting for the relatively high level of expression of LDL receptors in steroidogenic tissues. In the liver, however, LDL receptors serve to clear LDL particles from the plasma, targeting the cholesterol either for resecretion back into the plasma or excretion from the body as bile acids. Thus, the hepatic LDL receptor pathway is responsible for maintenance of steady-state plasma concentrations of LDL cholesterol.

Ligand specificity

The LDL receptor recognizes clusters of positive-charged basic amino acids (lysine, arginine, histidine) located within apo E and apo B_{100}, the primary form of apo B synthesized by the liver [2,3]. Apo B_{48} is a truncated form of apo B that is synthesized by the intestine and secreted in triglyceride-rich chylomicrons. This apo B lacks the receptor recognition domain and thus is not a ligand for the LDL receptor. The basic amino acids in the receptor-binding domains create positive charges that interact with negative-charged regions of the LDL receptor which are rich in glutamic and aspartic acids. Studies of the three-dimensional structure of the NH_2-terminal region of apo E have shown that the LDL receptor-binding domain (amino acids 136–150) is a solvent-exposed region of positive electrostatic potential that extends from the surface of the protein [4]. The positive-charged residues in this region do not form salt bridges within the apo E molecule and thus are free to interact with oppositely charged regions of the LDL receptor.

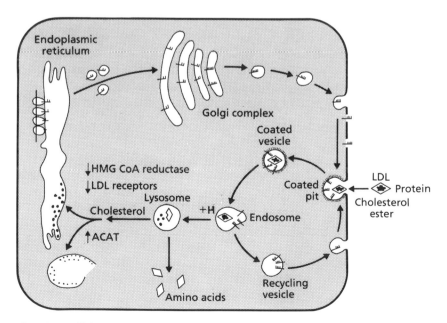

Fig. 10.1 Cellular route of the LDL receptor and its ligand. (Redrawn from [2].)

Human genetic variants have been identified that have a neutral or acidic residue substituted for a basic residue in the receptor-binding domain of apo E [3,5]. In each case, the substitution leads to defective LDL receptor binding of apo E-containing particles. There are three major natural isoforms of apo E (E-II, E-III, and E-IV), with apo E-III being the most common [3,5]. Apo E-II isoforms that have a cysteine in place of an arginine in position 158 have reduced binding to the LDL receptor when compared to the apo E-III isoform. Although this substitution lies outside the receptor-binding domain of apo E, it appears to influence the conformation of the molecule so as to affect its receptor recognition. A mutation in apo B has been described where a glutamine is substituted for an arginine in a region that is within or near the receptor-binding domain [5]. This mutation is also associated with defective binding of LDL with its receptor. Genetic defects or variability in the structure of apo E and B that lead to decreased LDL receptor binding are associated with hypercholesterolemia and premature atherosclerosis.

The LDL receptor pathway

The LDL receptor is synthesized in the rough endoplasmic reticulum as a precursor glycoprotein with an apparent molecular mass of 120 kDa [2]. The precursor rapidly undergoes a shift in apparent molecular mass from 120 to 160 kDa, which is due to compositional changes induced by modification of its carbohydrate residues. Within 1 hour after its synthesis, the mature LDL receptor appears on the cell surface where it binds lipoprotein particles (Fig. 10.1).

To function as a molecule that promotes both scavenging and nutrient delivery, the LDL receptor mediates uptake and degradation of its bound ligand by an endocytotic pathway (Fig. 10.1). The ligand—receptor complexes cluster in coated pits, specialized domains of the plasma membrane that contain a high concentration of a structural protein called clathrin. The coated pits pinch off from the surface to form coated vesicles, which mature into early endocytotic vesicles by losing their clathrin coat. After further maturation and fusion, late endosomes are formed that maintain an acidic environment because of the action of a membrane-associated proton pump. The lower pH of endosomes promotes dissociation of LDL from its receptor and directs unoccupied receptors back to the cell surface where they can rebind additional LDL particles and initiate another round of endocytosis. By this recycling process, an LDL receptor molecule can be reutilized several hundred times before being degraded, making one round trip every 10 minutes. The LDL particles that dissociate in endosomes are delivered to lysosomes when endosomal and lysosomal membranes fuse. Once within lysosomes, the LDL apolipoprotein is degraded to amino acids and its cholesteryl esters are hydrolyzed to produce unesterified cholesterol.

The cholesterol liberated by lysosomal hydrolysis of LDL is translocated across the lysosomal membrane into the "microsomal" compartment of the cell where it mediates several metabolic processes (Fig. 10.1). It suppresses synthesis of the LDL receptor and enzymes of the sterol biosynthetic pathway to shut off further delivery and production of cholesterol. These regulatory processes allow cells to obtain enough cholesterol for membrane synthesis and steroidogenesis, and they protect cells from overaccumulation of cholesterol, which can damage membranes when in excess. As an additional protection, excess lysosomal-derived cholesterol is esterified by the microsomal enzyme acyl CoA:cholesterol acyltransferase (ACAT) and is stored as lipid droplets within the cell. Overaccumulation of cholesterol within cells also activates the HDL receptor pathway that promotes excretion of excess cholesterol from cells (see below).

Knowledge about the mechanisms by which cholesterol suppresses synthesis of the LDL receptor and sterol biosynthetic enzymes is still incomplete. It is believed that the physiologic regulatory agent is an oxygenated sterol formed from cholesterol within the cell rather than cholesterol itself [6,7]. This oxysterol appears to suppress protein synthesis at the level of transcription, which is controlled in part by a sterol regulatory element within the promoter of the LDL receptor gene and the genes for two sterol biosynthetic enzymes, HMG-CoA reductase and HMG-CoA synthase [7]. A protein that binds to the sterol regulatory element has been identified, suggesting that it may be the transcriptional factor that regulates gene expression, but this protein does not appear to interact with oxysterols [8]. Conversely, an oxysterol-binding protein has been identified, but this protein does not interact with the sterol regulatory element [9]. It is unknown if these proteins interact with each other or additional proteins to mediate regulation of gene expression by oxysterols.

Structure of the LDL receptor

The LDL receptor precursor contains an NH_2-terminal signal sequence of 21 amino acids that is cleaved from the receptor immediately after translation. The mature receptor is a multiple-domain protein of 839 amino acids (Fig. 10.2) [2,10]. The first 292 NH_2-terminal amino acids contain seven 40-residue repeat units that are rich in cysteines. This

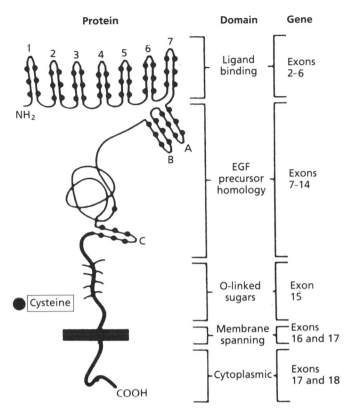

Fig. 10.2. Schematic model of the domain structure of the LDL receptor and its organization of gene exons. (Redrawn from [10].)

domain is located on the external surface of the plasma membrane and directly interacts with the positively charged receptor-binding domains of apo B_{100} and apo E. The second external domain of the LDL receptor consists of 400 amino acids and belongs to a family of membrane proteins that have homology to a precursor for epidermal growth factor (EGF). The third external domain contains 58 amino acids which are rich in O-linked sugars. The fourth domain consists of a stretch of 22 hydrophobic amino acids that span the plasma membrane. The fifth domain is the 50-amino-acid COOH-terminal region that projects into the cytoplasm. This domain plays a role in clustering of receptors within clathrin-coated pits and thus mediates endocytosis of receptor molecules.

The gene for the LDL receptor is located on chromosome 19 and contains 18 exons separated by 17 introns (Fig. 10.2). The first exon encodes the NH_2-terminal signal sequence. Exons 2–6 encode the cysteine-rich ligand-binding domain. The seven repeats in this domain are produced from a single exon that has been duplicated multiple times. The next eight exons encode the sequence that is homologous to the EGF precursor. The O-linked sugar domain is encoded by a single exon, whereas the membrane spanning and cytoplasmic domains are each encoded by parts of two exons.

The LDL receptor gene is a mosaic protein that is encoded by exons shared by members of a supergene family [10]. These proteins share distinct sets of sequences. Several complement factors contain sequences homologous to the ligand-binding domain of the LDL receptor. The EGF precursor sequences are present in a wide variety of proteins, including proteins of the blood clotting cascade, cell surface receptors, adhesion glycoproteins, and developmental proteins. Thus, the gene for the LDL receptor has evolved partially through the assembly of preexisting functional units shared by other genes.

Genetic defects in the LDL receptor pathway

Multiple mutations in the LDL receptor gene have been discovered, many of which cause functional impairment in the LDL receptor pathway that leads to decreased clearance of LDL from the plasma. These mutations fall into five classes [10]. The alleles for class 1 mutations (null alleles) produce either no or very little LDL receptor protein. The alleles for class 2 mutations synthesize receptor protein, but the receptor is transported slowly or not at all to the plasma membrane. These are either missense mutations or amino acid deletions that lead to misfolding of the molecule. The alleles of the class 3 mutations synthesize receptor protein that is processed normally and transported to the plasma membrane, but these receptors are defective in their ability to bind LDL. These mutations occur in the ligand-binding or epidermal growth factor (EGF) precursor domains of the receptor.

For the class 4 mutations, receptors are synthesized and appear on the cell surface where they bind LDL, but they fail to cluster in clathrin-coated pits. Thus, this mutation causes a defective endocytosis of LDL particles. All the class 4 mutations so far described are characterized by alterations of the cytoplasmic domain of the receptor. A variation of class 4 mutations has been identified in which the mutant genes produce LDL receptors that are missing both the cytoplasmic and membrane spanning domains. For these mutations, most of the truncated receptor molecules that reach the cell surface are secreted from the cell rather than incorporated into the plasma membrane.

Class 5 mutant alleles produce receptors that bind and internalize ligand in coated pits but fail to dissociate from ligand in endosomes and thus do not recycle to the cell surface. These mutations occur in the EGF precursor domain, which functions in part to mediate ligand–receptor dissociation in the acidic environment of endosomes. This defective recycling leads to increased degradation of receptor protein and deficient LDL binding.

The mutations described above lead to a disorder called familial hypercholesterolemia (FH) which is characterized by high levels of circulating LDL. Approximately two-thirds of the LDL that is cleared from the blood is removed by the LDL receptor pathway primarily in the liver. Not only does a defect in this pathway lead to reduced clearance of LDL from the blood, but it may also increase LDL production. The overproduction occurs largely because the removal of the immediate precursor for LDL is also impaired when the LDL receptor pathway is defective.

LDL is formed as an endproduct of a lipoprotein cascade that starts when very low-density lipoprotein (VLDL) is secreted from the liver (Fig. 10.3). This large lipoprotein is rich in triglycerides and provides a source of free fatty acids for adipose tissue in muscle. The triglycerides are removed in the capillaries by the action of lipoprotein lipase, and the VLDL is converted to a smaller particle, termed IDL, that has lost most of its triglycerides but has retained its cholesterol esters. IDL contains multiple copies of apo E, as well as apo B_{100}. The multiple copies of apo E allow IDL to bind to the LDL receptor with very high affinity. Thus, a fraction of the IDL is rapidly cleared by the hepatic LDL receptor pathway. The remaining fraction of IDL is converted to LDL, losing its apo E in the process but retaining apo B_{100}. Most defects in the LDL receptor pathway reduce clearance of both IDL and LDL, causing more IDL to be converted to LDL (Fig. 10.3). The combination of reduced clearance and overproduction of LDL leads to elevated steady-state plasma levels of cholesterol.

Some individuals with LDL receptor mutations have defective receptor binding of LDL, but their receptors retain the ability to bind apo E-containing lipoproteins [10]. Thus, these subjects are able to clear IDL particles from the plasma. In these cases, the production of LDL is not increased and there is a more moderate elevation in plasma LDL.

The major pathologic consequence of defective LDL receptors is related to its role as a scavenger-type receptor. The elevated level of LDL that results from decreased hepatic clearance is associated with an increased incidence of atherosclerosis. Numerous population studies have shown a positive correlation between LDL cholesterol levels and risk for heart disease. Subjects with the highest levels of LDL cholesterol

(a) **Normal**

(b) **FH**

Receptors
genetically
defective

(c) **High fat diet**

Receptors saturated
and suppressed

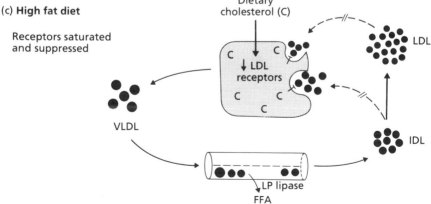

Fig. 10.3 Model of the mechanism by which hepatic LDL receptors control production and catabolism of plasma LDL in normal subjects (a), hypercholesterolemic subjects (b), and in subjects consuming a high saturated fat and cholesterol diet (c). (Redrawn from [2].)

have one or more mutant alleles for the LDL receptor, and many of these individuals have heart attacks at an early age. Thus, the LDL receptor pathway is not directly responsible for the overaccumulation of cholesterol in atherosclerotic cells of the artery wall but plays a secondary role by controlling the level of LDL in the plasma. Defective delivery of cholesterol as a nutrient for cell growth appears to have less of a pathologic impact, since cells are capable of providing sterols through their biosynthetic pathway.

Acquired defects in the LDL receptor pathway

Most subjects with elevated plasma levels of LDL cholesterol do not have apparent genetic defects in the LDL receptor pathway. Many of these hypercholesterolemic subjects may have an acquired suppression of the LDL receptor pathway in the liver, leading to decreased clearance of LDL [2]. The acquired hypercholesterolemia reflects the interplay of the scavenger and nutrient-delivery functions of the hepatic LDL receptor pathway. As with other tissues, the liver suppresses synthesis of LDL receptors when cells overaccumulate intracellular cholesterol. Since the plasma level of LDL cholesterol exceeds that needed to saturate receptors, the rate of clearance of LDL from the plasma is a function of the number of receptors in the liver. A diet rich in fats and cholesterol can suppress the receptor number by overloading the liver with cholesterol (Fig. 10.3). The entry of dietary cholesterol into the liver occurs through another receptor pathway, the chylomicron receptor (see below), that is unaffected by overaccumulation of cholesterol in cells. Thus, a build-up of dietary cholesterol through this pathway may suppress synthesis of LDL receptors and decrease LDL removal, leading to an acquired hypercholesterolemia. A high cholesterol and saturated fat diet may also promote synthesis of other sterol-rich lipoproteins, such as VLDL and IDL, which may exacerbate the acquired defect in receptor clearance of LDL. This acquired hypercholesterolemia also appears to be influenced by genetic as well as environmental factors, since individuals vary in their hypercholesterolemic response to dietary fat.

The LDL receptor as a target for drug therapy

Since the activity of the LDL receptor is rate-limiting for removal of LDL cholesterol from the plasma, pharmaceutic agents that raise LDL receptor activity should increase clearance of LDL and lower plasma cholesterol levels. Two classes of drugs have been developed that achieve this therapeutic effect [2,11]. These drugs alter hepatic cholesterol metabolism to cause a temporary state of cholesterol deficiency. The first class of drugs are bile acid sequestrants, which trap bile acids in the intestine and prevent their reabsorption. This increases conversion of cholesterol to bile acids and depletes hepatic cells of cholesterol, resulting in an activation of the LDL receptor gene. Treatment with bile acid sequestrants has been shown to lower plasma LDL levels by 10–20%.

A second class of drugs acts by inhibiting HMG-CoA reductase, the rate-limiting enzyme in the sterol biosynthetic pathway. As with bile acid sequestrants, reductase inhibitors create a relatively cholesterol-depleted state in hepatocytes by blocking the production of sterol through the biosynthetic pathway. These agents, however, are more efficacious than bile acid sequestrants and lower the plasma LDL cholesterol levels by 30–40%. Administration of reductase inhibitors in combination with bile acid sequestrants is more effective than administration of either type of drug alone and can reduce LDL cholesterol levels by more than half. Although the major mechanism of action of these drugs is through activation of the LDL receptor and increased clearance of LDL from the plasma, they may also reduce hepatic production of cholesterol-rich lipoproteins that are precursors to LDL, which would also contribute to the lowering of plasma LDL levels.

The development of cholesterol-lowering drugs is an important example of how understanding the regulatory mechanisms of a receptor pathway has led to a targeted strategy for prevention of a disease. Although population and genetic studies predict that lowering LDL cholesterol levels should be beneficial, it is too early to assess how effective such drug therapy will be in decreasing the incidence of myocardial infarction in patients with moderate to severe hypercholesterolemia.

The LDL receptor-related protein

Chylomicrons are large triglyceride-rich lipoproteins synthesized by the intestine for transport of dietary fat. These particles are degraded by lipoprotein lipase to form remnants that are enriched in cholesterol and apo E. Chylomicron remnants are cleared rapidly from the plasma by the liver. Evidence from metabolic studies suggest that this rapid clearance is mediated by a receptor distinct from the LDL receptor.

A membrane protein has been identified that is a strong candidate for a chylomicron receptor [12]. This 4525-amino-acid protein is present at the cell surface and in intracellular vesicles of a wide variety of cells, including hepatocytes. Because of its sequence homology to the LDL receptor, this protein has been designated as the LDL receptor-related protein (LRP). Shortly after its discovery it was determined that LRP is the receptor for α_2-macroglobulin, a protease inhibitor that is relatively abundant in the plasma [13]. The native form of α_2-macroglobulin contains four internal thiol ester bonds that prevent it from interacting with LRP. When native α_2-macroglobulin interacts with proteases, thiol ester bonds are cleaved and receptor-binding sites are exposed. As a result, the activated α_2-macroglobulin–protease complexes are cleared rapidly from the plasma by the liver.

Ligand specificity

Several lines of evidence suggest that LRP plays a role in clearing chylomicron remnants from the plasma through its interaction with apo E molecules on remnant particles. Ligand blotting and chemical cross-linking studies have shown that apo E-rich vesicles and lipoproteins can bind directly to LRP [14,15]. Studies with cultured cells suggest that the apo E molecules in lipoprotein particles must ,have a unique conformation to be accessible for binding to LRP. Mutant fibroblasts from subjects who lack LDL receptors but express LRP on their surfaces are unable to take up native β-VLDL, a subclass of remnant lipoproteins that accumulate in cholesterol-fed animals, despite the presence of multiple copies of apo E on each lipoprotein particle [16]. However, when exogenous apo E is added to β-VLDL, the particles interact with LRP and are taken up and degraded by cells. Studies with perfused livers also have demonstrated that enrichment of lipoproteins or lipid vesicles with apo E enhances clearance of these particles by hepatocytes. Addition of excess apo Cs, particularly C-I, interferes with the uptake of apo E-rich lipoproteins both by the LRP pathway of cultured cells [14,17] and by intact livers [18], presumably by displacing apo E from the particles and/or modifying apolipoprotein conformation. Binding of apo E to LRP is enhanced markedly in the presence of lipoprotein lipase [19]. This appears to be due to direct binding of the enzyme to LRP, which alters receptor conformation so as to increase its binding of apo E. Thus, the enzyme responsible for creating chylomicron remnants may also increase clearance of these particles by interacting with hepatic LRP.

Metabolic studies have suggested that LRP is responsible for clearing both chylomicron remnants and α_2-macroglobulin–protease complexes *in vivo* [20]. Injection of unlabeled chylomicron remnants into mice partially blocks clearance and hepatic uptake of radiolabeled activated α_2-macroglobulin. Conversely, injection of unlabeled activated α_2-macroglobulin retards clearance and hepatic uptake of radiolabeled chylomicron remnants. Chylomicron remnants and activated α_2-macroglobulin also compete for binding to LRP on cultured cells [20]. The properties of the receptor recognition sites in these two classes of ligands are currently unknown.

Why LRP functions to promote clearance of two such widely diverse macromolecules is still unclear, but the explanation may be related to the need to rapidly remove metabolic endproducts from the plasma. Thus, once lipoprotein lipase associates with chylomicrons and tri-glycerides are degraded, the conformation of apo E is altered so as to interact with LRP in the liver, leading to rapid clearance of remnant particles from the plasma. Similarly, once α_2-macroglobulin inactivates a protease, a complex is formed that is rapidly cleared by the hepatic LRP pathway. Additional studies are needed to define the precise role of LRP in clearing these two macromolecular complexes and to determine whether or not LRP is involved in the hepatic clearance of other metabolic products.

Structure of LRP

LRP is one of the largest cell-surface proteins identified to date. The mature protein contains 4525 amino acids, 4400 of which extend from the external side of the plasma membrane [12]. The molecule has four functional regions (Fig. 10.4). Most of the NH_2-terminal extracellular region has four domains that are homologous to the LDL receptor. Each domain contains variable copies of the 40-residue, cysteine-rich repeats that contain the ligand-binding sites in the LDL receptor. In addition, each of the four LDL receptor-like domains contains sequences that are homologous to the EGF precursor. Between the four LDL receptor-like domains and the plasma membrane is a stretch of six 40-amino-acid repeats that also are present in EGF but differ from the EGF precursor repeats that appear in the LDL receptor. This region replaces the O-linked sugar domain of the LDL receptor. The third region of the molecule is a stretch of 25 hydrophobic amino acids that represent the membrane spanning domain.

The COOH-terminal cytoplasmic tail of LRP is 100 amino acids in length, which is approximately twice as long as the corresponding region of the LDL receptor. This region contains two amino acid sequences homologous to a motif in the cytoplasmic tail of the LDL receptor that is responsible for clustering of LDL receptors into coated pits. Thus, it is likely that LRP takes up its ligand through an endocytotic pathway similar to the one used by the LDL receptor (Fig. 10.1). Recycling of LRP between endosomal compartments and the cell surface

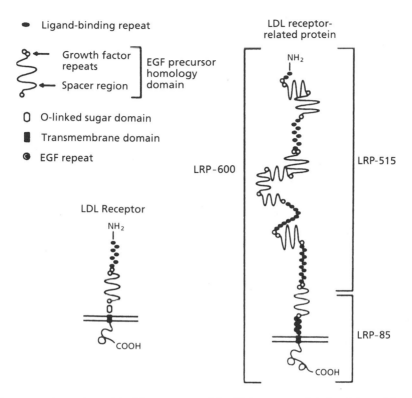

Fig. 10.4 Schematic model of the structure of the LDL receptor-related protein and its comparison to the structure of the LDL receptor. Brackets indicate molecular mass in kDa of the intact protein (*left*, LRP-600) and the two proteolytic cleavage products (*right*, LRP-515 and LRP-85). (Redrawn from [21].)

is suggested by the high abundance of LRP in membranes of early and late endosomes [22]. These properties and its ligand specificity suggest that LRP is a class II receptor that functions predominantly as a scavenger.

Expression of LRP

Unlike expression of the LDL receptor, expression of LRP is not regulated by changes in the cholesterol content of cells. The promoter region of the LRP gene lacks the sterol regulatory elements common to several cholesterol-regulated proteins [23]. LRP is synthesized as a glycosylated precursor and has an apparent molecular mass of 600 kDa. Upon reaching the Golgi complex, the precursor protein is clipped by an endoprotease to form two subunits of 515 and 85 kDa. This proteolytic clipping occurs within the eighth EGF precursor repeat (Fig. 10.4) at a site with the amino acid sequence arginine−histidine−arginine−arginine [21]. This tetrabasic amino acid sequence is nearly identical to the cleavage site of insulin and insulin-like growth factor-1 (IGF-1) receptors. Clipping of LRP occurs in the Golgi complex or post-Golgi secretory vesicles and is coincident with maturation of the N-linked carbohydrates.

After clipping occurs, the two subunits remain associated in a 1:1 stoichiometric ratio [21]. Unlike the subunits of the insulin and IGF-1 receptors, which are joined by covalent disulfide bonds, the LRP subunits stay tightly associated through noncovalent binding. The attachment regions have not yet been identified, but they are likely to represent amino acid sequences in each subunit that are complementary to each other. This posttranslational processing of LRP is distinctly unique, as proteolytic cleavage of a precursor peptide and noncovalent attachment of its subunits has not been described for any other receptor protein. The functional reason for this unique processing is unknown.

Possible genetic defects and drug therapy

Genetic defects in the LRP pathway have yet to be discovered. It would be predicted that such defects would lead to a decreased hepatic clearance of chylomicron remnants, as well as α_2-macroglobulin−protease complexes. However, subjects with elevated plasma levels of chylomicron remnants have not been identified, suggesting that such a phenotype is extremely rare or nonexistent. It is questionable whether the LRP pathway would be a useful target for drug therapy. An agonist that would stimulate such a pathway may have minimal benefits, since the clearance of chylomicron remnants by the liver is extremely fast in the basal state.

The scavenger receptor

The lipoprotein "scavenger" receptor is a class II receptor that promotes binding, uptake, and degradation of modified lipoproteins. This receptor is expressed almost exclusively on macrophages [24,25], a phagocytic cell type that functions to clear foreign molecules from tissues. Scavenger receptors may also be expressed *in vitro* under certain conditions by aortic endothelial cells, smooth-muscle cells, and fibroblasts [26,27].

The discovery of the scavenger receptor was prompted by studies showing that atherosclerotic lesions contain numerous cholesteryl ester-loaded macrophages. These cells ingest large quantities of circulating lipoproteins that penetrate the endothelium and infiltrate the artery wall. It appeared likely that this intracellular accumulation of cholesteryl esters occurred by receptor-mediated endocytosis similar to what had been described for the LDL receptor pathway. However, cell culture studies revealed that macrophages are incapable of taking up large amounts of lipoproteins by the LDL receptor pathway. Moreover, subjects with defective LDL receptors accumulate LDL-derived cholesteryl esters in macrophages of the artery wall and develop atherosclerosis at an early age. Thus, macrophages must have additional pathways that mediate rapid uptake of sterol-rich lipoproteins. It was postulated that macrophages selectively ingest LDL particles that have undergone some chemical or physical modification.

This hypothesis was tested by incubating cultured macrophages with LDL particles that had been chemically modified by acetylation [28]. It was discovered that macrophages avidly take up and degrade acetyl-LDL by receptor-mediated endocytosis. This uptake could not be mediated by the LDL receptor, since acetylation of LDL destroys its ability to bind to the LDL receptor. Unlike the LDL receptor, this scavenger receptor is not downregulated when cells accumulate excess cholesterol, and macrophages continue to take up and degrade acetyl-LDL during long-term exposure, resulting in massive deposition of cholesteryl esters. Thus, this receptor pathway could account for the appearance of cholesteryl ester-rich foam cells in the developing atherosclerotic lesion.

Ligand specificity

The scavenger receptor has broad specificity for a diverse group of ligands [24]. These include other modified lipoproteins and proteins, such as acetoacetylated LDL, maleylated LDL, succinylated LDL, malondialdehyde-treated LDL, and maleylated bovine serum albumin. All these modifications cause an increase in net negative charge of the protein by attaching carboxyl groups to the ε-amino groups of lysine residues. The scavenger receptor also interacts with compounds in which the negative charges reside on noncarboxylic moieties, such as sulfates (e.g., dextran sulfate and fucoidin) or phosphates (e.g., polyinositic acid). These and other studies indicate that binding to the acetyl-LDL receptor is dependent on the presence of a high density of negatively charged residues within specific regions of the molecule.

Evidence that the scavenger receptor functions *in vivo* was provided by studies showing that iodinated lipoproteins injected intravenously into animals was cleared rapidly from the plasma by macrophage-like Kupffer cells of the liver [24]. Although the scavenger receptor interacts with chemically modified lipoproteins, it is unlikely that these particles represent the physiologic ligands for the receptor and the source of excess cholesterol that accumulates in macrophages of the artery wall. With the possible exception of malondialdehyde-induced modifications, these types of chemical reactions probably do not occur *in vivo* to an extent sufficient to modify even small amounts of LDL.

One possible physiologic ligand for the scavenger receptor is oxidatively modified LDL [29]. Exposure of LDL to cultured endothelial cells or smooth-muscle cells can modify LDL so that it is recognized by the scavenger receptor [30,31]. This modification involves free-radical peroxidation of LDL lipids and can be mimicked in the absence of cells by exposure of LDL to redox-active metal ions such as copper. This oxidation process causes alterations in both the lipid and protein components of LDL, including peroxidation of lipids, fragmentation of apo B, and derivatization of apo B lysine residues. Oxidized LDL no longer interacts with the LDL receptor but is taken up by macrophages *in vitro* and promotes accumulation of excess cholesteryl esters within these cells. These and other observations led to the hypothesis that one of the initiating events in formation of atherosclerotic lesions is oxidation of LDL particles that penetrate the endothelium and become trapped in the artery wall [29].

Structure of the scavenger receptor

The scavenger receptor is an integral membrane glycoprotein with a molecular mass of approximately 220 kDa [32−34]. It is composed of three 77-kDa subunits. Molecular cloning of the scavenger receptor has uncovered two types of receptor subunits, designated Type I and Type II [33,34]. The scavenger receptor can be separated into six distinct domains (Fig. 10.5). The first five domains are common to both Type I and II receptors, but the sixth domain differs between the two subunit types.

Each subunit of the scavenger receptor spans the plasma membrane once with their first (NH_2-terminal) domains localized within the cytoplasm. This orientation is opposite to that for both the LDL receptor and LRP, which have their NH_2-terminal domains localized to the extracellular side of the plasma membrane. The 50-amino-acid cytoplasmic tails of the scavenger receptor subunits have amino acid sequence motifs that have been shown to promote endocytosis of the transferrin receptor, another integral membrane protein with an NH_2-terminal cytoplasmic tail. The second domain of the scavenger receptor is a transmembrane spanning region of 26 hydrophobic amino acids. The third domain is a

Type I (453 aa)   Type II (349 aa)

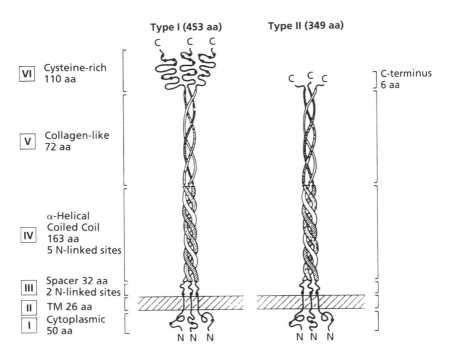

VI Cysteine-rich 110 aa

V Collagen-like 72 aa

IV α-Helical Coiled Coil 163 aa 5 N-linked sites

III Spacer 32 aa 2 N-linked sites

II TM 26 aa

I Cytoplasmic 50 aa

C-terminus 6 aa

Fig. 10.5 Schematic model of the structure of the Type I and Type II bovine scavenger receptor. (Redrawn from [34].)

32-amino-acid spacer that is rich in prolines and connects the trans-membrane domain to the remaining three extracellular domains.

The fourth domain contains 23 seven-amino-acid heptad repeats. The sequence of these repeats predicts a three-stranded α-helical coiled-coil structure held together by interhelical hydrophobic cores of aliphatic residues. Such a structure could play a role in assembling the three subunits to form a functioning trimeric receptor. The fifth domain contains 24 tandem tripeptide repeats similar to those found in collagen. These structures also promote triple helix formation. The tripeptide repeats are either uncharged or positively charged at neutral pH, and clusters of the positively charged tripeptides located near the COOH-terminal end of the fifth domain appear to mediate binding of the negatively charged ligands [25]. Together, the fourth and fifth domains form a long, fibrous stalk that extends outward from the plasma membrane. This α-helical coiled coil and collagen-like stalk has not been described for any other integral membrane protein.

The sixth (COOH-terminal) domain shows striking differences between Type I and II scavenger receptor subunits. The Type I subunits contain a 110-amino-acid sequence that is rich in glycines and contains six cysteines that could form interchain and/or intrachain disulfide bonds. This domain has been shown to be homologous to regions found in other membrane proteins, including sea urchin speract receptors and lymphocyte proteins CD5 and Ly-1 [35]. The function of this domain for each of these diverse membrane proteins is unclear. The sixth domain of the Type II scavenger receptor subunit lacks cysteines and contains only 6 (mouse and bovine) to 17 (human) amino acid residues.

Expression of the scavenger receptor

The two types of scavenger receptor subunits are generated by alternative splicing of a single gene product [25]. The functional reason for the existence of these two subunit types is unclear. Transfection of cells with cDNAs encoding either Type I or II subunits leads to expression of receptors that have very similar ligand saturation kinetics and specificities [36]. Both receptor types interact with acetyl-LDL and oxidized LDL, as well as other modified LDL proteins (e.g., maleylated albumin) and negatively charged molecules (e.g., fucoidin, polyinositic acid). Expression of both types of receptors promotes uptake and degradation of acetyl-LDL and intracellular accumulation of cholesteryl ester-rich lipid droplets. Studies using antibodies raised against synthetic peptides specific to each subunit type have detected both Types I and II subunits in human macrophages [25]. If both types are expressed in a single cell, it is possible that heterotrimers are formed that contain variable combinations of the two subunits, and this somehow influences receptor function.

The scavenger receptor gene is localized on chromosome 8 near the gene for lipoprotein lipase [25,37]. The structure of the scavenger receptor gene and its promoter region has not yet been described; thus, information about regulation of gene expression is not available. Expression of the scavenger receptor is not influenced by the cholesterol content of cells. However, several reports suggest that the relative activity of the scavenger receptor pathway may be modulated *in vitro* by cytokines or other agents that influence cell differentiation or activation. Monocyte colony stimulating factor, which stimulates proliferation and differentiation of monocyte progenitor cells, has been shown to increase the abundance of scavenger receptor protein in human monocyte-derived macrophages [39]. Treatment of cultured rabbit fibroblasts and smooth-muscle cells with platelet secretory products and phorbol esters was reported to cause a marked increase in scavenger receptor activity [27]. Treatment of human monocyte cell lines with phorbol esters to induce differentiation into macrophages causes appearance of scavenger receptor mRNA and active protein [33,37].

Both Type I and II scavenger receptor mRNAs have been detected in bovine and human lung, liver, placenta, and brain [25,37]. The bovine scavenger receptor protein appears to be localized exclusively to the macrophages in these tissues, including Kupffer cells of the liver and perivascular macrophages of the brain. Although aortic endothelial cells take up and degrade acetyl-LDL *in vitro*, these cells *in vivo* do not react with a scavenger receptor-specific antibody [25]. Scavenger receptor mRNA and protein have been detected in macrophages of athero-sclerotic lesions [37,38], consistent with their postulated role in formation of cholesteryl ester-rich foam cells.

Possible genetic defects and drug therapy

Genetic defects in the scavenger receptor pathway have not yet been reported. It can be predicted that such defects would impair the ability of macrophages to take up modified lipoproteins and thus prevent foam-cell formation in atherosclerotic lesions. However, genetic defects in the scavenger receptor pathway may also hamper the antiinflammatory action of macrophages and prevent them from clearing a variety of potentially harmful macromolecules from the plasma and tissues. Similarly, drug therapy targeted at blocking the scavenger receptor path-way may retard atherosclerotic lesion formation but create secondary complications. More information about the physiologic role of the scavenger receptor will be required before the potential benefits or side-effects in modulating this pathway are apparent.

The HDL receptor

The HDL receptor is a postulated but yet unidentified cell surface protein that functions to stimulate excretion of excess cholesterol from cells. Unlike the other lipoprotein receptors, the HDL receptor appears to be a class I receptor that transmits signals between extracellular and intra-cellular compartments.

Evidence for the existence of HDL receptors has been provided by three separate lines of investigation. First, many different types of cells have been shown to have high-affinity binding sites for HDL on their surfaces [40–43]. The number of these binding sites increases when cells are either overloaded with cholesterol [41–43] or growth arrested [44]. Thus, the HDL-binding sites are upregulated when supply of cholesterol exceeds demand for membrane synthesis, consistent with the hypothesis that these binding sites represent receptors that function to promote excretion of excess cholesterol. As a second line of evidence, a membrane protein of 110 kDa has been identified that binds HDL with similar specificity as the high-affinity binding sites on cells [45]. The relative abundance of this protein increases when cells are cholesterol loaded [45] or growth arrested [44], suggesting that it is a strong candidate for the HDL receptor molecule. The third line of evidence was provided by studies showing that the interaction of HDL apolipoproteins with cells stimulates translocation to the plasma membrane of intracellular cholesterol by a complex signalling pathway [46−48]. The latter observation strongly suggests that HDL-mediated removal of cholesterol from cells involves multiple cell proteins, including a cell-surface receptor that is capable of transmitting signals. It has not yet been ascertained if the cell-surface HDL-binding sites or the 110-kDa HDL-binding protein are components of this cholesterol removal pathway.

Ligand specificity

Both the high-affinity cell-surface binding sites and the isolated 110-kDa membrane protein exhibit broad specificity for HDL apolipoproteins. They interact strongly with apo A-I, apo A-II, and apo A-IV, and only weakly or not at all with apo E and apo B [41,42,45,49]. Thus, the HDL-binding sites and binding protein preferentially bind the major apolipoproteins of HDL, but they do not distinguish between the different apo As.

The receptor recognition sites in these different apolipoproteins are unknown. Chemical modifications of HDL particles that alter lysine, cysteine, and arginine residues do not inhibit HDL binding to cells [50], suggesting that these residues are not involved in receptor recognition. However, nonenzymatic glycation of HDL, which attaches sugar groups to free amino groups, markedly suppresses receptor interactions [51]. In addition, very mild treatment of HDL particles with the proteolytic enzyme trypsin, which attacks basic amino acids, abolishes receptor binding and biologic activity of HDL [47]. These latter two observations suggest that alterations of basic amino acids can affect receptor binding of HDL at least under some conditions. Treatment of HDL with tetranitromethane, which nitrates tyrosine residues, reduces high-affinity HDL binding to cells and the ability of HDL to promote cholesterol efflux from intracellular pools [46,48,50]. However, this procedure causes extensive cross-linking of apolipoproteins, and other cross-linking procedures have been shown to have similar effects [52]. Based on studies using monoclonal antibodies directed against apo A-I epitopes

[53], it has been suggested that HDL may bind to cellular receptors through the cooperative interaction of its apolipoprotein amphipathic helices.

The HDL receptor pathway

The HDL receptor appears to function to rid cells of excess cholesterol that accumulates within intracellular pools. When quiescent cells are overloaded with cholesterol *in vitro* in the absence of HDL, much of the excess cholesterol accumulates within intracellular compartments and is converted to cholesterol esters by the enzyme ACAT (Fig. 10.6). This storage mechanism presumably protects cells from incorporating too much cholesterol into the plasma membrane, which can have a deleterious effect on the activity of multiple cell-surface proteins. Even when cholesterol esterification is blocked by an ACAT inhibitor, much of the excess free cholesterol is stored within intracellular compartments [47], probably within newly synthesized membranous structures [53]. When these cholesterol-loaded cells are exposed to HDL, there is an increase in translocation of cholesterol from intracellular compartments to the plasma membrane (Fig. 10.6) [46–48]. Once at the cell surface, the cholesterol molecules can desorb into the extracellular fluid and be picked up by HDL particles. This stimulatory action of HDL is mediated by binding of HDL apolipoproteins to the cell surface. Modification of apolipoproteins by treatment with tetranitromethane or trypsin abolishes the ability of HDL to stimulate cholesterol translocation and efflux. Moreover, incubation of cells with lipid-free apo A-I can stimulate intracellular cholesterol translocation to the plasma membrane [48].

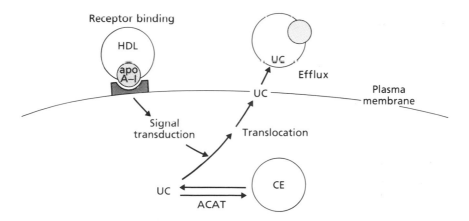

Fig. 10.6 Model for the cellular HDL receptor pathway.

HDL apolipoproteins stimulate cholesterol translocation by activating a signalling pathway that appears to modulate cholesterol trafficking [48]. Binding of HDL to cells liberates diacylglycerol from cellular phospholipids that in turn activate protein kinase C. This process is likely to cause phosphorylation of key intracellular proteins that promote transport of cholesterol from intracellular storage sites into an excretory pathway. The biochemical and morphologic details of this pathway are still unknown.

This model is unique among lipoprotein receptors, in that it predicts that HDL is exerting its biologic effect through interaction with a class I receptor. This interaction communicates to cells that appropriate cholesterol acceptors are present at the cell surface and that excess cholesterol should be transported to the plasma membrane for removal. Such a pathway may be the cellular mechanism that underlies some of the apparent antiatherogenic effects of HDL.

Possible genetic defects and drug therapy

Genetic defects in the HDL receptor pathway have not yet been identified. Population studies have shown an inverse correlation between HDL cholesterol levels and risk for atherosclerosis. It is possible that some of these subjects with low HDL cholesterol and premature atherosclerosis have a cellular defect in the HDL receptor pathway. Such defects could block clearance of excess cholesterol from peripheral cells, such as those of the artery wall, and lead to lower than normal levels of plasma HDL cholesterol. The HDL receptor pathway could also be an important target for drug therapy. An HDL receptor agonist could stimulate clearance of excess cholesterol from macrophages in the artery wall and retard lesion formation. The HDL receptor pathway, however, is the least understood of all the major lipoprotein receptor systems, and considerably more information is needed before its relevance to atherosclerosis is established.

Other lipoprotein receptors

Studies from several different laboratories have suggested that macrophages possess additional scavenger-type receptors that recognize unique lipoprotein subclasses, modified lipoproteins, or lipoproteins conjugated to other macromolecules. Membranes of cultured murine macrophages contain a 190-kDa protein that appears to preferentially bind hypertriglyceridemic VLDL but not normal VLDL or LDL [55]. It has been suggested that this candidate receptor protein may mediate high-affinity uptake of triglyceride-rich lipoproteins by macrophages. Murine macrophages may also have receptors that take up and degrade oxidized LDL by a process distinct from the scavenger receptor. This possibility was suggested by studies showing that exposure of cultured macrophages to high levels of acetyl-LDL could only partially block high-affinity uptake and degradation of oxidized LDL [56].

Even when different lipoprotein particles bind to the same receptors on macrophages, subsequent intracellular processing of the particles may be different. Both LDL and β-VLDL are taken up largely by the LDL receptor on murine macrophages, but these two classes of lipoprotein particles are targeted to separate intracellular organelles and are degraded at markedly different rates [57]. Thus, consistent with its role as a scavenger and phagocytic cell, the macrophage is likely to possess multiple pathways for ingestion and processing of modified and potentially atherogenic lipoprotein particles.

In addition to HDL receptors that function to remove excess cholesterol from cells, it has also been postulated that cells of certain tissues have receptors that promote internalization of intact HDL particles or selective uptake of HDL lipids. HDL interacts with specialized regions of the surface of steroidogenic cells that form "microvillar channels" [58], and this interaction may be mediated by a receptor that promotes uptake of HDL sterols for utilization as substrate for steroid hormone synthesis. Selective transport of HDL cholesteryl esters into cells has been demonstrated both *in vitro* and *in vivo* [59]. Although most of the evidence suggests that this process occurs independent of receptor binding, the possibility exists that receptors play at least a partial role in facilitating cellular uptake of HDL cholesteryl esters. Whether or not hepatic receptors mediate clearance from the plasma of HDL lipids and apolipoproteins has not been established. In general, very little is known about the mechanisms by which HDL is cleared from the blood, but receptor pathways are likely to be involved.

References

1 Kaplan J. Polypeptide-binding membrane receptors: analysis and classification. *Science* 1981;212:14–20.
2 Brown MS, Goldstein JL. A receptor-mediated pathway for cholesterol homeostasis. *Science* 1986;232:34–47.
3 Mahley RW, Innerarity TL, Weisgraber KH *et al*. Cellular and molecular biology of lipoprotein metabolism: characterization of lipoprotein-ligand interactions. In *Cold Spring Harbor Symposia on Quantitative Biology*, Vol. LI. Cold Spring Harbor, NY: Cold Spring Harbor Laboratory, 1986.
4 Wilson C, Wardell MR, Weisgraber KH, Mahley RW, Agard DA. Three-dimensional

structure of the LDL receptor-binding domain of human apolipoprotein E. *Science* 1991;252:1817–22.

5 Mahley RW, Weisgraber KH, Innerarity TL, Rall SC. Genetic defects in lipoprotein metabolism. Elevation of atherogenic lipoproteins caused by impaired catabolism. *JAMA* 1991;265:78–83.

6 Kandutsch AA, Chen HW, Heiniger HJ. Biological activity of some oxygenated sterols. *Science* 1978;201:498–501.

7 Goldstein JL, Brown MS. Regulation of the mevalonate pathway. *Nature* 1990;343: 425–30.

8 Rajavashisth TB, Taylor AU, Andalibi A, Svenson RL, Lusis AJ. Identification of a zinc finger protein that binds to the sterol regulatory element. *Science* 1989;245:640–3.

9 Dawson PA, Ridgway ND, Slaughter CA. Brown MS, Goldstein JL. cDNA cloning and expression of oxysterol binding protein; an oligomer with a potential leucine zipper. *J Biol Chem* 1989;264:16798–803.

10 Hobbs HH, Russell DW, Brown MS, Goldstein JL. The LDL receptor locus in familial hypercholesterolemia: mutational analysis of a membrane protein. *Annu Rev Genet* 1990;24:133–70.

11 Brown MS, Goldstein JL. Lipoprotein receptors: therapeutic implications. *J Hypertens* 1990;8(Suppl):533–6.

12 Herz J, Hamann U, Rogne S *et al.* Surface location and high affinity for calcium of a 500-kd liver membrane protein closely related to the LDL-receptor suggest a physiological role as lipoprotein receptor. *EMBO J* 1988;7:4119–27.

13 Kristensen T, Moestrup SK, Gliemann J *et al.* Evidence that the newly cloned low-density lipoprotein receptor related protein (LRP) is the α_2-macroglobulin receptor. *FEBS Lett* 1990;276:151–5.

14 Kowal RC, Herz J, Weisgrabe KM *et al.* Opposing effects of apolipoproteins E and C on lipoprotein binding to low density lipoprotein receptor-related protein. *J Biol Chem* 1990;265:10771–9.

15 Beisiegel U, Weber W, Ihrke G, Herz J, Stanley KK. The LDL-receptor-related protein, LRP, is an apolipoprotein E-binding protein. *Nature* 1989;341:162–4.

16 Kowal RC, Herz J, Goldstein JL, Esser V, Brown MS. Low density lipoprotein receptor-related protein mediates uptake of cholesteryl esters derived from apoprotein E-rich lipoproteins. *Proc Natl Acad Sci USA* 1989;86:5810–14.

17 Weisgraber KH, Mahley RW, Kowal RC *et al.* Apolipoprotein C-I modulates the interaction of apolipoprotein E with β-migrating very low density lipoprotein (β-VLDL) and inhibits binding of β-VLDL to low density lipoprotein receptor-related protein. *J Biol Chem* 1990;265:22453–9.

18 Windler E, Havel RJ. Inhibitory effects of C apolipoproteins from rats and humans on the uptake of triglyceride-rich lipoproteins and their remnants by the perfused rat liver. *J Lipid Res* 1985;26:556–65.

19 Beisiegel U, Weber W, Bengtsson-Olivecrona G. Lipoprotein lipase enhances the binding of chylomicrons to low density lipoprotein receptor-related protein. *Proc Natl Acad Sci USA* 1991;88:8342–6.

20 Hussain MM, Maxfield FR, Mas-Oliva J *et al.* Clearance of chylomicron remnants by the low density lipoprotein receptor-related protein/α_2-macroglobulin receptor. *J Biol Chem* 1991;266:13936–40.

21 Herz J, Kowal RC, Goldstein JL, Brown MS. Proteolytic processing of the 600 kd low density lipoprotein receptor-related protein (LRP) occurs in a *trans*-Golgi compartment. *EMBO J* 1990;9:1769–76.

22 Lund H, Takahashi K, Hamilton RL, Havel RJ. Lipoprotein binding and endosome itinerary of the low density lipoprotein receptor-related protein in rat liver. *Proc Natl Acad Sci USA* 1989;86:9318–22.

23 Kutt H, Herz J, Stanley K. Structure of the low-density lipoprotein receptor-related protein (LRP) promoter. *Biochim Biophys Acta* 1989;1009:229–36.

24 Brown MS, Goldstein JL. Lipoprotein metabolism in the macrophage: implications for cholesterol deposition in atherosclerosis. *Annu Rev Biochem* 1983;52:223–61.

25 Kurihara Y, Matsumoto A, Itakura H, Kodama T. Macrophage scavenger receptors. *Curr Opin Lipidol* 1991;2:295–300.

26 Stein O, Stein Y. Bovine endothelial cells display macrophage-like properties towards acetylated ^{125}I-labelled low density lipoprotein. *Biochim Biophys Acta* 1980;620:631–5.

27 Pitas RE. Expression of the acetyl low density lipoprotein receptor by rabbit fibroblast and smooth muscle cells. Up-regulation by phorbol esters. *J Biol Chem* 1990;265: 12722–7.

28 Goldstein JL, Ho YK, Basu Sk, Brown MS. Binding site on macrophages that mediate uptake and degradation of acetylated low density lipoprotein, producing massive cholesterol deposition. *Proc Natl Acad Sci USA* 1979;76:333–7.

29 Steinberg D, Parthasarathy SP, Carew TE, Khoo JC, Witzum JL. Modifications of LDL that increase its atherogenicity. *N Engl J Med* 1989;320:916–24.

30 Steinbrecher UP, Parthasarathy S, Leake DS, Witztum JL, Steinberg D. Modification of low density lipoprotein by endothelial cells involves lipid peroxidation and degradation of low density lipoprotein phospholipids. *Proc Natl Acad Sci USA* 1984;81:3883–7.

31 Heinecke JW, Baker L, Rosen H, Chait A. Superoxide-mediated free radical modification of low density lipoprotein by arterial smooth muscle cells. *J Clin Invest* 1986;77: 757–61.

32 Via DP, Dresel HA, Cheng SL, Gotto AM. Murine macrophage tumors are a source of a 260 000-dalton acetyl-low density lipoprotein receptor. *J Biol Chem* 1985;260: 7379–86.

33 Kodama T, Freeman M, Rohrer L *et al.* Type I macrophage scavenger receptor contains α-helical and collagen-like coiled coils. *Nature* 1990;343:531–5.

34 Rohrer L, Freeman M, Kodama T, Penman M, Krieger M. Coiled-coil fibrous domains mediate ligand binding by macrophage scavenger receptor II. *Nature* 1990;343:570–2.

35 Freeman M, Ashkenas J, Rees DJG *et al.* An ancient, highly conserved family of cysteine-rich protein domains revealed by cloning type I and type II murine macrophage scavenger receptors. *Proc Natl Acad Sci USA* 1990;87:8810–14.

36 Freeman M, Ekkel Y, Rohrer L *et al.* Expression of type I and type II bovine scavenger receptors in Chinese hamster ovary cells: lipid droplet accumulation and nonreciprocal cross competition by acetylated and oxidized low density lipoprotein. *Proc Natl Acad Sci USA* 1991;88:4931–5.

37 Matsumoto A, Naito M, Itakura H *et al.* Human scavenger receptors: primary structure, expression, and localization in atherosclerotic lesions. *Proc Natl Acad Sci USA* 1990;87: 9133–7.

38 Yla-Herttuala S, Rosenfeld ME, Parthasarathy S *et al.* Gene expression in macrophage-rich human atherosclerotic lesions. *J Clin Invest* 1990;87:1146–52.

39 Ishibashi S, Inaba T, Shimano H *et al.* Monocyte colony-stimulating factor enhances uptake and degradation of acetylated low density lipoproteins and cholesterol esterification in human monocyte-derived macrophages. *J Biol Chem* 1990;265:14109–17.

40 Eisenberg S. High density lipoprotein metabolism. *J Lipid Res* 1984;25:1017–58.

41 Oram JF, Brinton EA, Bierman EL. Regulation of HDL receptor activity in cultured human skin fibroblasts and human arterial smooth muscle cells. *J Clin Invest* 1983;72: 1611–21.

42 Brinton EA, Kenagy R, Oram JF, Bierman EL. Regulation of high density lipoprotein binding activity of aortic endothelial cells by treatment with acetylated low density lipoprotein. *Arteriosclerosis* 1985;5:329–35.

43 Schmitz G, Niemann R, Brennhausen B, Krause R, Assman G. Regulation of high density lipoprotein receptors in cultured macrophages: role of acyl CoA:cholesterol acyltransferase. *EMBO J* 1985;4:2773–9.

44 Oppenheimer MJ, Oram JF, Bierman EL. Up-regulation of high density lipoprotein receptor activity by gamma-interferon associated with inhibition of cell proliferation.

J Biol Chem 1988;263:19318−23.

45 Graham DL, Oram JF. Identification and characterization of a high density lipoprotein-binding protein in cell membrane by ligand blotting. *J Biol Chem* 1987;262:7439−42.

46 Slotte JP, Oram JF, Bierman EL. Binding of high density lipoprotein to cell receptors promotes translocation of cholesterol from intracellular membranes to the cell surface. *J Biol Chem* 1987;262:12904−7.

47 Oram JF, Mendez AJ, Slotte JP, Johnson TF. High density lipoprotein apolipoproteins mediate removal of sterol from intracellular pools but not from plasma membranes of cholesterol-loaded fibroblasts. *Arterioscler Thromb* 1991;11:403−14.

48 Mendez AJ, Oram JF, Bierman EL. Protein kinase C as a mediator of high density lipoprotein receptor-dependent efflux of intracellular cholesterol. *J Biol Chem* 1991; 266:10104−11.

49 Fidge NH, Nestel PJ. Identification of apolipoproteins involved in the interaction of human high density lipoproteins with receptors on cultured cells. *J Biol Chem* 1985; 260:3570−5.

50 Brinton EA, Oram JF, Chen C-H, Albers JJ, Bierman EL. Binding of high density lipoprotein to cultured fibroblasts after chemical alteration of apoprotein amino acid residues. *J Biol Chem* 1986;261:495−503.

51 Duell PB, Oram JF, Bierman EL. Nonenzymatic glycosylation of HDL resulting in inhibition of high-affinity binding to cultured human fibroblasts. *Diabetes* 1990;39: 1257−63.

52 Chacko GK, Mahlberg FH, Johnson WJ. Cross-linking of apoproteins in high density lipoprotein by dimethysuberimidate inhibits specific lipoprotein binding to membranes. *J Lipid Res* 1988;29:319−24.

53 Leblond L, Marcel YL. The amphipathic alpha-helical repeats of apolipoprotein A-I are responsible for binding of high density lipoproteins to HepG2 cells. *J Biol Chem* 1991; 266:6058−67.

54 McGookey DJ, Anderson RGW. Morphological characterization of the cholesteryl ester cycle in cultured mouse macrophage cells. *J Cell Biol* 1983;97:1156−68.

55 Gianturco SH, Lin AH-Y, Hwang S-LC *et al*. Distinct murine macrophage receptor pathway for human triglyceride-rich lipoproteins. *J Clin Invest* 1988;82:1633−43.

56 Sparrow CP, Parthasarathy S, Steinberg D. A macrophage receptor that recognizes oxidized low density lipoprotein but not acetylated low density lipoprotein. *J Biol Chem* 1989;264:2599−604.

57 Tabas I, Lim S, Xu X-X, Maxfield IR. Endocytosed β-VLDL and LDL are delivered to different intracellular vesicles in mouse peritoneal macrophages. *J Cell Biol* 1990;111: 929−40.

58 Reaven E, Shi X-Y, Azhar S. Interaction of lipoproteins with isolated ovary plasma membranes. *J Biol Chem* 1990;265:19100−11.

59 Rinninger F, Pittman RC. Regulation of the selective uptake of high density lipoprotein-associated cholesteryl esters. *J Lipid Res* 1987;28:1313−25.

Section III
Quantification of Lipoproteins

Chapter 11
Lipoprotein Classes and Subclasses

DAVID W. GARBER

Introduction

Plasma lipoproteins are heterogeneous in size, composition, and metabolism. As our knowledge of the role of lipid-containing plasma particles in disease processes has expanded, our need to better understand the role of individual lipoprotein classes in that disease process has also grown. Indeed, separation and quantification of lipoprotein classes and subclasses has played a critical role in the development of that understanding.

The clinician and the researcher often have very different needs for separation and quantification of lipoprotein classes and subclasses. High resolution of multiple subclasses requires techniques which are neither appropriate nor necessary for clinical work, but are essential to the researcher. Obviously, both clinicians and researchers require accuracy and reproducibility, but the clinical laboratory requires procedures which are simple, fast, relatively low in cost, and can be done in volume. Lengthy techniques, such as sequential-density ultracentrifugation, are inappropriate for most clinical use. Thus, precipitation and ultracentrifugation techniques (and combinations of the two), such as the Vertical Auto Profile (VAP) and Beta-Quantification procedures (discussed below), are currently most appropriate to the clinician, especially since some resolution of lipoprotein subclasses can be made.

Although this chapter will primarily consider separation techniques in the analysis of lipoprotein classes and subclasses, methods of quantification are equally important. Lipoprotein levels can be measured in many ways, including protein content, cholesterol content, triglyceride content, total mass, etc. When comparing methods of analysis, or selecting a method, it is essential to consider the accuracy, sensitivity, reproducibility, and applicability of the analysis method to the needs of the investigator. Quality control and use of appropriate standards are as important in the quantification of plasma lipoproteins as in any other laboratory procedure.

Early studies separated lipoprotein classes by electrophoretic mobility on agarose gel electrophoresis. In this technique, plasma proteins were separated electrophoretically and then stained for the presence of lipids. Several lipid-containing bands were uniformly recognized, and were designated as having α-mobility, β-mobility, or pre-β-mobility. In some cases, especially following a fatty meal, a nonmigrating lipid-containing band was evident as well. Although this method allowed for definition of several distinct types of hyperlipidemia, it provided little information regarding the structure or metabolism of the migrating material. As such, this method provided qualitative, rather than quantitative, information. However, the nomenclature resulting from this method has persisted in such terms as hyperalphalipoproteinemia or dysbetalipoproteinemia.

Separation of lipoprotein classes by density was made possible using ultracentrifugation techniques, as first described by Gofman et al. [1] and Havel et al. [2]. This procedure led to a nomenclature based on the

Table 11.1 Summary of methods for separation of lipoprotein classes and subclasses

Centrifugation
Sequential-density ultracentrifugation
  Use: research
  Applications: lipoprotein classes, subclasses
Density-gradient ultracentrifugation
  Uses: clinical and research
  Applications: lipoprotein classes, subclasses

Chromatography
Size-exclusion
  Use: research
  Applications: lipoprotein classes, subclasses
Immunoaffinity
  Use: research
  Applications: lipoprotein subclasses
Heparin-affinity
  Use: research
  Applications: lipoprotein subclasses

Nondenaturing gradient gel electrophoresis
  Use: research
  Applications: lipoprotein classes, subclasses

Precipitation methods
  Uses: clinical and research
  Applications: removal of apo B-containing lipoproteins, determination of HDL subclasses

Nuclear magnetic resonance
  Use: research
  Applications: lipoprotein classes

Combination methods
  Uses: clinical and research
  Applications: lipoprotein classes, subclasses

relative density of the lipoproteins. Thus, pre-β-migrating lipid-containing material corresponds to very low-density lipoprotein (VLDL), β-migrating lipid-containing material corresponds to low-density lipoprotein (LDL), and α-migrating lipid-containing material corresponds to high-density lipoprotein (HDL). Chylomicrons are turbid particles in the plasma which float to the surface without centrifugation, and correspond to material which remained at the origin in agarose gel electrophoresis. Additional minor lipoprotein classes have also been identified, including intermediate-density lipoprotein (IDL) and lipoprotein(a), or Lp(a). The individual lipoprotein classes are also heterogeneous, and can be further subdivided into subclasses. The role of these lipoprotein classes and subclasses in coronary artery disease is considered in detail elsewhere in this volume.

The ability to differentiate classes and subclasses of lipoproteins has led to a major increase in our knowledge regarding lipoprotein structure and function. The basic tools of centrifugation and electrophoresis have been modified and extended to include chromatography, immunologic, and other techniques. A summary of the techniques which will be discussed is presented in Table 11.1.

Separation and quantification of the major lipoprotein classes

Centrifugation

SEQUENTIAL-DENSITY ULTRACENTRIFUGATION

The most direct method of separating major lipoprotein species is sequential-density ultracentrifugation [3]. Lipoproteins are separated by flotation using ultracentrifugation. The density of the remaining infranatant is increased by the addition of salt, and lipoproteins are again isolated by ultracentrifugal flotation. The process is repeated for each lipoprotein density range desired; the generally accepted lipoprotein density ranges are shown in Table 11.2.

This procedure has the advantage of technical simplicity and reproducibility, but has the major disadvantage of extended time of preparation (4 or more days for a complete separation). It is generally used for preparation of isolated lipoprotein species for use in research or compositional analysis, but is not commonly employed for clinical purposes. However, it provides for direct quantification of lipoproteins by measurement of the cholesterol, triglyceride, or protein content of each isolated lipoprotein fraction.

Table 11.2 Lipoprotein density ranges

Lipoprotein	Density range (g/ml)
VLDL	<1.006
IDL	1.006−1.019
LDL	1.019−1.063
HDL	1.063−1.210

DENSITY-GRADIENT ULTRACENTRIFUGATION

Lipoprotein classes can be separated in a single-step ultracentrifugation using discontinuous-density salt gradients [4]. Although separation of individual lipoproteins may not be as complete as with the sequential-flotation method described above, this procedure has the advantage of speed, in that lipoproteins are separated in a single ultracentrifugation.

Typically, a two- or three-step density gradient is produced in an ultracentrifuge tube by adjusting the sample to a relatively high density with KBr and overlaying with a lower-density salt solution. The method can be optimized for preparative isolation of lipoproteins using larger-sized centrifuge tubes and three-step gradients in fixed-angle rotors, or for rapid analysis of lipoprotein content using a two-step gradient and smaller centrifuge tubes in vertical rotors. The density gradient and ultracentrifugation conditions can be modified to optimize separations of specific lipoproteins, or to separate lipoprotein subclasses as described below.

The VAP procedure combines density-gradient vertical ultracentrifugation with computer acquisition and analysis of cholesterol content across the lipoprotein density profile [5]. In this method, lipoproteins are separated in a two-step density gradient in a vertical rotor, and the centrifuge tubes are placed in a fractionator. The tube is emptied from the bottom, and the sample is continuously mixed with an enzymatic cholesterol reagent in a Technicon Autoanalyzer. Output from the Autoanalyzer is digitized to produce a lipoprotein cholesterol profile, which is decomposed into individual lipoprotein species, giving direct measurement of all lipoprotein classes in a one-step process. The VAP method is currently the only clinical procedure which provides direct measurement of LDL, IDL, and Lp(a) cholesterol.

Size-exclusion column chromatography

Lipoproteins differ in both density and size. Although a rough correlation exists between these two parameters, several particles, most notably Lp(a), do not follow this relationship. Lipoproteins can be separated on the basis of size using size-exclusion (or molecular-sieve) column chromatography [6]. This procedure is generally not used in the clinical setting, since separation and analysis are slow relative to other procedures. Use of fast-protein liquid chromatography (FPLC) or high performance liquid chromatography (HPLC) has improved the analysis time considerably, but clinical use of size-exclusion column chromatography remains relatively minor.

Like ultracentrifugation, this technique can be used to isolate lipoproteins for experimental or analytical purposes. Samples separated using this technique can be analyzed for lipid and protein content using methods similar to those employed for sequential-density or density-gradient ultracentrifugation.

Nondenaturing gradient gel electrophoresis

Like size-exclusion column chromatography, nondenaturing gradient polyacrylamide-gel electrophoresis separates lipoproteins on the basis of size [7]. This method has the advantage of reduced sample volume and faster analysis time compared with column chromatography, but the reduced sample volume largely precludes preparative isolation of lipoproteins. This method is not commonly used clinically for lipoprotein quantification, but can be useful for the determination of Lp(a) levels. Lipoproteins are generally visualized in the electrophoretic gel using protein stains such as Coomassie Blue, but lipid stains such as Oil Red O can also be employed. This method is most useful as a qualitative assessment of the presence and size of lipoprotein species, rather than as a measurement of the levels of lipoproteins in the sample.

Precipitation methods

Lipoproteins, especially those containing apolipoprotein B (apo B), can be selectively precipitated from solution by adding combinations of polyanions and divalent cations, such as heparin–$MnCl_2$ [8], dextran sulfate–$MgCl_2$ [9], or other precipitating agents. After precipitation, HDL remains in the supernatant and can be measured directly. HDL cholesterol levels reported by most clinical laboratories are derived from such precipitation methods.

The major advantage of this method is its relative technical simplicity, as demonstrated by its widespread use in clinical laboratories. However, precipitation methods have a number of significant problems which can lead to somewhat inaccurate results. Ideally, all of the apo

B-containing lipoprotein and none of the nonapo B-containing lipo-protein should precipitate. However, this is often not the case, with varying amounts of apo B-containing lipoprotein remaining in the supernatant and nonapo B-containing lipoprotein precipitating. Thus, the measurement of the nonprecipitation material as HDL cholesterol depends on either perfect precipitation, or offsetting errors in precipi-tation. Although this method has proven to be useful in the clinical laboratory, separation of HDL by sequential-density or density-gradient ultracentrifugation provides a more reliable method of measurement of HDL cholesterol.

Combination methods

A number of procedures have been developed for rapid clinical quan-tification of lipoproteins using a combination of methods previously described. For instance, the Beta-Quantification method [10] employed by the Lipid Research Clinics Program involves both precipitation and ultracentrifugation. Briefly, VLDL is removed from whole plasma by ultracentrifugation, and LDL is precipitated from the infranatant by dextran sulfate-magnesium. Whole plasma, VLDL ultracentrifugation infranatant, and LDL precipitation supernatant are measured for cho-lesterol concentration. VLDL cholesterol is determined by both direct measurement and the difference between the VLDL infranatant and whole plasma; HDL is determined by direct measurement of the LDL precipitation supernatant; and LDL is determined by the difference between the VLDL infranatant value and the HDL supernatant value.

Besides complexity alone, there are a number of disadvantages to this approach. The use of the precipitation method to determine HDL cholesterol is subject to the inaccuracies described above. LDL values are not measured directly, but are determined by the difference between VLDL infranatant and HDL supernatant. Therefore, the reported LDL value includes other lipoprotein species, such as IDL and Lp(a). How-ever, this procedure does provide reproducible values, and is widely used in the clinical analysis of cholesterol in lipoproteins.

Nuclear magnetic resonance

Water-suppressed proton nuclear magnetic resonance (NMR) of plasma samples produces signals based on resonance peaks corresponding to methyl and methylene groups in lipids of lipoproteins [11–14]. For reasons not currently understood, each major lipoprotein class has methyl and methylene proton resonances at slightly different positions. Thus, the envelope of lipoprotein NMR resonances can be decomposed to give quantitative information about lipoprotein levels in each major class. Although this procedure has potential clinical application, the novelty and relative unavailability of the method places it out of the reach of most clinical practitioners. The ability of this method to reliably resolve lipoprotein species and subclasses has not yet been demonstrated.

Separation and quantification of lipoprotein subclasses

With further refinement of analytical techniques, it has become obvious that the major lipoprotein classes are themselves heterogeneous, with each lipoprotein having several to numerous subclasses. These subclasses vary in their composition, metabolism, and influence on atherogenesis.

Measurements of lipoprotein subclasses have generally been of more use in research applications, rather than clinical ones. However, with further understanding of the role of various subclasses in the development or prevention of atherosclerosis, these measurements will become increasingly important to the practicing physician. For instance, the relationship of LDL subclasses with risk of atherosclerosis [15] may become an important predictive tool.

High-density lipoprotein

HDL levels are inversely correlated with atherosclerotic disease [16–21], suggesting that HDL has a protective effect against atherogenesis. However, all HDL subclasses do not appear to be equally protective, with the less dense subclass, HDL_2, having the greatest protective effect [22–27]. Thus, measurement of HDL subclasses may be important in assessing risk of atherosclerotic disease.

ULTRACENTRIFUGATION

HDL was first shown to be heterogeneous by density-gradient analytical ultracentrifugation [28,29], with three components: HDL_1 (in humans, a minor component with density overlapping with LDL) [30], HDL_2 (d 1.063–1.125 g/ml) [31], and HDL_3 (d 1.125–1.21 g/ml) [31]. Zonal ultracentrifugation provides somewhat greater resolution of these subclasses [32,33].

NONDENATURING GRADIENT GEL ELECTROPHORESIS

While ultracentrifugation methods for determination of HDL subclasses depend primarily on differences in density, subclasses can be separated on the basis of size and shape using nondenaturing gradient gel electrophoresis (GGE). This technique resolves a larger number of subclasses. For instance, Nicols *et al.* [34,35] describe five subclasses designated (from largest to smallest) HDL_{2b}, HDL_{2a}, HDL_{3a}, HDL_{3b}, and HDL_{3c}. Cheung *et al.* [25] describe nine subclasses, designated (from smallest to largest) HDL(1) through HDL(9). Using the latter nomenclature, HDL_2 contains primarily subclasses (7) and (6) with some (5) and (4), and HDL_3 contains primarily subclasses (3) through (5) with some (6).

SIZE-EXCLUSION COLUMN CHROMATOGRAPHY

Size-exclusion column chromatography, like nondenaturing polyacrylamide gradient gel electrophoresis, separates subclasses on the basis of size and shape. The most commonly reported techniques use low pressure agarose columns, or TSK HPLC columns, especially the G3000SW and G4000SW columns alone or in combination [36]. However, resolution of HDL subclasses is not markedly better than that obtained using density-gradient ultracentrifugation.

IMMUNOAFFINITY CHROMATOGRAPHY

Separation of HDL subclasses on the basis of apolipoprotein composition can be done using immunoaffinity chromatography or heparin-affinity chromatography (described below). For immunoaffinity chromatography [37], antibodies specific to either apo A-I or A-II are isolated by HDL affinity chromatography, and conjugated to CNBr-activated Sepharose 4B. Since all apo A-containing lipoproteins have apo A-I present [37], whole plasma can be used in this separation. The antiapo A-I immunosorbent is packed in a glass chromatography column, and fresh plasma is applied, washed, then eluted. The samples can be rechromatographed with antiapo A-II immunosorbent, with the nonbinding material containing only apo A-I and the bound material containing both apo A-I and apo A-II. The resulting classes can be analyzed for composition, or by nondenaturing polyacrylamide gradient gel electrophoresis for size distribution [25].

Although this technique has provided considerable information about HDL subclass structure and composition, it has not been used to directly investigate the role of HDL in protection against atherosclerosis.

HEPARIN-AFFINITY CHROMATOGRAPHY

Heparin-affinity chromatography is similar to immunoaffinity chromatography in that subclasses are separated on the basis of their apolipoprotein composition. HDL samples are passed over a heparin–agarose column, and particles containing apo E bind to the column, while those with no apo E pass through. Apo E-containing subclasses can then be eluted with solutions of increasing salt concentration, to purify several HDL subclasses. This technique has been used to characterize multiple subclasses of rat HDL [38–40], but is not generally used to study human samples.

PRECIPITATION

As previously discussed, total HDL levels can be measured by first precipitating apo B-containing lipoproteins from plasma using polyanions and divalent cations. Precipitation methods can also be used to separate HDL_2 and HDL_3 [41–44]. In general, the apo B-containing lipoproteins are first precipitated using a standard method, and the cholesterol concentration of the HDL-containing supernatant is determined. The HDL_2 subclass is then precipitated by adding a higher concentration of the polyanion–divalent cation solution, and the cholesterol content of the remaining HDL_3 is measured, with the HDL_2 concentration presumed to be the difference of the two values.

Although these procedures separate the HDL subclasses on a basis other than density, the techniques gives results in good agreement with those derived by ultracentrifugation [44]. Precipitation has the advantage of speed and high sample capacity, but shares the disadvantage of total HDL precipitation in that separation of the subclasses may be incomplete, or that small changes in reagent concentration may alter the results.

COMBINATION METHODS

The above techniques can be combined to analyze HDL subclasses. For instance, Cheung et al. [25] used immunoaffinity chromatography, nondenaturing gradient gel electrophoresis, and gradient ultracentrifugation to investigate HDL subclass size, distribution, and composition.

Apo B-containing lipoproteins (VLDL, IDL, and LDL)

The apo B-containing lipoproteins, VLDL, IDL, and LDL, are also each structurally and metabolically heterogeneous. The simple concept that VLDL is secreted by the liver and processed by interaction with lipoprotein lipase and other enzymes to IDL, which is further processed to LDL, has proved to be very incomplete, with multiple pathways and particle interactions [45]. These lipoproteins have been separated into subclasses by various techniques, as described below.

VLDL has been fractionated into four subclasses by sequential ultra-centrifugation [29,46], on the basis of the following decreasing S_f (flotation constant in Svedberg units) values: >400, 175−400, 100−175, and 20−100. These subclasses differ in their apolipoprotein and lipid composition, and in their affinity to receptors. Other flotation cuts have been made; for instance, S_f 100−400, 60−100, and 20−60 [47]. These subclasses are somewhat arbitrary, as no VLDL subclasses can be directly visualized by ultracentrifugation. They do, however, provide a useful tool for studying particle structure and affinity to receptors through the VLDL catabolic cascade.

IDL subclasses cannot be completely separated by ultracentrifugation methods [48]; nondenaturing polyacrylamide gradient gel electro-phoresis has been the primary tool for separation, as noted below.

LDL can be separated by ultracentrifugation into up to six subclasses by using a shallow density gradient [48−51]. The subclasses can be quantified by Schlieren optics in the analytical ultracentrifuge, or can be fractionated and analyzed for cholesterol or protein content. This procedure shares the disadvantage of other ultracentrifugation pro-cedures in that the number of samples is limited by rotor capacity, and separation time can be quite lengthy in standard rotors. However, isolation of lipoprotein subclasses by nondenaturing polyacrylamide gradient gel electrophoresis generally requires a preliminary ultracen-trifugation step to separate the major lipoprotein classes.

Nondenaturing 2−16% polyacrylamide gradient gel electrophoresis separates VLDL and IDL into two main peaks each [52], and LDL into four subclasses, LDL-I through IV [48,53]. However, the LDL subclasses can be roughly grouped into two phenotypes, characterized by either a predominance of larger, more buoyant particles, or smaller, denser particles [54]. This technique does not provide complete separation of the subclasses, but is rapid and reproducible. It does, however, require that the lipoproteins be first isolated by ultracentrifugation.

Analysis of apo B-containing lipoprotein subclasses by nondena-turing polyacrylamide gradient gel electrophoresis has provided con-siderable information about the metabolic pathways of the VLDL−IDL−LDL catabolic cascade, and has led to the observation that the smaller, more dense LDL subclass is significantly associated with an increased risk of myocardial infarction [55]. The two major subclasses of LDL appear to be produced from different precursor VLDL and IDL particles [48], and the pattern of LDL subclasses appears to be inherited [54].

IMMUNOAFFINITY CHROMATOGRAPHY

Triglyceride-rich lipoproteins are secreted by both the liver and the intestine. Except for chylomicrons, which are intestinally synthesized and can be removed from other lipoproteins by ultracentrifugation, hepatically and intestinally derived particles cannot be separated by normal procedures. This is not usually necessary, since chylomicron remnants containing apo B_{48} are normally cleared from the plasma very rapidly and therefore no particles containing apo B_{48} are generally found in VLDL, IDL, or LDL. In certain disease states, such as Type III hyperlipoproteinemia, normal clearance of chylomicron and VLDL remnants is deficient, resulting in an accumulation of both hepatically and intestinally derived particles. These particles can be separated by immunoaffinity chromatography, as lipoproteins produced by the liver contain primarily apo B_{100}, while those produced by the intestine contain primarily apo B_{48}. Monoclonal antibodies can be produced which are specific to regions of apo B_{100} which are not part of B_{48} [56]. Immunosorbent columns prepared using these monoclonal antibodies can be used to separate the particles containing apo B_{48} from those with apo B_{100} for studies of particle size and composition.

Conclusions

It should be obvious from the previous discussion that there may be as many ways to separate and quantify lipoprotein classes and subclasses as there are laboratories studying lipoproteins. The proliferation of techniques has been very useful in expanding our knowledge of lipoprotein structure and function, but has provided some confusion in the clinical situation. It has become difficult for the clinician to know how much information is necessary about lipoprotein classes and subclasses, and how reliable the measurement procedures are. Currently available clinical procedures such as the VAP procedure and Beta-Quantification are providing reliable information on cholesterol distribution in lipoprotein classes and subclasses which can be of great use to the clinician. As we fully grasp the involvement of lipoprotein subclasses in the development of atherosclerotic disease, other analytical procedures from the research laboratory should begin to enter the clinical arena as well.

References

1 Gofman JW, Lindgren FT, Elliott H. Ultracentrifugal studies of lipoproteins of human serum. *J Biol Chem* 1949;179:973–9.

2 Havel RJ, Eder HA, Bragon JH. The distribution and chemical composition of ultracentrifugally separated lipoproteins in human serum. *J Clin Invest* 1955;34:1345–53.

3 Schumaker VN, Puppione DL. Sequential flotation ultracentrifugation. *Methods Enzymol* 1986;128:155–70.

4 Chung BH, Segrest JP, Ray MJ et al. Single vertical spin density gradient ultracentrifugation. *Methods Enzymol* 1986;128:181–209.

5 Cone, JT, Segrest JP, Chung BH et al. Computerized rapid high resolution quantitative analysis of plasma lipoprotein based upon single vertical spin ultracentrifugation. *J Lipid Res* 1982;23:923–935.

6 Rudel LL, Marzetta CA, Johnson FL. Separation and analysis of lipoproteins by gel filtration. *Methods Enzymol* 1986;129:45–57.

7 Nichols AV, Krauss RM, Musliner TA. Nondenaturing polyacrylamide gradient gel electrophoresis. *Methods Enzymol* 1986;128:417–31.

8 Burstein M, Samaille J. Sur un dosage rapide du cholesterol lié aux α- et aux β-lipoprotéines du serum. *Clin Chim Acta* 1960;5:609.

9 Warnick GR, Benderson J, Albers JJ. Dextran sulfate-Mg^{2+} precipitation procedure for quantitation of high density lipoprotein cholesterol. *Clin Chem* 1982;28:1279–88.

10 Hainline A, Karon J, Lipple K. (eds) *Manual of Laboratory Operations, Lipid Research Clinics Program, Lipid and Lipoprotein Analysis*, 2nd edn. Bethesda: Public Health Service, National Institutes of Health, 1983.

11 Bell JD, Sadler PJ, Macleod A, Turner P, LaVille A. H-1 NMR studies of human blood plasma: assignment of resonances for lipoproteins. *FEBS Lett* 1987;219:239–43.

12 Hamilton JA, Morrisett JD. Nuclear magnetic resonance studies of lipoproteins. *Methods Enzymol* 1986;128:472–515.

13 Otvos JD, Jeyarajah EJ, Hayes LW et al. Relationships between the proton nuclear magnetic resonance properties of plasma lipoproteins and cancer. *Clin Chem* 1991;37:369–76.

14 Otvos JD, Jeyarajah EJ, Bennet DW. Quantification of plasma lipoproteins by proton nuclear magnetic resonance spectroscopy. *Clin Chem* 1991;37:377–86.

15 Krauss RM. Relationship of intermediate and low-density lipoprotein subspecies to risk of coronary artery disease. *Am Heart J* 1987;113:578–82.

16 Gordon DJ, Probstfield JL, Garrison RJ et al. High-density lipoprotein cholesterol and cardiovascular disease. *Circulation* 1989;79:8–15.

17 Wilson PWF, Abbott RD, Castelli WP. High density lipoprotein cholesterol and mortality: The Framingham Heart Study. *Arteriosclerosis* 1988;8:737–41.

18 Abbott RD, Wilson PWF, Kannel WB, Castelli WP. High density lipoprotein cholesterol, cholesterol screening, and myocardial infarction: The Framingham Study. *Arteriosclerosis* 1988;8:207–11.

19 Schaefer EJ, Moussa PB, Wilson PWF et al. Plasma lipoproteins in healthy octogenarians: Lack of reduced high density lipoprotein cholesterol levels. *Metabolism* 1989;38:293–6.

20 Bodurtha J, Schieken R, Segrest JP, Nance WE. High-density lipoprotein cholesterol subfractions in adolescent twins. *Pediatrics* 1987;79:181–9.

21 Grundy SM, Goodman DW, Rifkind BM, Cleeman JL. The place of HDL in cholesterol management: A perspective from the National Cholesterol Education Program. *Arch Intern Med* 1989;149:505–10.

22 Gofman JW, Young W, Tandy R. Ischemic heart disease, atherosclerosis, and longevity. *Circulation* 1966;34:679–97.

23 Miller NE, Hammett F, Saltissi S et al. Relation of angiographically defined coronary artery disease to plasma lipoprotein subfractions and apolipoproteins. *Br Med J* 1981;282:1741–4.

24 Ballantyne FC, Clark RS, Clark HD, Simpson HS, Ballantyne D. High density and low density lipoprotein subfractions in survivors of myocardial infarction and in control subjects. *Metabolism* 1982;31:433—7.

25 Cheung MC, Segrest JP, Albers JJ *et al.* Characterization of high density lipoprotein subspecies: structural studies by single vertical spin ultracentrifugation and immunoaffinity chromatography. *J Lipid Res* 1987;28:913—29.

26 Segrest JP, Ray MJ. HDL subspecies: Structural basis and relationship to atherosclerosis. In *Proceedings of the (NIH) Workshop on Lipoprotein Heterogeneity.* (ed. K Lippel). Bethesda: Public Health Service, National Institutes of Health, 1987:351—61.

27 Manninken V, Elo MO, Frick MH *et al.* Lipid alterations and decline in the incidence of coronary heart disease in the Helsinki Heart Study. *JAMA* 1988;260:641—51.

28 Krauss RM, Lindgren FT, Ray RW. Interrelationships among subgroups of serum lipoproteins in normal human subjects. *Clin Chim Acta* 1980;104:275—90.

29 Lindgren FT, Jensen LC, Hatch FT. The isolation and quantitative analysis of serum lipoproteins. In *Blood Lipids and Lipoproteins: Quantitation, Composition, and Metabolism* (ed. GJ Nelson). New York: John Wiley-Interscience, 1972:181—274.

30 Schmitz G, Assmann G. Isolation of human serum HDL$_1$ by zonal ultracentrifugation. *J Lipid Res* 1982;23:903—10.

31 Patsch W, Schonfeld G, Gotto AM Jr, Patsch J. Characterization of human high density lipoproteins by zonal ultracentrifugation. *J Biol Chem* 1980;255:3178—85.

32 Patsch JR, Sailer S, Kostner G *et al.* Separation of the main lipoprotein density classes from human plasma by rate-zonal ultracentrifugation. *J Lipid Res* 1974;15:356—66.

33 Patsch JR, Patsch W. Zonal ultracentrifugation. *Methods Enzymol* 1986;129:3—26.

34 Blanche PH, Gong EL, Forte T, Nichols AV. Characterization of human high density lipoproteins by gradient gel electrophoresis. *Biochim Biophys Acta* 1981;665:408—19.

35 Nichols AV, Blanche PH, Gong EL. Gradient gel electrophoresis of human plasma high density lipoproteins. In *CRC Handbook of Electrophoresis*, Vol III (ed. LA Lewis). Boca Raton: CRC Press Inc., 1983:29—47.

36 Hara I, Okazaki M. High-performance liquid chromatography of serum lipoproteins. *Methods Enzymol* 1986;129:57—78.

37 Cheung MC. Characterization of apolipoprotein A containing lipoproteins. *Methods Enzymol* 1986;129:130—45.

38 Lee CC, Koo SI. Effect of copper deficiency on the composition of three high-density lipoprotein subclasses as separated by heparin-affinity chromatography. *Biochim Biophys Acta* 1988;963:278—87.

39 Lee CC, Koo SI. Separation of three compositionally distinct subclasses of rat high density lipoproteins by heparin-affinity chromatography. *Atherosclerosis* 1988;70:205—15.

40 Koo SI, Lee CC. Cholesterol and apolipoprotein distribution in plasma high-density-lipoprotein subclasses from zinc-deficient rats. *Am J Clin Nutr* 1989;50:73—9.

41 Whitaker CF, Srinivasan SR, Berenson GS. Simplified methods for measuring cholesterol concentrations of high-density lipoprotein subclasses in serum compared. *Clin Chem* 1986;32:1274—8.

42 Gidez LI, Miller GJ, Burstein M, Slagle S, Eder HA. Separation and quantitation of subclasses of human plasma high density lipoproteins by a simple precipitation procedure. *J Lipid Res* 1982;23:1206—23.

43 Bachorik PS, Albers JJ. Precipitation methods for quantification of lipoproteins. *Methods Enzymol* 1986;129:78—100.

44 Burstein M, Fine A, Atger V, Wirbel E, Girard-Globa A. Rapid method for the isolation of two purified subfractions of high density lipoproteins by differential dextran sulfate-magnesium chloride precipitation. *Biochimie* 1989;71:741—6.

45 Krauss RM. Relationship of intermediate and low-density lipoprotein subspecies to risk of coronary artery disease. *Am Heart J* 1987;113:578—82.

46 Kuchinskiene Z, Carlson LA. Composition, concentration, and size of low density lipoproteins and of subfractions of very low density lipoproteins from serum of normal

men and women. *J Lipid Res* 1982;23:762−9.

47 Bradley WA, Gotto AM Jr, Gianturco SH. Expression of LDL receptor binding determinants in very low density lipoproteins. *Ann N Y Acad Sci* 1985;454:239−47.

48 Musliner TA, Krauss RM. Lipoprotein subspecies and risk of coronary disease. *Clin Chem* 1988;34:B78−B83.

49 Shen MMS, Krauss RM, Lindgren FT, Forte TM. Heterogeneity of serum low density lipoproteins in normal human subjects. *J Lipid Res* 1981;22:236−44.

50 Chapman MJ, Laplaud PM, Luc G *et al.* Further resolution of the low density lipoprotein spectrum in normal human plasma: physicochemical characteristics of discrete subspecies separated by density gradient ultracentrifugation. *J Lipid Res* 1988;29:442−58.

51 Griffin BA, Caslake MJ, Yip B *et al.* Rapid isolation of low density lipoprotein (LDL) subfractions from plasma by density gradient ultracentrifugation. *Atherosclerosis* 1990;83:59−67.

52 Musliner TA, Giotas C, Krauss RM. Presence of multiple subpopulations of lipoproteins of intermediate density in normal subjects. *Arteriosclerosis* 1986;6:79−87.

53 Krauss RM, Burke DJ. Identification of multiple subclasses of plasma low density lipoproteins in normal subjects. *J Lipid Res* 1982;23:97−104.

54 Austin MA, King MC, Vranizan KM, Newman B, Krauss RM. Inheritance of low density lipoprotein subclass patterns: results of complex segregation analysis. *Am J Hum Genet* 1988;43:838−46.

55 Austin MA, Breslow JL, Hennekens CH *et al.* Low-density lipoprotein subclass patterns and risk of myocardial infarction. *JAMA* 1988;260:1917−21.

56 Milne RW, Weech PK, Blanchette L *et al.* Isolation and characterization of apolipoprotein B-48 and B-100 very low density lipoproteins from type III hyperlipoproteinemic subjects. *J Clin Invest* 1984;73:816−23.

Chapter 12
Apolipoprotein Measurements

JOHN J. ALBERS & SANTICA M. MARCOVINA

Introduction

The protein component of the lipoproteins, called apolipoproteins, represent a heterogeneous group of proteins that play an essential role in maintaining the structural integrity and stability of the lipoprotein particles. In addition to their role to solubilize and transport the neutral lipids (cholesteryl ester and triglyceride) and the polar lipids (phospholipid and unesterified cholesterol), the apolipoproteins play an important role in the metabolic interconversion of lipoproteins. They act as recognition ligands for cell surface receptors, activate the lipolytic enzymes to promote uptake and catabolism, and can also retard catabolism by inhibiting lipolytic action or binding to receptor sites.

The nomenclature for the lipoprotein classes was originally based on physical properties defined by the separation methods, i.e., hydrated density in the ultracentrifuge or electrophoretic mobility on paper. The high-density lipoproteins (HDL) obtained by ultracentrifugation are called α-lipoproteins by electrophoretic criteria and the low-density lipoproteins (LDL) are called β-lipoproteins. Alaupovic [1] proposed that the apolipoprotein content of the lipoproteins be used for identifying and classifying lipoproteins and designated the apolipoproteins by letter. Thus, the major HDL apolipoprotein (apo) constituent was designated apo A, and the protein of LDL or β-lipoprotein was designated apo B. The other apolipoproteins were subsequently assigned letter designations, e.g., C, D, E, F, G, H. Due to their clinical relevance, we will restrict our discussion to apo A-I, apo B, and lipoprotein(a).

In tissue fluids or serum, the apolipoproteins are found in association with lipids to form lipid–protein macromolecular complexes called lipoproteins. Apo A, as it was originally called to identify the protein content of HDL [1], comprises two distinct proteins, apo A-I and apo A-II. These proteins are synthesized primarily by the liver and intestine. Apo A-I, the major protein of HDL representing about 66% of the total HDL protein, is a single polypeptide chain of 243 amino acids with a molecular mass of 28 kDa [2]. It facilitates the solubilization of lipids and activates the enzyme lecithin cholesterol acyltransferase (LCAT) [3]. From the primary structure of apo A-I it has been deduced to contain numerous amphipathic α-helical domains [4]. Apo A-II is formed by two identical polypeptide chains of 77 amino acids each linked by a disulfide bridge with a combined molecular mass of 17 kDa. While apo A-I is present in all HDL particles (two to four apo A-I molecules per particle), apo A-II is present in about 50–75% of the particles [5,6]. Thus, HDL contains two populations of particles, those that contain only apo A-I and those containing apo A-I and apo A-II. Each apo-specific population is heterogeneous in size, hydrated density, and composition, and appears to have distinct metabolic pathways and functional roles in lipoprotein metabolism [7–9]. LCAT and cholesteryl ester transfer protein, which are involved in modulating the chemical composition and physical properties of HDL, are preferentially associated with particles containing apo A-I without A-II [10].

Extrahepatic cells possess specific high-affinity receptors for HDL [11]. Specific binding of apo A-I-containing particles stimulates the translocation of cholesterol from intracellular storage pools to the plasma membrane of cells, where it becomes accessible for removal by HDL particles [12]. The reversible binding of HDL to its cell-surface receptor provides a mechanism to facilitate the removal of cholesterol from extrahepatic cells and subsequent transport back to the liver.

Apo B exists in two structurally distinct forms, B_{100} and B_{48} [13]. Apo B_{100}, with a molecular mass of 513 kDa, is primarily found in LDL and very low-density lipoproteins (VLDL). Apo B_{100} is principally of hepatic origin and is required for synthesis and secretion of VLDL. LDL is the metabolic product of VLDL and apo B_{100} accounts for over 95% of its protein mass. The second form of apo B, B_{48}, with a molecular mass of about 214 kDa and so named because it is about 48% the size of apo B_{100} on SDS polyacrylamide gels, is homologous with the amino-terminal portion of B_{100}. It is associated with chylomicrons and chylomicron remnants and is of intestinal origin. Apo B_{48} is obligatory for the synthesis and secretion of chylomicrons and the intestinal absorption of fat.

The primary structure of apo B has defied chemical elucidation because lipid-free apo B is insoluble in aqueous solution. For this reason, for over 20 years only small portions of this large protein were sequenced by conventional techniques. Direct analysis of tryptic peptides has provided sequence analysis of a large portion of this protein [14], but the complete amino acid sequence has been deduced by sequence analysis of complementary DNA clones [15–17]. Examination of the primary structure indicates that it contains repeated amphipathic helical domains and repeated hydrophobic proline-rich domains [18]. These latter domains serve as strong lipid-binding domains and provide the basis for the fact that unlike the other apolipoproteins, apo B does not exchange between lipoproteins. Also, because apo B-containing lipoproteins contain only one apo B per particle, the measurement of apo B reflects lipoprotein particle number. Apo B contains specific LDL receptor-binding domains located in the carboxyl-terminal portion of the molecule [19]. Apo B_{100} of LDL therefore serves as the ligand for LDL receptor-mediated uptake of LDL particles by the liver and extra-hepatic tissues and provides a mechanism for the transport of cholesterol to cells.

Lipoprotein(a), or Lp(a), unlike LDL and HDL, is not classified on the basis of its physical–chemical properties defined by the classical lipoprotein separation methods, but is defined on the basis of the presence of apo(a), a unique glycoprotein linked by a disulfide bond to apo B_{100}, which is associated with lipid, to form a single macromolecule. Lp(a) has a buoyant density that spans both the LDL and HDL range with most of the Lp(a) usually found within the 1.050–1.100 g/ml density range [20]. Some Lp(a) is also found to be associated with VLDL (d <1.006 g/ml), particularly in postprandial plasma or in subjects with hypertriglyceridemia [21]. Like VLDL, Lp(a) has pre-β-mobility. Thus, Lp(a) does not fit in any of the conventional lipoprotein classes based upon either hydrated density or electrophoretic mobility. Also, the nomenclature for apo(a) does not follow the A, B, C nomenclature of Alaupovic. The (a) refers to an antigenic determinant in a lipoprotein fraction, first described by Berg [22]. It is now known to represent antigen determinants on apo(a).

Lp(a) exhibits considerable density and size heterogeneity [23]. The difference in Lp(a) particle size is due primarily to the different sizes of the apo(a) isoforms which range from 280 to 838 kDa. The structure of apo(a) is very different from the other apolipoproteins in that it binds rather poorly to lipids and does not contain the amphipathic repeat units characteristic of the other apolipoproteins. In addition, apo(a) has a high structural homology with plasminogen [24]. It contains two types of plasminogen-like kringle domains: a single Kringle 5 domain with 82% amino acid homology with plasminogen, and multiple repeats of a Kringle 4 domain with 61–75% amino acid homology with the Kringle 4 of plasminogen. Thus, the different sizes in apo(a) relate primarily to the number of Kringle 4 repeat units in apo(a). Most Lp(a) particles are believed to contain one molecule of apo B_{100} and one molecule of apo(a). A detailed review of the properties of Lp(a) and its immuno-chemical measurement has been published [25].

Clinical significance of the apolipoprotein measurements

In the late 1960s clinical and epidemiologic studies clearly showed that the risk of coronary artery disease (CAD) was directly related to the concentration of plasma cholesterol. Subsequently, in the early 1970s, these basic findings were extended from the cholesterol hypothesis to the lipoprotein hypothesis, when it was shown that the risk of CAD is directly related to plasma LDL cholesterol and inversely related to plasma HDL cholesterol concentrations. Unfortunately, as yet, a direct measurement of LDL cholesterol is not practical in the clinical laboratory. Also accurate, precise, and standardized HDL cholesterol measurements have been difficult to achieve.

Numerous clinical studies have suggested that the protein component of the lipoproteins, specifically apo B of LDL and apo A-I of HDL, are better indices of risk of CAD than lipoprotein cholesterol [26–28]. The vast majority of studies relating apolipoproteins to CAD have been of the case-control design, with the cases defined as subjects surviving a myocardial infarction or subjects having angina and angiographically proven CAD. The control subjects without overt CAD have been matched for age and sex and occasionally other variables. Most case-control studies report significantly higher apo B and lower apo A-I levels in cases of CAD compared to noncases. Of the 28 studies we examined [27], 25 studies reported lower apo A-I levels in the group with CAD compared to controls; whereas 19 of 26 studies we examined reported lower HDL cholesterol in cases as compared to controls. These cross-sectional studies have not clarified, however, whether or not apo A-I is a better discriminator than HDL cholesterol.

In all but two of the 24 studies in which apo B levels have been examined, the cases had significantly higher levels of apo B than controls. Also, there is a substantially larger number of coronary patients with an apo B concentration above the 90th or 95th percentile compared to those with an LDL cholesterol above this level [27,29]. Multivariant analysis indicated that apo B is superior to total or LDL cholesterol in discriminating cases from controls in seven of the eight studies after exclusion of subjects with familial hypercholesterolemia. The suggestion that apo B level is a better predictor of CAD than LDL cholesterol has been made by Sniderman *et al.* [30]. These investigators described a group of patients with high levels of LDL apo B in the absence of significantly elevated LDL cholesterol, a condition referred to as hyper-apobetalipoproteinemia, which is associated with the development of premature CAD. A similar relationship between the calculated LDL cholesterol and total plasma apo B was found in Seattle in 311 consecutive males under 60 years of age who underwent coronary angiography [27]. Among the patients with apo B levels above the 95th percentile of the control group formed by their spouses, more than half had LDL cholesterol levels below the 95th percentile. The subjects with an elevation of apo B but relatively normal LDL cholesterol levels and enriched in small dense LDL have the characteristics of familial combined hyperlipidemia, which is associated with premature CAD. Hypertriglyceridemic subjects who have a concomitant elevation of apo B appear to be at greater risk of coronary disease than those who do not have an apo B elevation [31,32]. Elevated apo B is also one of the most common lipid-associated abnormalities among patients undergoing coronary artery bypass surgery or angioplasty. Nearly half of these patients have elevated apo B [33]. Among subjects who underwent coronary bypass surgery, apo B and HDL cholesterol were shown to be the best predictors of disease progression in native coronary arteries or the appearance of lesions in saphenous vein bypass grafts [34]. Finally, in a clinical trial of men with elevated apo B and established coronary disease, angiographic and clinical improvement correlated best with the amount of decrease in apo B and increase in HDL cholesterol [35].

Because LDL apo B usually represents more than 90% of total plasma apo B, even in subjects with moderate hypertriglyceridemia, there is close agreement between measurement of plasma apo B and apo B in LDL. Therefore, the measurement of apo B in plasma, which is much more readily determined in clinical practice than apo B in LDL, should provide information not available from the measurement of LDL cholesterol and allow identification of subjects with increased LDL particle number associated with increased risk of coronary disease.

There is growing evidence that high concentrations of Lp(a) are good biochemical markers for both cardiovascular disease and cerebral vascular disease. Numerous studies have demonstrated that higher concentrations of Lp(a) are associated with both coronary and cerebral vascular disease [20,36–39]. Lp(a) levels are predictive of coronary disease severity among men with premature CAD and elevated apo B [27] and vein graft stenosis after coronary artery bypass surgery [40]. Subjects with familial hypercholesterolemia have Lp(a) concentrations at least twofold that found in healthy control subjects [41]. Among subjects with familial hypercholesterolemia, those with CAD have significantly higher Lp(a) concentrations than those without coronary disease [42]. Increased concentrations of Lp(a) concomitant with elevation of apo B may act synergistically to promote atherosclerosis, and appears to be a strong risk factor for coronary artery disease (CAD) in patients with familial hypercholesterolemia.

The weakness of the case-control studies is that CAD is already present. For primary prevention those at high risk must be identified prior to overt disease. Thus, from case-control studies it is not possible to determine whether apolipoproteins are better predictors of the risk of developing CAD than lipoprotein cholesterol. Another approach to address this question is the use of family studies to elucidate the predictive value of apolipoproteins and their relationship to other lipoprotein parameters. Five of six family studies which have compared the levels of apolipoproteins and lipids in relatives of subjects with CAD have shown that apo B or apo A-I or both predict parental history of CAD better than lipids or lipoprotein cholesterol [27]. In one study Lp(a) concentration accounted for much of the familial predisposition to cardiac ischemia [43], and in another study white children with serum Lp(a) concentrations above 0.25 g/l had an increased prevalence of parental myocardial infarction [44]. These studies suggest that apolipoprotein measurements are more useful than lipoprotein cholesterol in identifying the young at risk for CAD.

What is really needed to clearly document that apolipoprotein measurements are better predictors of the risk of developing CAD are large-scale prospective studies. Although several small-scale preliminary studies have been reported [27], no large-scale prospective studies have been published to date. Recently, a prospective case-control study from a general population sample of 776 men from Sweden who had sustained a myocardial infarction has demonstrated that the men who suffered CAD had significantly higher serum Lp(a) concentrations than controls, supporting the conclusion that serum Lp(a) concentration in middle-aged men is an independent risk factor for subsequent myocardial infarction or death from CAD [45].

Immunoassay methods

Peculiar properties of apolipoproteins

The conformation of the purified apolipoprotein in the absence of lipids differs significantly from the conformation of the protein in the lipid–protein complex. Purified apolipoproteins undergo self-association and form oligomeric complexes and under some circumstances form irreversible aggregates. Antigenic determinants can be masked after delipidation of the lipoproteins or in the purified form in aqueous solution because delipidated apolipoproteins readily self-associate [46].

In the presence of lipids, the apolipoproteins have the peculiar property of forming amphipathic helices, such that the polar and non-polar regions of the amino acids of the protein are on the opposite side of the helix. The nonpolar amino acids penetrate into the lipid surface, and the polar residues face the lipoprotein surface in contact with the aqueous environment. The conformation of a given apolipoprotein in lipoprotein particles can vary significantly depending on the specific composition and nature of the particle and the environment or specific experimental conditions. A change in apolipoprotein conformation can significantly alter its immunoreactivity. Also, other apolipoproteins and the lipid constituents of lipoproteins can conceal the antigenic sites or epitopes of apolipoproteins.

Antisera preparation, selection, and characterization

Antisera should be selected that recognize native and conserved epitopes that are expressed on all particles containing a given apolipoprotein. Antisera to modified epitopes are not suitable for measuring native apolipoproteins or lipoproteins. By their very nature, polyclonal antisera are not highly specific for a single epitope and often it is not possible to remove antibodies against nonnative epitopes.

All apolipoproteins are multivalent in the sense that they contain multiple antigenic determinants. Polyclonal antibodies raised against apolipoproteins by conventional techniques react with multiple epitopes and are therefore heterogeneous with respect to affinity and specificity to the multiple epitopes expressed in apolipoproteins. They often contain unwanted antibodies reactive with contaminating proteins that are usually removed by adsorption.

Although both polyclonal and monoclonal antibodies have been used extensively in apolipoprotein assays, monoclonal antibodies offer a number of advantages not available with the use of polyclonal anti-bodies. Monoclonal antibodies are, in contrast to polyclonal antibodies, highly specific, chemically uniform, and can be produced in large quantities. As a result, several recently introduced commercially available methods are based on monoclonal antibodies. However, the generation and selection of monoclonal antibodies appropriate for the measurement of apolipoproteins is a difficult and time-consuming process because monoclonal antibodies have peculiar properties that require careful consideration of the specific assay parameters [47]. For example, some monoclonal antibodies are quite sensitive to detergents or the ionic strength and pH of the buffers and the temperature of the reaction mixture. If such monoclonal antibodies are selected, then those assay parameters which are likely to alter the monoclonal antibodies' binding properties need to be carefully controlled.

One of the most critical requirements for selection of monoclonal antibodies is that the antibody must be capable of identifying the apolipoprotein in the test sample and the calibrator in exactly the same manner, i.e., with the same affinity. The affinity for the apolipoprotein should not only be high, e.g., 10^9-10^{10} l/mol, but also be independent of the physical and chemical properties of the lipoprotein in which it is found. The antibody should detect an epitope that is expressed in all lipoproteins in which the apolipoprotein is present. The selected antibodies should bind native epitopes rather than modified epitopes and they should not distinguish common genetic variants. In cases where monoclonal antibodies which bind all of the lipoprotein particles containing a given apolipoprotein cannot be selected, it is possible that a combination of monoclonal antibodies could be used in an immunoassay for apolipoprotein measurement [48,49].

Principles, advantages, and disadvantages of the different immunochemical methods

Single radial immunodiffusion (RID) refers to the radial diffusion of an antigen from a well into a uniform layer of antibody-containing agarose, thereby forming an antibody–antigen precipitin ring. The final area reached by the precipitate is directly proportional to the amount of antigen [50]. Particle size can affect the rate of diffusion and ultimately the size of the precipitin ring and thus the apparent concentration. Therefore, in order to minimize the effect of differences in particle size on the concentration, it is best that diffusion be allowed to proceed to completion, although this often will take 2–3 days. The RID method is relatively easy to perform and does not require dilution of the samples and can be used with either polyclonal antibodies or a mixture of defined monoclonal antibodies [48,49]. Because the RID procedure cannot be automated it is not suitable for screening large populations, it has limited sensitivity, and a between-assay coefficient of variation (CV) of about 6–8% if conditions and experimental technique are carefully controlled. Because it is sensitive to differences in size of the particles being measured, the smaller size particles may be potentially overestimated and the larger size particles underestimated. This consideration is particularly relevant for the measurement of apo B and apo(a) because these apolipoproteins are found associated with lipoproteins that vary widely in size.

Electroimmunodiffusion (EID) resembles RID in that it depends upon a quantitative relationship between the extent of visible antigen–antibody complex precipitated in an antibody-containing agarose matrix and the amount of antigen present. It differs from RID in that, rather than allowing for passive diffusion, the antigen is actively driven through the antibody-containing agarose by an electrical potential. The length of the precipitin patterns, or "rockets," is proportional to the antigen concentration [51]. In general, EID is more rapid than RID, yielding precipitin arcs within hours rather than days, and has greater sensitivity than RID. However, EID is technically more demanding than RID, requires the use of an electrophoresis chamber and power supply, and, as in RID, it cannot be automated. EID is also, to a certain extent, sensitive to size and charge differences in the antigen.

Highly automated methods such as immunoturbidimetric assays (ITA) and immunonephelometric assays (INA) have largely replaced the quantitative gel methods of RID and EID in the clinical laboratory. Nephelometry is the measurement of scattered light in a dilute suspension of particles formed by the antigen–antibody complex, whereas turbidimetry is the measurement of the decrease in light transmitted through a suspension of particles. INA and ITA are most suitable for the clinical laboratory because they have a high throughput, do not require isotopes, are easy to perform, and are highly automated. Nephelometric methods are sensitive to differences in size of the analyte being measured because the percentage of light scattered in the forward direction increases with the size of the particle. Thus, the measurements of apo B can be inaccurate because the light scattering of the immune complexes containing the large triglyceride-rich apo B-containing particles can differ from that of LDL particles in the calibrator. Secondly, large triglyceride-rich particles, such as chylomicrons and VLDL, inherently scatter light, which can result in high background scatter or high blank value. However, the magnitude of these potential problems can be minimized if a detergent is included in the diluent and assay conditions are optimized.

In radioimmunoassay (RIA), increasing concentrations of an analyte are reacted with a limiting amount of antibody in the presence of a fixed concentration of radiolabeled analyte. RIA is a highly sensitive technique that can be automated and can use either polyclonal or monoclonal antibodies. The disadvantages of RIA are that measurement of the analyte must be performed in either duplicate or triplicate to achieve satisfactory precision, and it uses radioisotopes which have a limited shelf-life. Furthermore, fluid phase RIA requires repeated purification of the antigen because of the relatively short-term stability of antigens such as LDL or Lp(a).

Enzyme-linked immunoadsorbent assay (ELISA) can be carried out in the different formats, double-antibody solid phase immunoassay and competitive solid phase immunoassay. In double-antibody ELISA specific antibody is bound to the solid phase, such as a microtiter plate. Antigen is then incubated in the presence of adsorbed antibody. Following a wash sequence, antibody conjugated to the enzyme is added to the reaction vessel. Following another wash period, substrate is added and the reaction product is measured spectrophotometrically. This procedures requires that at least two distinct epitopes are present per molecule of antigen. Because apolipoproteins are multivalent, this requirement is fulfilled. For the competitive solid phase immunoassay, the antigen is adsorbed to the solid phase, then enzyme-labeled antibody is added to a set of control wells, and enzyme-labeled antibody plus the unlabeled antigen are simultaneously added to the other wells. After incubation, the reaction vessels are washed, substrate provided, and the reaction product measured. Alternatively, the competitive assay can be carried out by binding the antibody to the solid phase and adding, simultaneously, enzyme-labeled and unlabeled antigen.

ELISA has the same advantages and disadvantages as RIA except that no radioisotopes are required and the enzyme-labeled reagents generally have a longer shelf-life than radiolabeled reagents. The competitive ELISA format, which utilizes the binding of the antigen to the microtiter plates, can lead to artifacts attributable to diminished epitope recognition. Alteration of epitope expression by adsorption of Lp(a) or LDL to plastic has been reported and presumably involves conformational changes in the lipoprotein upon binding to plastic [52,53].

Earlier work from this laboratory [54,55] has emphasized the difference in apo A-I and apo B values obtained by different methods. Although most of the differences were related to differences in calibration, some of the differences were clearly method dependent. More recently, we compared three methods for measuring apo A-I and apo B, monoclonal antibody-based RID [48,49], fixed time nephelometric assay (Behring nephelometer analyzer), and rate nephelometric assay (Beckman Array), on normotriglyceridemic ($n = 102$, triglyceride $<1.5\,g/l$) and hypertriglyceridemic samples ($n = 93$, triglyceride $>1.5\,g/l$). In addition apo B was also measured by an RIA method [56]. A common frozen serum pool was used to calibrate the different methods. Excellent agreement in apo A-I values was obtained by the different methods regardless of the triglyceride concentration of the samples (r ranging from 0.90 to 0.95) with the mean values obtained by the different methods differing by no more than 3%. Comparison of apo B value obtained on all samples with triglyceride $<5\,g/l$ indicated excellent agreement between the four methods (*r* value ranging from 0.92 to 0.97). However, for samples with triglyceride >5 g/l much poorer agreement was obtained between the methods. Thus, apo B measurements on samples with triglyceride >5 g/l cannot be considered reliable.

Initially, Lp(a) was quantified by either RID [57] or RIA [20] using polyclonal antisera. The major disadvantage of the RID procedure for Lp(a) was its relative insensitivity or inability to measure accurately Lp(a) in plasma or serum samples with levels of Lp(a) mass <0.08 g/l, which represented about one-half of the general population. In contrast, the RIA with its increased sensitivity permitted measurement of Lp(a) in all samples. However, because apo(a) has a high degree of homology with plasminogen [24] it is essential to demonstrate that the polyclonal antibodies used to measure apo(a) do not cross-react with plasminogen as we have shown for the previously reported RIA [21]. The potential problem of antibody specificity can most appropriately be solved by the generation and selection of monoclonal antibodies specific to apo(a) that do not cross-react with plasminogen. With adequately selected and characterized monoclonal antibodies, Lp(a) can be reliably measured by either ELISA or RIA. It is possible, however, even with the use of specific monoclonal antibodies that the immunoreactivity or epitope expression of apo(a) varies with the number of kringle units in apo(a) and the size of apo(a) in the Lp(a) particle. Furthermore, agreement has not yet been reached on how to express Lp(a), e.g., in terms of total Lp(a) mass, total protein mass, or apo(a) mass.

Reliable measurements of apo A-1, apo B, and Lp(a) are currently available. However, it is essential that only those methods whose calibration can be traced back to an international reference (see section on Secondary Reference Material) should be used. Among those methods whose accuracy and good precision have been documented, the selection of the most appropriate method depends upon the specific requirements of the laboratory in terms of the daily workload, the skill of the technologist, the availability of instrumentation, the required turn around time, and the cost per sample.

Sources of variation in apolipoprotein measurements

Major sources of variation other than analytic variation can be arbitrarily grouped into the following categories: preanalytic variation attributed to conditions of sample collection and storage, biologic variation, and differences in lifestyle. To minimize preanalytic variation, repeat determinations of apolipoproteins are recommended to minimize misclassification. At least two measurements should be performed at a 2–8 week interval. Variable conditions of specimen collection and shipment, posture, and fasting can all contribute to preanalytic variation. For example, individuals tested in a standing position may have analyte levels 5–10% higher than those in a sitting position, and differences can occur if blood is drawn in a supine position as compared to a sitting position. Prolonged venous stasis can result in an apparent increase of as much as 10% in apolipoprotein concentration. Hemolysis can also lead to artifacts in the measurements. Variations in storage and improper shipping can affect the measurements because of bacterial contamination, evaporation, or chemical modification of apolipoproteins during storage or handling. Anticoagulants can cause different degrees of shifts of water from the blood cells into the plasma, from <1% to >10%, and thus lead to variation in the dilution of plasma. Although on average apo A-I and apo B values obtained under fasting conditions have been reported not to be significantly different compared to nonfasting conditions [58], on an individual basis significant differences in apolipoprotein values can be obtained as a result of postprandial conditions. Furthermore, postprandial conditions give rise to chylomicrons and often lead to turbid samples which can interfere with the apolipoprotein analysis as performed in the INA or ITA procedures.

Another major source of variation is intraperson biologic variation. As yet, there is no evidence that apolipoproteins exhibit significant circadian variations. The biologic or physiologic variation of apo A-I and apo B in healthy adults is on average relatively small, in the order of 5–8%. As there are seasonal variations in cholesterol and HDL cholesterol it is likely that apo A-I and apo B exhibit seasonal changes similar to LDL cholesterol and HDL cholesterol, respectively. Other physiologic and behavioral variables, such as dietary alterations, obesity, alcohol intake, vigorous exercise, cigarette smoking, concurrent illness, and medications known to alter lipoprotein levels such as beta-blockers, diuretics, steroids, oral contraceptives, and lipid-lowering agents, can significantly affect apolipoprotein concentration in plasma.

Apolipoprotein standardization

Blood collection, handling, and storage

Patient preparation and blood collection procedures should follow strict guidelines such as those recommended for cholesterol analysis [59]. The patient should be fasted for 12–14 hours and should be seated for 10 minutes before venipuncture. If a tourniquet is used, the blood should be drawn within 60 seconds of tourniquet application and the tourniquet released as soon as possible during venipuncture. The subject should refrain from alcohol and vigorous exercise 12–14 hours and cigarette smoking 1–2 hours before phlebotomy. For serum, venous blood should be collected, after brief application of the tourniquet, into an evacuated glass tube without anticoagulant. The sample should be allowed to stand at room temperature for 30–45 minutes or until the clot has retracted and the serum separated from the clot by brief centrifugation.

For plasma, venous blood should be collected into an evacuated glass tube or system that contains solid EDTA (fixed concentration after filling the tube of 1.0 mg/ml). EDTA is the preferred anticoagulant for measurement of apolipoproteins in plasma. All tubes should be filled to the same level. The blood and anticoagulant are mixed by gentle inversion and then the cells immediately cooled to 2–4°C and centrifuged in a refrigerated centrifuge (30 minutes at 1500 g). Either serum or EDTA-treated plasma is suitable for apolipoprotein measurements but it must be recognized that plasma values are approximately 3–5% lower than serum values due to dilution with water from the cells because of the osmotic effects of EDTA. It is important to fill the plasma tube completely to avoid variable dilution of the samples. EDTA-treated plasma also has the potential for forming fibrin which can present problems in diluting the samples, particularly when small volumes are used with automatic pipetting equipment. Also, because fibrin is often evident in plasma samples that have been thawed, serum is recommended for samples that need to be frozen [60].

Serum or plasma samples can be stored at 4°C for up to 2 weeks. However, to minimize the physical and chemical changes in lipoproteins during storage, it is recommended that apolipoprotein measurements be done as soon as possible, preferably within 1 week. If long-term storage is required, the samples should be stored at −70°C and the time between blood collection and freezing of the samples should be as short as possible [60]. Because potential changes with storage may be method and antibody dependent, the maximum allowable time the samples can be stored at −70°C has not been clearly established but the available evidence would suggest that for many methods serum may be stored for several years at −70°C.

Reference methods

Reference procedures are needed to assign target values to reference materials, calibrators and quality control materials, and to compare values of new methods with those obtained by the reference method

[61]. Unfortunately, there are no reference methods currently available for any of the apolipoproteins. In the absence of a reference method, a selected method can be used to assign values to reference materials. However, the selected method should meet strict guidelines and criteria. As for reference methods, ideally the selected method should be demonstrated to be precise, accurate, stable over time, and minimally affected by interferences or matrix effects [60]. Only defined primary standards in which the absolute mass has been accurately determined should be used for calibration of the selected methods. In the selected method, the primary standard must have the same immunochemical behavior as the native apolipoprotein in plasma. Finally, the method should have clearly defined performance limits.

Primary reference materials

To achieve an accuracy-based measurement of apolipoproteins, primary reference materials with absolute mass determined by chemical methods are an essential requisite. Highly purified proteins in aqueous solution are generally used as primary reference materials for plasma proteins. However, the association of apolipoproteins with lipid in their native state and consequently the altered immunochemical and physical properties of apolipoproteins in purified form significantly enhances the problem of preparation of primary reference materials for apolipoproteins.

Apo A-I in purified form, isolated by chromatography from delipidated HDL, can be used as primary reference material for apo A-I immunoassays. The isolation procedure should be carefully performed to avoid apo A-I undergoing chemical alteration such as deamidation, oxidation, or proteolytic degradation. After purification, apo A-I in aqueous solution of low ionic strength should be immediately stored at −70°C in order to prevent any alteration [61].

The epitope expression of purified apo A-I does not reflect that of apo A-I in native lipoprotein particles as demonstrated by monoclonal antibodies [62]. For this reason, when purified apo A-I is used as standard, the samples need to be treated with dissociating agents in order that the apo A-I in the sample is in the same physical state as the purified protein.

Delipidated apo B aggregates irreversibly in lipid-free form. Thus, isolated LDL is used as a primary reference material for apo B, because apo B represents nearly all the protein component of LDL. To avoid contaminating proteins, it has been recommended [60,61] that freshly prepared LDL of narrow density range (1.030−1.050 g/ml) obtained from normolipidemic donors with low Lp(a) concentrations be used as primary standard for apo B. Purified LDL can be stored in a buffered aqueous solution, pH 8.0, at 4°C for no longer than 3 weeks. As with apo A-I, LDL can also undergo chemical alteration during isolation or storage. For this reason carefully designed common protocols are required for the isolation of apolipoproteins when they are used as primary reference material. Purity of the proteins should be demonstrated by sensitive immunochemical tests.

Like apo B, the protein component of Lp(a), the apo(a)–apo B complex, undergoes a high degree of self-association and is unstable in aqueous solution upon delipidation. Thus, the isolated Lp(a) particle is commonly used as primary reference material. Although isolated LDL is used as primary standard for apo B and the value is assigned in terms of apo B mass, no such agreement has been reached for Lp(a) [25].

The assignment of protein mass to primary reference materials is usually performed by amino acid analysis. However, this method is difficult to apply in practice, has a high degree of variability, and is time consuming. The length of time required for the analysis is particularly critical for LDL that are known to be highly sensitive to storage. For these reasons, the use of a Lowry–sodium dodecyl sulfate (SDS) procedure can be considered as an alternative [63]. However, this apparently simple method is also difficult to standardize even when common protocols and source of standard are used [63].

Secondary reference materials

Primary reference materials, being proteins or lipoproteins in isolated form, do not have the same immunochemical behavior as plasma samples in all the immunoassays. For this reason, a direct transfer of the mass value to the calibrators of the different immunosystems would result in lack of comparability of the data. Additionally, apolipoproteins or lipoproteins have a limited shelf-life and this is particularly true for both LDL and Lp(a). Thus, secondary reference materials, usually formed by a pool of sera from normolipidemic donors, are required to achieve and monitor the accuracy of the measurements.

While primary reference materials must be demonstrated to behave immunochemically the same as plasma samples in the reference or selected method, a prerequisite of the secondary reference materials is an immunochemical behavior similar to that of the samples in all the tested methods, i.e., it must not exhibit matrix effect among methods.

Because of the long-term stability and ease of shipment, the secondary reference materials are usually in lyophilized form. While lyophilized materials for apo A-I do not exhibit matrix effect among methods, it has been demonstrated that lyophilization and subsequent reconstitution change the immunochemical behavior of apo B [64]. As a result, lyophilized material exhibits matrix effect among methods for measurement of apo B, the magnitude being method dependent.

The lack of internationally available secondary serum reference materials has been a major stumbling block in the standardization of apolipoproteins and accounts for most of the large variability of apo A-I and B values determined by different methods. In order to achieve accuracy and comparability of apo A-I and B measurements, the Committee on Apolipoproteins of the International Federation of Clinical Chemistry (IFCC) initiated in 1989 an international collaborative study with the participation of 27 manufacturers of instruments and/or reagents for the determination of apolipoproteins and five research laboratories under the coordination of the Northwest Lipid Research Laboratories of the University of Washington, Seattle, USA. The general aims of this study were to select and evaluate reference materials suitable to be proposed as international reference materials and to standardize commercially available methods by a common accuracy-based calibration.

Thic IFCC multistep collaborative study was carried out in three separate phases. The specific objectives of the first phase were to: (i) evaluate calibration differences among the test systems; (ii) evaluate whether comparability of the measurements can be achieved with the use of frozen serum pools to recalibrate the different test systems; and (iii) evaluate and select suitable candidate reference material. Relatively modest differences were found in calibration for apo A-I among 26 test systems, but wide differences were observed for the 28 apo B methods evaluated. By using frozen serum pools to recalibrate the different test systems, the CV between laboratories as assessed on 10 normolipidemic samples was 5% for apo A-I and 6% for apo B, demonstrating the key role of suitable reference materials in the standardization process. Among the materials (15 for apo A-I and 11 for apo B) proposed by several manufacturers enrolled in the study, three preparations in lyophilized form for apo A-I and three in liquid-stabilized form for apo B were considered suitable on the basis that they lacked matrix effect between methods as demonstrated by low CV between methods and they were optically clear, homogeneous, and yielded a low blank [65]. As two of these materials were prepared by the same company, only two lyophilized preparations for apo A-I (SP1 and SP2) and two liquid preparations for apo B (SP3 and SP4) were evaluated in the second phase of this study as candidate international reference materials.

The objective of the second phase was to evaluate the linearity and parallelism of the candidate reference materials selected in Phase 1 and to determine if any of the reference materials could be proposed as international reference material. The candidate reference materials SP1 and SP3 exhibited linearity and parallelism similar to that of a fresh-frozen serum pool and had between-laboratory CVs less than or similar to those obtained with normolipidemic serum samples. Therefore, these materials were proposed as candidate international reference materials.

The objectives of the third phase were to: (i) validate directly the selected reference materials in the different systems; (ii) transfer the target values from the reference materials to the in-house calibrators; and (iii) validate the comparability of the data among the different systems. Thus far, the reference material SP1 for apo A-I with an assigned value of 150 mg/dl was used as common calibrator in 29 different systems. The uniform calibration resulted in comparable values in three frozen serum pools with between-method CVs of 3–5%, confirming the lack of matrix effect of SP1 and its suitability as candidate international reference material. In the second step, the participants were requested to transfer the mass value from SP1 to their individual calibrators in order to achieve uniformity of the calibration of the different commercially available systems. Preliminary results indicate that uniformity of calibration results in comparability of apo A-I values on serum samples. Based on all the results obtained, SP1 exhibits all the properties [60] to be considered a suitable reference material. A complete documentation on SP1 along with the request to become International Reference Material for apo A-I has been recently submitted to the World Health Organization.

When SP3, the liquid-stabilized reference material for apo B, was used as common calibrator in the first step of Phase 3, an unusually high CV between methods was observed on the three frozen serum pools. Because the material was 1 year old and was shipped to the participants by the producer at room temperature, degradation of the material was suspected and subsequently confirmed. To confirm that the use of a common material can lead to uniformity of the data also for apo B, a frozen serum pool was used as interim reference material. Although preliminary, the results thus far indicate that uniformity of calibration results in comparability of apo B values on serum samples.

This IFCC study represents an important step forward to the achievement of standardization of apolipoprotein measurements and stresses the importance of a direct collaboration between experts from academic organizations and experts from manufacturers in order to achieve standardization of commercially available methods. At the end of this study a carefully planned quality assurance program with suitable quality control materials is required to monitor the performance of the clinical chemistry laboratories and to ensure that uniformity of the apolipoprotein data is maintained.

Quality control

A quality control system is needed to assess inherent random variation of results or precision and the deviation of results from the target value or bias. A quality assurance program ensures that accuracy and precision are maintained in the day-to-day performance of the laboratory. Both internal and external quality control programs are necessary to assure appropriate laboratory performance [66]. The internal quality control program assesses the accuracy and precision of the analytic method in order to determine the acceptability of daily results and it is also used for weekly or monthly retrospective evaluation of the results to determine potential drift in the analytic procedure. The external quality control program consists of blinded retrospective evaluation of the analytic performance in order to determine the performance of the laboratory in relationship to that of other laboratories.

The problems related to the quality control materials for apolipoprotein measurements are very similar to those which we have described for secondary reference material [60,61]. Quality control material should have many of the same features that are needed for secondary reference materials, including long-term stability, homogeneity, and immunochemical behavior similar to that of the test specimens. The quality control material should not exhibit matrix interactions among the different methods, and therefore should simulate as much as possible the matrix of the test sample. To evaluate precision and bias three quality control pools at low, normal, and high concentrations of the analyte that extend throughout the normal range of subject values are recommended. The target values of the quality control materials should be properly assigned. The accuracy of standards and/or calibrators should be assured by the manufacturer. Adequate numbers of quality control materials should be used in order to assess performance on patient samples. The quality control system should define limits for bias or nearness to the target value and precision. Apo A-I and apo B bias within 5% of the target value would be a reasonable guide. At this time, a CV between runs of <6% may be considered acceptable and <5% optimal. Required performance limits depend upon the physiologic range of values. Because the physiologic values of Lp(a) are very broad it is possible to accept less precise performance limits for Lp(a) than for apo A-I or apo B. In order for the laboratory to monitor accuracy it may not be sufficient to compare results on the quality control materials. The accuracy on patient samples can be assessed by comparing the apolipoprotein values with those obtained on the same samples by a reference laboratory.

Population-based reference values

For apo A-I, apo B, and Lp(a) there are relatively few population-based age-specific values. The available data up to 1988 have been previously reviewed [27]. Consistent with this review, we have recently found that apo A-I levels in healthy male subjects exhibit little change, if any, from age 40 to 70. Men in their 20s and 30s generally have slightly lower apo A-I levels than older men. For women, apo A-I levels change little with age from 20 to 40, with slightly higher values found for women in their fifties and sixties. For males aged 40–69, the median value is about 1.4 g/l and the 25th and 10th percentile values are 1.26 and 1.10 g/l, respectively, with younger men having lower values. As for HDL cholesterol levels below the 10th percentile value, subjects with apo A-I levels <1.10 g/l would have an increased risk for coronary disease. For females aged 20–49, the median value was 1.47 g/l and even higher median values were obtained for women in their fifties and sixties. A recent study of the distribution of apo A-I and B in young adults (age 18–30) indicates that black men have apo A-I levels about 5% higher on average than white men, but that white women and black women have similar apo A-I levels [67].

As we have previously reported [27] similar apo B values have been obtained in five independent studies in five different predominantly white populations using different measurement methods. Examination of these data shows that although apo B levels increase significantly with age in both men and women, the profile of the relationship of age with apo B values is quite different between the sexes. In men, apo B levels increase with age about 0.8 mg/dl per year from age 20 to about age 45 and then gradually level off in the fifties, with older men in the seventies and eighties having lower levels than those in their fifties and sixties. In contrast, the apo B levels in women change little in the twenties and thirties but increase significantly (about 1.3 mg/dl) in the forties, fifties, and sixties. Middle-aged men generally have higher levels of apo B than middle-aged women. For a 45-year-old man, the 50th, 75th, and 90th percentile values are estimated to be 1.05, 1.22, and 1.40 g/l, respectively. For comparison, the 50th, 75th, and 95th percentile values for a 45-year-old woman are estimated to be 0.98, 1.17, and 1.33 g/l, respectively. Consistent with the above data for men and the National Cholesterol Education Program guidelines for clinical cutpoints for LDL cholesterol, it would be desirable to have apo B values below the 50th percentile value of 1.05 g/l. Values between the 50th and 75th percentile, 1.05–1.22 g/l, would be considered borderline high, and values >1.40 g/l would be designated high and impart an increased risk for coronary disease. These values are nearly identical to the suggested clinical apo B cutpoints reported by Vega and Grundy [68].

Reference values for Lp(a) are not yet available. Historically, Lp(a) levels have been expressed in terms of total Lp(a) mass [20,57], although more recently some authors have reported either protein mass or estimated apo(a) mass. Uniform cutpoints for Lp(a) must await agreement on expressing the data and the availability of common reference material. The distribution of Lp(a) in healthy adults of predominantly Caucasian origin is highly skewed [21,25]. Lp(a) concentrations change little with age in adults and do not differ significantly between men and women [57]. Blacks have Lp(a) levels about double that of whites [69,70] with the population distribution much less skewed.

Clinical guidelines for apolipoprotein measurements

Apolipoprotein measurements can further aid in the detection of CAD risk and the diagnosis of hyperlipoproteinemia in the context of the National Cholesterol Education Program's patient-based strategy to identify and treat subjects with the highest coronary disease risk through the measurement of the blood cholesterol. The measurement of apo B provides a reliable clinical tool to identify subjects with an increased risk for coronary disease that may not be readily identified by the conventional cholesterol or lipoprotein cholesterol measurements. Thus, candidates for measurement of apo B include those with the National Cholesterol Education Program's borderline range for LDL cholesterol, and subjects with hypertriglyceridemia without an LDL cholesterol elevation in order to identify subjects who have an overproduction of hepatic apo B particles. It would be potentially beneficial to measure Lp(a) in subjects in which CHD is present or suspected, or in subjects with two or more CHD risk factors, particularly in those who have an elevation of apo B or cholesterol. Also, patients with an elevated apo B and/or Lp(a) undergoing hyperlipidemic therapy should have these apolipoproteins measured to monitor the effectiveness of therapy. However, standardization of the apolipoprotein measurements, uniformity of the data among laboratories, and the establishment of common clinical cutpoints are essential before general application of these measurements can be recommended.

Apo B, apo A-I, and Lp(a) measurements can serve as important predictors of CHD risk and can thereby provide additional information to that obtained from blood lipid and lipoprotein lipid levels. In addition, apolipoprotein measurements can be used to provide information about therapeutic response to lipid-lowering drugs. The decision to use apolipoprotein measurements depends upon the clinical setting, the availability of standardized measurements that can be related to population-based reference values, and the cost of the measurements. Standardized apolipoprotein measurements have potentially wide application in a variety of clinical settings.

Acknowledgments

The original work reported in this chapter was supported in part by grants HL 30086 and HL 44105 from the National Heart, Lung, and Blood Institute, National Institutes of Health, USA.

References

1 Alaupovic P. Conceptual development of the classification systems of plasma lipoproteins. *Protides Biol Fluids Proc Colloq* 1972;19:9–19.
2 Brewer HB, Fairwell T, LaRue A *et al.* The amino acid sequence of human apo A-I, an apolipoprotein isolated from high density lipoproteins. *Biochem Biophys Res Commun* 1978;80:623–30.
3 Fielding CJ, Shore VG, Fielding PE. A protein cofactor of lecithin: cholesterol acyltransferase. *Biochem Biophys Res Commun* 1972;46:1493–8.
4 Segrest JP, Jackson RL, Morrisett JD, Gotto AM. A molecular theory of lipid–protein interactions in the plasma lipoproteins. *FEBS Lett* 1974;38:247–53.
5 Cheung MC, Nichols AV, Blanche PJ *et al.* Characterization of A-I-containing lipoproteins in subjects with A-I Milano variant. *Biochim Biophys Acta* 1988;960:73–82.
6 Cheung MC, Wolf AC, Brunzell JD. Metabolic pathways of HDL subpopulations: physiological implications of *in vitro* observations. In *Disorders of HDL* (ed. LA Carlson). London: Smith-Gordon, 1990:89–97.
7 Cheung MC, Albers JJ. Characterization of lipoprotein particles isolated by immunoaffinity chromatography: particles containing A-I and A-II and particles containing A-I but not A-II. *J Biol Chem* 1984;259:12201–9.
8 Cheung MC, Wolf AC. *In vitro* transformation of A-I-containing lipoprotein subpopulation: role of lecithin cholesterol acyltransferase and B-containing lipoproteins. *J Lipid Res* 1989;30:499–509.
9 Cheung MC, Brown BG, Wolf AC, Albers JJ. Altered particle size distribution of apolipoprotein A-I containing lipoproteins in subjects with coronary artery disease. *J Lipid Res* 1991;32:383–94.
10 Cheung MC, Wolf AC, Lum KD, Tollefson JH, Albers JJ. Distribution and localization of lecithin–cholesterol acyltransferase and cholesteryl ester transfer activity in A-I-containing lipoproteins. *J Lipid Res* 1986;27:1135–44.

11 Biesbroeck R, Oram JF, Albers JJ, Bierman JL. Specific high-affinity binding of high density lipoproteins to cultured human skin fibroblasts and on trial smooth muscle cells. *J Clin Invest* 1982;71:525−39.

12 Oram JF, Mendez AJ, Bierman EL. HDL receptor function in cholesterol transport. In *Disorders of HDL* (ed. LA Carlson). London: Smith-Gordon, 1990:99−104.

13 Kane JP, Hardman DA, Paulus HE. Heterogeneity of apolipoprotein B: isolation of a new species from human chylomicrons. *Proc Natl Acad Sci USA* 1980;77:2464−9.

14 Yang C-Y, Gu Z-W, Weng S-A *et al.* Structure of apolipoprotein B-100 of human low density lipoproteins. *Arteriosclerosis* 1989;9:96−108.

15 Chen-SH, Yang C-Y, Chen P-F *et al.* The complete cDNA and amino acid sequence of human apolipoprotein B-100. *J Biol Chem* 1986;261:12918−21.

16 Knott TJ, Pease RJ, Powell LM *et al.* Complete protein sequence and identification of structural domains of human apolipoprotein B. *Nature* 1986;323:734−8.

17 Law SW, Grant SM, Higuchi K *et al.* Human liver apolipoprotein B-100 cDNA: complete nucleic acid and derived amino acid sequence. *Proc Natl Acad Sci USA* 1986;83:8142−6.

18 De Loof H, Rosseneu M, Yang C-Y *et al.* Human apolipoprotein B: analysis of internal repeats and homology with other apolipoproteins. *J Lipid Res* 1987;28:1455−65.

19 Yang C-Y, Chen S-H, Gianturco SH *et al.* Sequence, structure, receptor-binding domains and internal repeats of human apolipoprotein B-100. *Nature* 1986;323:738−42.

20 Albers JJ, Adolphson JL, Hazzard WR. Radioimmunoassay of human plasma Lp(a) lipoprotein. *J Lipid Res* 1977;18:331−8.

21 Albers JJ. The measurement of Lp(a) and its clinical application. In *Lipoprotein(a)* (ed. AM Scanu). San Diego: Academic Press, 1990:141−9.

22 Berg K. A new serum type system in man—the Lp system. *Acta Pathol Microbiol Scand* 1963;59:369−82.

23 Fless GM, Rolih CA, Scanu AM. Heterogeneity of human plasma lipoprotein(a). Isolation and characterization of the lipoprotein subspecies and their apoproteins. *J Biol Chem* 1984;259:11470−8.

24 McLean JW, Tomlinson JE, Kuang W-J *et al.* cDNA sequence of human apolipoprotein(a) is homologous to plasminogen. *Nature* 1987;330:132−7.

25 Albers JJ, Marcovina SM, Lodge MS. The unique lipoprotein(a): properties and immunochemical measurement. *Clin Chem* 1990;36:2019−26.

26 Brunzell JD, Sniderman AD, Albers JJ, Kwiterovich PO Jr. Apoproteins B and A-I and coronary artery disease in humans. *Arteriosclerosis* 1984;4:79−83.

27 Albers JJ, Brunzell JD, Knopp RH. Apoprotein measurements and their clinical application. *Clin Lab Med* 1989;9:137−52.

28 Marcovina SM, Zoppo A, Graziani MS, Vassanelli C, Catapano AL. Evaluation of apolipoproteins A-I and B as markers of angiographically assessed coronary artery disease. *Ric Clin Lab* 1988;18:319−28.

29 Blank D, Silberberg J, Sniderman AD. Trade-offs on cutpoints for the treatment of hyperlipidemia. *Coron Art Dis* 1990;1:455−9.

30 Sniderman A, Shapiro S, Marpole D *et al.* Association of coronary atherosclerosis with hyperapobeta lipoproteinemia (increased protein but normal cholesterol levels in human plasma low density (ß) lipoproteins). *Proc Natl Acad Sci USA* 1980;77:604−8.

31 Sniderman AD, Wolfson C, Teng B *et al.* Association of hyperapobetalipoproteinemia with endogenous hypertriglyceridemia and atherosclerosis. *Ann Intern Med* 1982;7:833−9.

32 Durrington PN, Hunt L, Ishola M, Kane J, Stepheno WP. Serum apolipoproteins A-I and B and lipoproteins in middle-aged men with and without previous myocardial infarction. *Br Heart J* 1986;56:206.

33 Zhao X-Q, Flygenring BP, Stewart DK *et al.* Increased potential for regression of post-PTCA restenosis using intensive lipid-altering therapy: comparison with matched

non-PTCA lesions. *J Am Coll Cardiol* 1991;17:203A.

34 Campeau L, Enjalbert M, Lesperance J *et al.* The relation of risk factors to the development of atherosclerosis in saphenous-vein bypass grafts and the progression of disease in the native circulation: a study 10 years before aortocoronary bypass surgery. *N Engl J Med* 1984;311:1329−32.

35 Brown G, Albers JJ, Fisher LD *et al.* Regression of coronary artery disease as a result of intensive lipid-lowering therapy in men with high levels of apolipoprotein B. *N Engl J Med* 1990;323:1289−98.

36 Kostner GM, Avogaro P, Cazzolato G *et al.* Lipoprotein Lp(a) and the risk of myocardial infarction. *Atherosclerosis* 1981;38:51−61.

37 Murai A, Miyahara T, Fujimoto N, Matsuda M, Kameyama M. Lp(a) lipoprotein as a risk factor for coronary heart disease and cerebral infarction. *Atherosclerosis* 1986; 59:199−204.

38 Armstrong VW, Cremer P, Eberle E *et al.* The association between serum Lp(a) concentrations and angiographically assessed coronary atherosclerosis. Dependence on serum LDL levels. *Atherosclerosis* 1986;62:249−57.

39 Zenker G, Koltringer P, Bone G *et al.* Lipoprotein(a) as a strong indicator for cerebrovascular disease. *Stroke* 1986;17:942−5.

40 Hoff HF, Beck GJ, Skibinski CI *et al.* Serum Lp(a) level as a predictor of vein graft stenosis after coronary artery bypass surgery in patients. *Circulation* 1988;77:1238−44.

41 Utermann G, Hoppichler F, Dieplinger H *et al.* Defects in the low density lipoprotein receptor gene affect lipoprotein Lp(a) levels: multiplicative interaction of two gene loci associated with premature atherosclerosis. *Proc Natl Acad Sci USA* 1989;86:4171−4.

42 Seed M, Hoppichler F, Reaveley D *et al.* Relation of serum lipoprotein (a) concentration and apolipoprotein (a) phenotype to coronary heart disease in patients with familial hypercholesterolemia. *N Engl J Med* 1990;322:1494−9.

43 Durrington PN, Ishola M, Hunt L, Arrol S, Bhatnagar D. Apolipoproteins(a), A1, and B and parental history in men with early onset ischaemic heart disease. *Lancet* 1988;ii:1070−3.

44 Srinivasan SR, Dahlen GII, Jarpa RA, Webber LS, Berenson GS. Racial (black−white) differences in serum lipoprotein(a) distribution and its relation to parental myocardial infarction in children. *Circulation* 1991;84:160−7.

45 Rosengren A, Wilhelmsen L, Eriksson E, Risberg B, Wedel H. Lipoprotein(a) and coronary heart disease: a prospective case-control study in a general population sample of middle aged men. *Br Med J* 1990;301:1248−51.

46 Osborne JC Jr, Lee NS, Powell GM. Solution properties of apolipoproteins. In *Methods in Enzymology*, Vol. 128, *Plasma Lipoproteins, Part A Preparation, Structure, and Molecular Biology* (eds JP Segrest, JJ Albers). Orlando: Academic Press, 1986:375.

47 Marcovina SM, Curtiss LK, Milne R, Albers JJ. Selection and characterization of monoclonal antibodies for measuring plasma levels of apolipoproteins A-I and B. *J Aut Chem* 1990,12:195−8.

48 Marcovina SM, DiCola G, Catapano AL. Radial immunodiffusion assay of human apolipoprotein A-I with use of two monoclonal antibodies combined. *Clin Chem* 1986;32:2155−9.

49 Marcovina SM, DiCola G, Rapetto C. Development of a radial immunodiffusion technique employing monoclonal antibodies for apolipoprotein B determination in human plasma. *Clin Chim Acta* 1985;114:117−25.

50 Mancini G, Carbonara AO, Heremans JF. Immunochemical quantitation of antigens by single radial immunodiffusion. *Immunochemistry* 1985;2:235−54.

51 Laurell CB. Quantitative estimation of proteins by electrophoresis in agarose gel containing antibodies. *Anal Biochem* 1966;15:45−52.

52 Guo H-C, Armstrong VW, Luc G *et al.* Characterization of five mouse monoclonal antibodies to apolipoprotein(a) from human Lp(a): evidence for weak plasminogen reactivity. *J Lipid Res* 1989;30:23−37.

53 Milne RW, Blanchette L, Theolis R, Weech PK, Marcel YL. Monoclonal antibodies distinguish between lipid-dependent and reversible conformational states of human apolipoprotein B. *Mol Immunol* 1987;24:435−47.

54 Albers JJ, Adolphson JL. Comparison of commercial kits for apoprotein A-I and apoprotein B with standardized apoprotein A-I and B radioimmunoassays performed at the Northwest Lipid Research Center. *J Lipid Res* 1988;29:102−8.

55 Adolphson JL, Albers JJ. Comparison of two commercial nephelometric methods for apoprotein A-I and apoprotein B with standardized apoprotein A-I and B radioimmunoassays. *J Lipid Res* 1989;30:597−606.

56 Albers JJ, Cabana VG, Hazzard WR. Immunoassay of human plasma apolipoprotein B. *Metabolism* 1975;24:1339−51.

57 Albers JJ, Hazzard WR. Immunochemical quantification of human plasma Lp(a) lipoprotein. *Lipids* 1974;9:15−26.

58 Rifai N, Merrill JR, Holly RG. Postprandial effect of a high fat meal on plasma lipid, lipoprotein cholesterol and apolipoprotein measurements. *Ann Clin Biochem* 1990;27:489−93.

59 Recommendations for improving cholesterol measurement. A report from the Laboratory Standardization Panel of the National Cholesterol Education Program. NIH Publication No. 90−2964, February 1990.

60 Marcovina SM, Albers JJ. Standardization of the immunochemical determination of apolipoproteins A-I and B: a report on the International Federation of Clinical Chemistry meeting on standardization of apolipoprotein A-I and B measurements (basis for future consensus), Vienna, Austria, April 18−19, 1989. *Clin Chem* 1989;35:2009−15.

61 Albers JJ, Marcovina SM. Standardization of apolipoprotein B and A-I measurements. *Clin Chem* 1989;35:1357−61.

62 Marcovina SM, Fantappie S, Zoppo A, Franceschini G, Catapano AL. Immunochemical characterization of six monoclonal antibodies to human apolipoprotein A-I: epitope mapping and expression. *J Lipid Res* 1990;31:375−84.

63 Henderson LO, Powell MK, Smith SJ *et al.* Impact of protein measurements on standardization of apolipoproteins A-I and B assays. *Clin Chem* 1990;36:1911−17.

64 Marcovina SM, Adolphson JL, Parlavecchia M, Albers JJ. Effects of lyophilization of serum on the measurement of apolipoproteins A-I and B. *Clin Chem* 1990;36:366−9.

65 Marcovina SM, Albers JJ, Dati F, Ledue TB, Ritchie RF. International Federation of Clinical Chemistry Standardization Project for measurements of apolipoproteins A-I and B. *Clin Chem* 1991;37:1676−82.

66 Marcovina SM, Albers JJ. Apolipoprotein assays: standardization and quality control. *Scand J Clin Lab Invest Suppl* 1990;198:58−65.

67 Donahue RP, Jacobs DR Jr, Sidney S *et al.* Distribution of lipoproteins and apolipoproteins in young adults. *Arteriosclerosis* 1989;9:656−64.

68 Vega GL, Grundy SM. Does measurement of apolipoprotein B have a place in cholesterol management? *Arteriosclerosis* 1990;10:668−71.

69 Parra H-J, Luyeye I, Bouramoue C, Demarquilly C, Fruchart J-C. Black−white differences in serum Lp(a) lipoprotein levels. *Clin Chim Acta* 1987;167:27−31.

70 Labeur C, Michiels G, Bury J, Usher DC, Rosseneu M. Lipoprotein(a) quantified by an enzyme-linked immunosorbent assay with monoclonal antibodies. *Clin Chem* 1989;35:1380−4.

Chapter 13 —————————————————————————
The Genetics of Premature Coronary Atherosclerosis

JOHN C. CHAMBERLAIN & DAVID J. GALTON

Introduction

For such a major cause of death in Western society the etiology of coronary atherosclerosis is surprisingly obscure. There would appear to be no one agent responsible for all atherosclerotic disease and premature coronary atherosclerosis would seem to be a multifactorial disorder under the influence of both genetic and environmental factors.

The aggregation of premature coronary artery disease (CAD) within families is well known [1]. In 1966 Slack and Evans analyzed first degree relatives of 121 men and 96 women with CAD [2] and showed the increased risk of death from CAD in these relatives. Since then many excellent studies have confirmed this trend [3,4] and further evidence comes from twin studies showing the concordance rates for angina pectoris or myocardial infarction in monozygotic twins to be higher than for dizygotic twins (0.65 vs. 0.25) [5]. If twins with premature CAD appearing before age 60 years are alone considered these differences are then even more marked (0.83 vs. 0.22) [6].

The use of linkage markers in the analysis of polygenic disease

One of the major problems of understanding polygenic disorders such as atherosclerosis is to distinguish between the inherited and secondary components of the disease. Before the advent of recombinant DNA technology there were no means to identify a mutant gene unless it produced a variant protein. Now there is a possibility of directly studying the genes thought to be involved in the etiology of the disorder (the so-called candidate genes) without recourse to a phenotypic intermediate.

The modes of inheritance of premature atherosclerosis are, if we exclude the rarer monogenic disorders, complex and multifactorial, with inherited "susceptibility" genes interacting with environmental factors to produce the phenotypic disease. Only when genetic liability coincides with environmental risk factors does the disease phenotype emerge.

Realizing this can help to explain the more puzzling features of the genetics of atherosclerosis. Its relatively high incidence may for example be due to the fact that under more favorable and natural environmental conditions the susceptibility genes are under no selective disadvantage and may instead offer other secondary advantages. In the face of such complexities the failure of classical genetics to elucidate recognizable patterns of inheritance is not surprising.

Our eventual goal must be the identification of these susceptibility loci for atherosclerosis and the quantification of their effect and environmental interaction, in the hope of predicting an individual's relative risk of developing the phenotypic disease.

Candidate genes

Defining the etiology of a polygenic disease is a straightforward but laborious task. The essential question is: Which of the 1.4 million potential genes that make up the human genome are involved in the pathogenesis of the disease being studied? Answers are usually achieved by either or both of two differing but complementary techniques.

1   *Candidate gene targeting.* This assumes that those genes known to code for a protein suspected as being involved with the disease pathology are the most worthy of study. In the case of atherosclerosis this might involve concentrating on a gene producing a protein known to be central to lipid metabolism, on the assumption that hyperlipidemia represents an intermediate phenotype for the development of atheroma, searching for mutation at that locus, and then examining for allelic association at that site with the disease.

2   *Complete genomic mapping.* This is based on the production of complementary DNA (cDNA) and genomic DNA (gDNA) libraries, which allow the isolation of random unique DNA fragments with regular spacing along each and every chromosome and the subsequent use of these fragments as hybridization probes to detect polymorphism within the genome. Pedigree studies may then be pursued using these alleles and should any disease association be found the gene fragment can be mapped to the genome and the underlying etiologic mutation tracked down by "walking" along the chromosomal segment with further probes [7].

Genetics of atherosclerosis

The identification of candidate genes for atherosclerosis has thus been based on data regarding proteins thought to be implicated in

Table 13.1 Candidate genes for atherosclerosis

Phenotype	Protein	Chromosomal location	PIC
Lipoproteins	Apolipoproteins		
	A-I−C-III−A-IV	11q23-24	0.73/0.36/0.55
	E−C-I−C-II	19q13	0.36/0.28/0.79
	B	2p24-23	0.66
Receptors	LDL receptor	19p13	0.60
	Remnant receptor	—	—
	Insulin receptor	19p13	0.80
Enzymes	LCAT	16q22	—
	CETP	—	—
	Lipoprotein lipase	8p22	0.57
Vessel/wall proteins	Fibronectin	2p34-36	0.36
	Collagen	17q21-22	0.43
Growth factors	PDGF B	22q12-13	0.37
	PDGF A	7p21-p22 or 7q11-12	—
	EGF	—	—
	Insulin	11p15	0.57
Coagulation factors	Fibrinogen A	4q28	0.34
	Fibrinogen B	4q28	0.28
	Prothrombin	—	—
	Factor VII	13q34	—

PIC, polymorphism information content, which is a function of genotype heterozygosity and allele frequencies at a particular locus, LCAT, lecithin cholesterol acyltransferase, CETP, cholesteryl ester transfer protein; PDGF, platelet-derived growth factor; EGF, epidermal growth factor.

atherogenesis. Examples of such include the apolipoproteins, the low-density lipoprotein (LDL) receptor, and many others. A list of such candidate genes is presented in Table 13.1. Some of those showing protein polymorphism have already been studied with regard to associations with atherosclerosis.

Protein polymorphism

APOLIPOPROTEIN E

Apolipoprotein (apo) E is a 34-kDa protein constituent of several plasma lipoproteins, which serves as a high-affinity ligand for the LDL receptor. The apo E gene is known to be located on chromosome 19, linked to several apolipoprotein genes in a 50-kb cluster [8]. Its well described protein polymorphism has three common alleles known as E-II, E-III, and

Table 13.2 Apo E polymorphisms

Apo E alleles	Protein	Polymorphism
E-II	Apo E-II (arg-158 to cys)	Receptor-binding activity <2% of apo E-III
E-III	Apo E-III	—
E-IV	Apo E-IV (cys-112 to arg)	E-nhanced *in vivo* catabolism

Frequencies of alleles of apo E-

Apo E- alleles

	Finland[1] (n = 408)	Finland[2] (n = 615)	Japan (n = 319)
E-II	0.029	0.041	0.081
E-III	0.750	0.733	0.849
E-IV	0.221	0.227	0.067
	Germany[1] (n = 1031)	Germany[2] (n = 1000)	USA (n = 152)
E-II	0.077	0.078	0.120
E-III	0.773	0.783	0.760
E-IV	0.150	0.139	0.110
	Canada (n = 102)	New Zealand (n = 426)	Scotland (n = 400)
E-II	0.078	0.120	0.080
E-III	0.770	0.739	0.770
E-IV	0.152	0.141	0.150

[1,2] Represent distinct population samples from two different hospitals.

E-IV (Table 13.2) and a series of rarer alleles more often found in patients with Type III hyperlipidemia [9].

The three common isoforms are known to differ by specific amino acid replacements in two positions of the peptide chain and thus by their functional properties. For example, apo E-II (arg-158 to cys) is defective in binding to its lipoprotein receptors and thus, when homozygous, predisposes to Type III hyperlipidemia. Most E-II/E-II subjects, however, never develop hyperlipidemia, but on the contrary have subnormal plasma cholesterol levels (mean effect of −0.367 mmol/l) due to reduced concentrations of LDL. Conversely, subjects with the E-IV allele have a raised plasma cholesterol (+0.181 mmol/l). The apo E gene locus is claimed to account for 4% and 20% of the phenotypic variance of plasma cholesterol and apo E concentrations, respectively in German populations [10]. This is reflected in the differing levels of LDL cholesterol found among survivors of myocardial infarction with differing apo E phenotypes (apo E-III/E-IV 5.15 mmol/l ± 1.16 and apo E-II/E-III 4.21 mmol/l ± 1.29) [11]. Another study has examined polymorphism of apo E in relation to the risk of premature CAD [12]. The isotype frequencies were determined in a random sample of 400 people, aged 45–60 years, living in northeast Scotland and compared to those found in a group of survivors of myocardial infarction, aged less than 56 years, collected from diverse sources. The isotype mix E-IV/E-III was seen more frequently in the CAD group than in the controls at the expense of E-III/E-II (0.32 vs. 0.25 and 0.075 vs. 0.127) and for survivors aged under 60 years this heterogeneity was even more marked.

Comparison of the average age of first myocardial infarction in male survivors also suggested that this may have occurred earlier in those of phenotype E-IV/E-III (E-III/E-III 53.95 ± 0.68, E-IV/E-III 51.20 ± 0.98, E-III/E-II 53.21 ± 2.02). This does raise the possibility that the E-IV allele may play a role in the etiology of premature coronary heart disease (CHD) but the frequency of alternate phenotypes among the survivors of myocardial infarction could also be explained as arising from a reduced survival of infarction in the subjects with alternate phenotypes.

Lp(a) LIPOPROTEIN

The Lp(a) antigen was originally described almost 30 years ago, using heterologous rabbit antibodies raised against human high-density lipoprotein (HDL) cholesterol [13]. Essentially, it appears to consist of an LDL particle in which the apo B_{100} moiety is linked by a disulfide bond to apo(a), a glycoprotein with some structural homology to plasminogen [14]. Lp(a) is a heterogeneous molecule varying in size and density as the apo(a) moiety varies in size (from 280 to 700 kDa). This heterogeneity is explicable in terms of varying numbers of repeating domains with high homology to Kringle 4 of plasminogen and high internal homology [15] which comprise the bulk of the Lp(a) molecule [16]. The structure of these domains can also vary to a slight degree. Such variation is encoded by the apo(a) gene, found on chromosome 6 [17]. In addition to this hypervariable region apo(a) contains one kringle with homology to plasminogen Kringle 5. The protease domain of apo(a) has a 94% homology with that of plasminogen [15]. More than seven Lp(a) isoforms have been described to date and their size appears to be inversely related to the Lp(a) concentration in the plasma [18].

The cysteine involved in the disulfide linkage is thought to be located in Kringle 36 of apo(a) but where this linkage occurs and the other steps in the assembly of apo(a) are not currently known. The liver, however, is known to represent the major source of Lp(a) in the plasma and Lp(a) phenotypes are known to change after liver transplantation [19]. The mode of clearance of Lp(a) is also obscure, though it is thought to be at least in part dependent on the hepatic LDL receptor, as some workers have noted raised levels of Lp(a) in patients with familial hypercholesterolemia (FH).

The molecular heterogeneity of Lp(a) and its similarity to plasminogen greatly complicates its effective assay, raising difficulties for clinical studies. Although the most reliable assay for Lp(a), the enzyme-linked immunosorbent assay (ELISA) technique, appears to be free of interference by plasminogen, few clinical studies have yet made use of this. Studies using other less reliable methods of assay have shown that in case-control studies Lp(a) levels of more than approximately 30 mg/dl are associated with an increased risk of myocardial or cerebrovascular infarction [20,21]. A recent study has shown that individuals with a plasma concentration of greater than 25 mg/dl exhibit a twofold higher risk of myocardial infarction than controls [22]. Apo(a) alleles resulting in a raised level of Lp(a) in the individual also appear to associate strongly with CHD [23].

As to the mechanism of this association, it has been suggested that Lp(a) may be affecting the fibrinolytic system and blocking the action of plasminogen thus predisposing to thrombogenesis. This possibility is suggested by the structural homologies between plasminogen and Lp(a). It should, however, be noted that apo(a) contains mainly the Kringle 4 domain of plasminogen which is known to bind fibrin only weakly, unlike Kringle 1 domains. The issue is complicated by the existence of many variant forms of Kringle 4 within Lp(a) molecules and the varying numbers of these units. There is a strong possibility that the larger isoforms of Lp(a) may have differing effects from the smaller ones. All isoforms of Lp(a) need to be studied before the thrombogenic potential of Lp(a) can be assessed and this is a prerequisite to assessing the atherogenic role of the apolipoprotein.

Genetic polymorphism

Alongside this information about protein polymorphism has begun to emerge a parallel body of data relating to genetic polymorphisms and atherosclerosis.

APO A-I–C-III–A-IV GENE CLUSTER

These three genes are congregated on the long arm of chromosome 11, covering a segment of DNA of approximately 4 kb in length [24,25]. The organization of the cluster shows the following features.

1   The apo C-III gene is transcribed in the opposite direction to the apo

A-I and A-IV genes despite their proximity.

2 More than nine restriction enzyme dimorphisms occur within the cluster [26,27]. Many population studies have been performed examining the frequencies of alleles at these restriction sites to examine for association with premature CAD and its lipoprotein intermediates and the results are discussed below.

UK

Two groups of patients have been studied, young survivors of myocardial infarction [28] and patients with coronary and extracoronary atheroma demonstrated by angiography [29]. In the former group the frequency of an uncommon allele (the S2 allele) at the *Sst*I restriction site, within the fourth exon of the apo C-III gene, was approximately 4% in healthy controls ($n = 47$) compared to 21% in young survivors of myocardial infarction ($n = 48$). When other restriction site polymorphisms were included in the analysis, thereby constructing DNA haplotypes [30], it was found that one particular haplotype containing the uncommon allele at both the *Msp*I and *Sst*I site was increased from 2% in normolipemic controls ($n = 48$) to 21% in survivors of myocardial infarction ($n = 47$) giving a relative incidence of 12.7 ($p < 0.01$). It was not, however, possible to identify haplotypes with any greater association with premature CAD than the S2 allele alone. In a study from Edinburgh, looking at 713 men aged 30–59 years [31], the *Sst*I site S2 allele, combined with rare alleles at the *Xmn*I, *Pst*I, and *Msp*I sites, showed an increased frequency in patients with coronary atherosclerosis who had a positive family history of the disease, as compared to those without a family history (relative incidence 3.34, $p < 0.0005$).

Since atherosclerosis has a variable age of onset, control groups may contain individuals who will later go on to develop the disease. For example, the frequency of the S2 allele in the control group for the Scottish study was 18% ($n = 64$) as compared to 4% for the London-based studies ($n = 47$). This may of course represent a real difference in allelic frequencies of the restriction fragment length polymorphism (RFLP) between ethnically differing populations but it may merely represent the differences in selection criteria applied to create the two groups (i.e., presence or absence of hyperlipidemia or other risk factors for CHD).

In the light of such considerations particular weight may be laid on studies providing for angiographic assessment in both patient and control groups. In one such study by Rees *et al.* the frequency of the rarer S2 allele of the *Sst*I site was found to be 22% in patients with severe obstructive coronary atheroma ($n = 61$) as compared to 6% in subjects with minimal disease ($n = 68$, $p <0.02$) [29].

Analysis of this group, including a fifth restriction site as revealed with PvuII, allowed the identification of a group of rare haplotypes based on the minor alleles of these polymorphisms which even after adjustment for major risk factors such as age, smoking, social class, blood pressure, lipids, and apolipoproteins was associated with a higher familial prevalence of CHD (relative incidence 2.73, $p <0.023$) [32].

Caution must, however, be exercised in attempting to interpret these results, as CAD is not a disease of homogeneous pathology, nor are such population groups free from ethnic heterogeneity. To achieve the best results the patient groups must be clearly defined and standardized as much as is possible with regard to racial origin and clinical diagnostic features.

Such associations of markers at the apo A-I–C-III–A-IV gene cluster with CAD are supported by a recent study looking at families with very carefully defined familial combined hyperlipidemia, a known phenotypic intermediate for premature coronary atherosclerosis [33]. In this instance familial combined hyperlipidemia was defined on the basis of an existing proband with two fasting plasma cholesterol and triglyceride values greater than the 95th centile for the population, with at least one other first degree relative with two fasting plasma cholesterol and/or triglyceride values similarly raised. Significant association was found between the rarer X2 (6.6 kb) allele of the XmnI restriction polymorphism and the disease phenotype ($p <0.012$).

USA

Studies from Boston, Seattle, and New York have been reported. In the first [34], Caucasian patients ($n = 88$) with severe CAD were compared to a Framingham control population ($n = 64$) matched for ethnic origin and with other clinical criteria carefully standardized. The frequency of the uncommon allele revealed by the enzyme PstI at a restriction site 34 bp 3' to the apo A-I gene was 32% in patients compared with 4% in the controls ($p <0.01$) and 3% in 30 subjects with no angiographic evidence of CAD, giving a relative risk of at least 10. The same rare allele was found at increased frequency in subjects with familial hypoalphalipoproteinemia. Frequencies of alleles at other polymorphic sites at this locus were not reported. In Seattle, however, frequencies of alleles revealed by PstI were found to be similar in random normal groups and patient groups with CAD defined by angiography ($n = 140$) [35]. The background frequency of the allele P2 was, however, markedly different from that reported in the Boston study. Clearly this kind of discrepancy would tend to minimize observable disease associations. *Sst*I alleles compared in the same Seattle study were found to differ significantly (p <0.05) between controls and patients (S2 allele, 0.06 vs. 0.12, $n = 101$ and $n = 140$, respectively).

Germany

A study from Munster [11] examined eight polymorphic sites at the apo A-I—C-III—A-IV gene cluster. These included those of the restriction enzymes *Apa*I, *Msp*I, *Pst*I, *Bam*II, and *Pvu*II. Pseudohaplotypes were constructed for 314 patients suffering from premature CAD (myocardial infarct before age 45) and compared with those of 267 student controls. Given considerations of the age of expression of the disease phenotype in atherosclerosis and the importance of group homogeneity, the similar allelic frequencies reported in the respective study groups may not exclude association between these linkage markers and atherosclerosis.

Japan

A study from northern Japan compared 69 subjects surviving myocardial infarction with 82 controls. The haplotype S1-M2 was significantly increased in the patient group (0.24 vs. 0.11, p <0.05). As might be expected control frequencies differed markedly from caucasoid norms.

Kuwait

A study from Kuwait compared the frequency of the *Sst*I polymorphism of the apo C-III gene in 79 Arab patients with proven myocardial infarction and in both 75 age- and sex-matched healthy controls and 34 normotriglyceridemic controls. Once again the S2 allelic frequency was raised in the patient group as compared with either control group (0.25 vs. 0.11 and 0.01; p <0.005 and p <0.01, respectively) [36].

All the studies examined here, apart from the Munster study, seem to support the hypothesis that within the apo A-I—C-III—A-IV gene cluster there exists an etiologic locus for atherosclerosis which accounts for several linkage disequilibrium phenomena observable with different RFLPs in separate and unique populations. This linkage disequilibrium is illustrated for the most studied RFLP, the *Sst*I site, in Table 13.3. The varying degree of association observed would be in keeping with a situation in which linkage with a separate etiologic mutation underlies the reported associations. The association of differing linkage markers

Table 13.3 *Sst*I allele frequencies

	Allelic frequencies			
	n	S1	S2	References
Control groups				
Random medical outpatients	37	0.96	0.04	Rees *et al.* [26]
Health screen clinics				
Sample 1	42	1.0	0.00	Rees *et al.* [29]
Sample 2	74	0.98	0.02	Ferns *et al.* [28]
Sample 3	56	0.98	0.02	O'Connor *et al.* [56]
Normal coronary arteries	68	0.97	0.03	Rees *et al.* [29]
Random medical outpatients	35	0.99	0.01	Trembath *et al.* [57]
Normolipidemic controls	71	0.94	0.06	Kessling *et al.* [58]
Random normals	101	0.94	0.06	Deeb *et al.* [35]
Controls	66	0.98	0.02	Hegele *et al.* (unpublished)
Random normals (Arabic)	75	0.89	0.11	Tas [36]
Normotriglyceridemic (Arabic)	34	0.99	0.01	Tas [36]
Patient groups				
Hyperlipidemic (IV/V)	28	0.80	0.20	Rees *et al.* [26]
Survivors of MI	48	0.88	0.12	Ferns *et al.* [59]
Coronary atheroma	61	0.89	0.11	Rees *et al.* [29]
Peripheral atheroma	49	0.88	0.12	O'Connor *et al.* [56]
Diabetic survivors of MI	47	0.86	0.14	Trembath *et al.* [57]
Hyperlipidemia with gout	22	0.88	0.12	Ferns *et al.* [59]
CHD	140	0.88	0.12	Deeb *et al.* [35]
Survivors of MI	66	0.96	0.04	Hegele *et al.* (unpublished)
Survivors of MI (Arabic)	79	0.75	0.25	Tas [36]

MI, myocardial infarction; CHD, coronary heart disease.

for equivalent etiologic mutations occurring in differing populations has been well documented in other situations [37].

LDL RECEPTOR GENE

The elevation in LDL cholesterol resulting from FH is known to lead to premature CAD and this may account for up to 6% of myocardial infarction occurring before the age of 60 years [38]. The human LDL receptor gene has been cloned and localized to chromosome 19 and shown to consist of 18 exons, 13 of which have marked sequence homology to the genes for the C9 component of complement and for epidermal growth factor [39,40].

RFLP studies at this locus have demonstrated segregation with FH in several isolated families [41,42] and within certain well characterized hypercholesterolemic groups the defect underlying LDL receptor failure is known to be genetic and has been elucidated [43−45]. In certain instances this knowledge has led to homozygous FH patients being identified as possessing either similar or dissimilar gene defects on each parentally derived chromosome. Single gene defects can be often shown to account for high levels of FH present in populations with marked founder effects, such as the Quebecois, the Lebanese, and the Afrikaaners.

APO B GENE

The gene for human apo B has been cloned and localized to chromosome 2 in the region p24 [46,47]. It extends over 43 kb containing 29 exons and 28 introns. The distribution of these introns is somewhat asymmetric with most occurring in the 5′-terminal third of the gene. The sequence of the coding portion of the gene is known and the protein structure has been deduced from this [48]. A domain rich in basic amino acids has been identified as important for the cellular uptake of cholesterol by the LDL receptor pathway. Many RFLPs have been observed at the locus including those of the enzymes *Xba*I, *Eco*RI, and *Msp*I and several studies have addressed the question of possible disease associations. In one such UK study the allelic frequencies of the *Xba*I polymorphism were not noted to be significantly different in 52 survivors of myocardial infarction and 33 healthy controls [49]. This was also noted in a study in the USA where very similar allele frequencies were reported [35]. In this latter study there was, however, found to be a change in the frequency of an *Msp*I-revealed insertional−deletional polymorphism, which increased in frequency in patient groups (from 0.06 to 0.15, $n = 62$ and $n = 103$). This finding was supported in another study where the frequency of the insertional polymorphism was increased from 0.142 in controls to 0.267 in patients ($n = 84$ and $n = 84$) [50]. In addition the latter study reported an increased frequency of the rarer allele of the *Xba*I polymorphism in patients compared to controls. The authors concluded that such polymorphisms were acting as genetic markers in linkage disequilibrium with etiologic mutations nearby. A summary of the data regarding association of alleles at the *Xba*I restriction site and atherosclerosis is provided in Table 13.4. Genetic variants of the apo B gene have not yet been reported to consistently associate with the phenotypic intermediates of atheroma. The small fluctuations of allelic frequencies seen across the board for such linkage markers would seem to suggest a role for the apo B gene as an intermediate or minor gene for the development of premature CAD.

Table 13.4 Apo B mutation: frequency of the *Xba*I allelic variants in control and patient populations

	n	X1	X2	References
Control groups				
Controls	84	0.50	0.50	Hegele *et al.* [50]
Random normals	102	0.54	0.46	Deeb *et al.* [35]
Controls	52	0.48	0.52	Wiklund *et al.* [60]
Random normals	146	0.47	0.53	Myant *et al.* [61]
Controls	33	0.44	0.56	Ferns *et al.* [62]
Patient groups				
Survivors of MI	84	0.64	0.76	Hegele *et al.* [50]
CHD	117	0.50	0.50	Deeb *et al.* [35]
Survivors of MI	52	0.39	0.61	Wiklund *et al.* [60]
CHD	124	0.54	0.46	Myant *et al.* [61]
Survivors of MI	52	0.51	0.49	Ferns *et al.* [62]

MI, myocardial infarction; CHD, coronary heart disease.

LIPOPROTEIN LIPASE (LPL)

The gene for human lipoprotein lipase has been cloned and localized to chromosome 8 in the region p22 [51] and its gene product is known to play a central role in lipid catabolism, catalyzing the rate-limiting step in the removal of triglyceride-rich particles from the plasma. Two RFLP studies at this locus [52,53] have demonstrated a promising association with CAD for a polymorphic *Hind*III site thought to lie between exons 8 and 9 at the 3' end of the gene. The H2 allele associating with premature CAD would also appear to associate with the intermediate phenotype of hypertriglyceridemia in at least two separate populations (Caucasian and Japanese) [54]. The *Pvu*II site of LPL has been similarly associated with the variation of fasting plasma triglyceride in a random UK Caucasian population [54].

In support of this observation another linkage marker has recently been reported as associating with hypertriglyceridemia. In this case hypertriglyceridemia is seen to be associated with the absence of a premature stop codon in exon 9 of the LPL gene (C to G 1595), this premature stop codon being a common mutation in the Utah population under study (33% of controls) resulting in the synthesis of a truncated but seemingly fully active protein lacking the last two carboxy-terminal amino acids [55].

Although an excess of triglyceride-rich lipoproteins may not be an independent risk factor from HDL for the development of coronary atherosclerosis, the close metabolic interrelationship between HDL$_2$ and triglyceride makes it very difficult to evaluate their separate roles. Hypertriglyceridemia with low HDL would seem to constitute an important risk factor for the development of coronary atherosclerosis and this association of linkage markers at the LPL gene and both hyper-triglyceridemia and CAD suggests that this gene is a causal determinant of atherosclerosis, though its relative importance has yet to be assessed.

Conclusion

It would thus seem that atherosclerosis is an archetypal multifactorial disease with a strong genetic component. As the techniques of recombinant DNA technology are increasingly applied to its analysis the roles of linkage markers for the disease and intermediate lipoprotein phenotypes will hopefully become correspondingly well understood. A handful of genes, mostly those coding for the apolipoproteins and proteins associated with the metabolism of such apolipoproteins, have already been identified as minor or intermediate genes in the multigenic background of atherosclerosis; these include the apo E gene, the apo A-I−C-III−A-IV gene cluster, the LDL receptor gene, the apo B gene, and the gene for LPL. There remains, however, a great deal more of this genetic background to be studied in the search for possible major etiologic genes for premature atherosclerosis and CAD.

References

1 Yater WM, Traum AH, Brown WG et al. Coronary artery disease in men eighteen to thirty-nine years of age. Am Heart J 1948;36:334−72.
2 Slack J, Evans KA. The increased risk of death from ischaemic heart disease in first-degree relatives of 121 men and 96 women with ischaemic heart disease. J Med Genet 1966;3:239−57.
3 Rissanen AM. Familial aggregation of coronary heart disease in a high incidence area (North Karelia, Finland). Br Heart J 1979;42:294−303.
4 Nora JJ, Lortscher RH, Spangler RD. Genetic epidemiology study of early onset ischaemic heart disease. Circulation 1980;61:503−8.
5 Berg K. Twin studies of coronary heart disease and its risk factors. Acta Genet Med Gemellol Roma 1984;33:349−61.
6 Berg K. Genetics of coronary heart disease. Prog Med Genet 1983;5:36−9.
7 Wiessman SM. Molecular genetic techniques for mapping the human genome. Mol Biol Med 1987;4:133−43.
8 Lauer SJ, Walker DH, Elshourbagy NA et al. Two copies of the human apolipoprotein C-I gene are linked closely to the apolipoprotein E gene. J Biol Chem 1988;263:7277−86.
9 Utermann G, Hess M, Steinmetz A. Polymorphism of apolipoprotein E and occurrence of dysbetalipoproteinaemia in man. Nature 1977;269:604−7.
10 Utermann G. Apolipoproteins, quantitative lipoprotein traits and multifactorial hyperlipidaemia. Ciba Found Symp 1987;130:52.
11 Assmann G, Schulte H, Funke H, Schmitz G, Robenck H. High density lipoproteins and

atherosclerosis. In *Atherosclerosis VIII* (eds G Crepaldi, AM Gotto, E Manzato, G Baggio). Amsterdam: Elsevier, 1989:341–51.

12 Cumming AM, Robertson FW. Polymorphism at the apoprotein E locus in relation to risk of coronary disase. *Clin Genet* 1984;25:310.

13 Berg K. A new serum type system in man: The Lp- system. *Acta Pathol Microbiol Scand* 1963;59:369–82.

14 Scanu AM, Fless GM. Lp(a) a lipoprotein particle with atherogenic and thrombogenic potential. In *Atherosclerosis VIII* (eds G Crepaldi, AM Gotto, E Manzato, G Baggio). Amsterdam: Elsevier, 1989:189–91.

15 Tomlinson JE, McClean JW, Lawn RM. Rhesus monkey apolipoprotein (a): sequence, evolution and sites of synthesis. *J Biol Chem* 1989;264:5965–7.

16 Lindahl G, Gersdorf GE, Menzel HJ *et al.* Variation in the size of human apolipoprotein (a) is due to hypervariable region in the gene. *Hum Genet* 1990;84:563–7.

17 McClean JW, Tomlinson JE, Kuang WJ *et al.* cDNA sequence of human apolipoprotein (a) is homologous to plasminogen. *Nature* 1987;330:132–7.

18 Gavish D, Azrolan N, Breslow JL. Plasma Lp(a) concentration is inversely correlated with the ratio of Kringle IV/Kringle V encoding domains in the apo(a) gene. *J Clin Invest* 1989;84:2021–7.

19 Kraft HG, Menzel HJ, Hopplicher F, Vogel W, Utermann G. Changes of genetic apolipoprotein phenotypes caused by liver transplantations: implications for apolipoprotein synthesis. *J Clin Invest* 1989;83:137–42.

20 Kostner GM, Avogaro P, Gazzolato G, Marth E, Bittolobon G. Lipoprotein Lp(a) and the risk of myocardial infarction. *Atherosclerosis* 1981;38:51–61.

21 Armstrong VW, Walli AK, Sendel D. Isolation, characterization and uptake in human fibroblasts of an apo(a) free lipoprotein obtained on reduction of lipoprotein (a). *J Lipid Res* 1985;26:1314–17.

22 Kostner GM. Lipoprotein Lp(a) and HMG-CoA reductase inhibitors. In *Atherosclerosis VIII* (eds G Crepaldi, AM Gotto, E Manzato, G Baggio). Amsterdam: Elsevier, 1989:405–8.

23 Seed M, Hopplicher F, Reavely D *et al.* Relation of serum lipoprotein (a) concentration and apolipoprotein (a) phenotype to coronary heart disease in patients with FH. *N Engl J Med* 1990;322:1494–9.

24 Karathanasis SK, McPherson J, Zanthis VI, Breslow JL. Linkage of human apolipoprotein AI and CIII genes. *Nature* 1983;304:371–3.

25 Karathanasis SK. Apolipoprotein multigene family: tandem organisation of human apolipoprotein AI, CIII and AIV genes. *Proc Natl Acad Sci USA* 1985;82:6374–8.

26 Rees A, Shoulders CC, Stocks J, Galton DJ, Baralle FE. DNA polymorphism adjacent to the human apoprotein AI gene in relation to hypertriglyceridaemia. *Lancet* 1983;i:444–6.

27 Seilhammer JJ, Protter AA, Frossard P, Levy-Wilson B. Isolation and DNA sequence of full length cDNA of the entire gene for human apolipoprotein AI. Discovery of a new genetic polymorphism. *DNA* 1984;3:309–17.

28 Ferns GA, Stocks J, Ritchie C, Galton DJ. Genetic polymorphisms of apolipoprotein C-II and insulin in survivors of myocardial infarction. *Lancet* 1985;ii:300–3.

29 Rees A, Jowett NI, Williams LG *et al.* DNA polymorphisms flanking the insulin and apolipoprotein CIII genes and atherosclerosis. *Atherosclerosis* 1985;58:269.

30 Ferns GA, Galton DJ. Haplotypes of the human apoprotein AI–CIII–AIV gene cluster in coronary atherosclerosis. *Hum Genet* 1986;73:245–9.

31 Price WH, Morris SW, Kitchin AH *et al.* DNA restriction fragment length polymorphisms as markers of familial coronary artery disease. *Lancet* 1989;i:1407–11.

32 Price WH, Morris SW, Kitchin AH *et al.* Genetic markers of familial coronary heart disease. *Lancet* 1990;336:629.

33 Wojciechowski AP, Farall M, Cullen P *et al.* Familial combined hyperlipidaemia linked to the apolipoprotein AI–CIII–AIV gene cluster on chromosome 11q23-q24. *Nature*

1991;349:161−4.

34 Ordovas JM, Schaeffer EJ, Salem D *et al.* Apolipoprotein A-I gene polymorphism associated with premature coronary artery disease and familial hypoalphalipoproteinaemia. *N Engl J Med* 1986;314:671−7.

35 Deeb S, Failor A, Brown BG *et al.* Molecular genetics of apolipoproteins and coronary heart disease. *Cold Spring Harbor Symp Quant Biol* 1987;51:403−9.

36 Tas S. Genetic predisposition to coronary heart disease and gene for apolipoprotein-CIII. *Lancet* 1991;337:113.

37 Humphries SE, Williams LG, Myklebost O *et al.* Familial apolipoprotein CII deficiency: a preliminary analysis of the gene defect in two independent families. *Hum Genet* 1984; 65:151−5.

38 Goldstein JL, Hazzard WR, Schrott HG. Hyperlipidaemia in coronary heart disease. Lipid levels in 500 survivors of myocardial infarction. *J Clin Invest* 1973;52:1533−43.

39 Sudhof TC, Goldstein JL, Brown MS, Russell DW. The LDL receptor gene: a mosaic of exons shared with different proteins. *Science* 1985;228:815−22.

40 Francke U, Brown MS, Goldstein JL, Assignment of the human gene for the low density lipoprotein receptor to chromosome 19: Synteny of a receptor, a ligand and a genetic disease. *Proc Natl Acad Sci USA* 1986;81:2826−30.

41 Humphries SE, Kessling AM, Hortshemke B *et al.* A common DNA polymorphism of the LDL receptor gene and its use in diagnosis. *Lancet* 1985;i:1003−5.

42 Leppert MF, Hasstedt SJ, Holm T *et al.* A DNA probe for the LDL receptor gene is tightly linked to hypercholesterolaemia in a pedigree with early coronary disease. *Am J Hum Genet* 1986;39:300−6.

43 Tolleshaug H, Hobgood KK, Brown MS, Goldstein JL. The LDL receptor locus in familial hypercholesterolaemia. Multiple mutations disrupt the transport and processing of a membrane receptor. *Cell* 1983;32:941−51.

44 Lehrmann MA, Schneider WJ, Sudhof TC *et al.* Mutation in LDL receptor: Alu-Alu recombination deletes exons encoding transmembrane and cytoplasmic domains. *Science* 1985;227:140−6.

45 Hortshemke B, Kessling AM, Seed M *et al.* Identification of a deletion in the low density lipoprotein (LDL) receptor gene in a patient with familial hypercholesterolaemia. *Hum Genet* 1985;71:75−8.

46 Knott TJ, Rall SC Jr, Innerarity TL *et al.* Human apolipoprotein B: structure of carboxy-terminal domain sites of gene expression and chromosomal localisation. *Science* 1985;230:37−43.

47 Shoulders CC, Myant N, Sidoli A *et al.* Molecular cloning of human LDL apolipoprotein B cDNA. *Atherosclerosis* 1985;58:277−89.

48 Knott TJ, Pease RJ, Powell LM *et al.* Human apolipoprotein B: complete cDNA sequence and identification of domains of the protein. *Nature* 1986;323:734−8.

49 Ferns GA, Galton DJ. Frequency of the *Xba* I polymorphisms of the apolipoprotein B gene in myocardial infarct survivors. *Lancet* 1986;II:572.

50 Hegele RA, Huang LS, Herbert AN *et al.* Apolipoprotein B-gene DNA polymorphisms associated with myocardial infarction. *N Engl J Med* 1986;315:1509−15.

51 Sparkes RS, Zollman S, Klisak I *et al.* Human genes involved in lipolysis of plasma lipoproteins: mapping of loci for lipoprotein lipase to 8p22 and hepatic lipase to 15q21. *Genomics* 1987;1:138−44.

52 Thorn J, Chamberlain JC, Stocks J, Galton DJ. RFLPs at the lipoprotein lipase and hepatic lipase gene loci in coronary atherosclerosis. *Atherosclerosis* 1989;79:94.

53 Chamberlain JC, Thorn JA, Morgan R *et al.* A linkage marker at the human lipoprotein lipase gene locus associates with coronary atherosclerosis in a Welsh population. *Adv Med Exp Biol* 1991;285:275−9.

54 Chamberlain JC, Thorn JA, Oka K, Galton DJ, Stocks J. DNA polymorphisms at the lipoprotein lipase gene: associations in normal and hypertriglyceridaemic subjects. *Atherosclerosis* 1989;79:85−91.

55 Hata A, Robertson M, Emi M, Lalouel J-M. Direct detection and automated sequencing of alleles after electrophoretic strand separation: identification of a common nonsense mutation in exon 9 of the human lipoprotein lipase gene. *Nucleic Acids Res* 1990;18:5407−11.

56 O'Connor G, Stocks J, Lumley J, Galton DJ. A DNA polymorphism of the apolipoprotein C-III gene in extracoronary atherosclerosis. *Clin Sci* 1988;74:289−92.

57 Trembath RC, Thomas DJ, Hendra TJ *et al.* Deoxyribonucleic acid polymorphism of the apolipoprotein AI-CIII-AIV gene cluster and coronary heart disease in non-insulin dependant diabetics. *Br Med J Clin Res* 1987;294:1577−8.

58 Kessling AM, Horsthemke B, Humphries SE. A study of DNA polymorphisms around the human apolipoprotein AI gene in hyperlipidaemic and normal individuals. *Clin Genet* 1985;28:296−306.

59 Ferns GA, Lanham J, Dieppe P, Galton DJ. A DNA polymorphism of an apoprotein gene associates with the hypertriglyceridaemia of primary gout. *Hum Genet* 1988;78:55−9.

60 Wiklund O, Damfors C, Bjursell G *et al.* Xba I restriction fragment length polymorphism of apolipoprotein B in Swedish myocardial infarction patients. *Eur Clin Invest* 1989;19:255−8.

61 Myant NB, Gallagher J, Barbir M *et al.* Restriction fragment length polymorphisms in the apo B gene in relation to coronary artery disease. *Atherosclerosis* 1989;77:193−201.

62 Ferns GA, Galton DJ. Frequency of the Xba I polymorphism of the apolipoprotein B gene in myocardial infarct survivors. *Lancet* 1986;2:572.

Section IV
Therapy

Chapter 14
Therapy of Hypercholesterolemia

D. ROGER ILLINGWORTH

Treatment of patients identified to have hyperlipidemia is directed at modifying plasma concentrations of lipoproteins with two goals: (i) to reduce the plasma concentrations of known atherogenic lipoproteins, particularly low-density lipoproteins (LDL), very low-density lipoprotein (VLDL) remnants, and Lp(a); and (ii) to potentially increase plasma concentrations of high-density lipoproteins (HDL), thereby exerting a favorable effect upon lipid deposition in the arterial wall. Treatment of patients with increased plasma concentration of triglyceride-rich lipoproteins (chylomicrons and VLDL) aims to prevent the development of hepatomegaly, splenomegaly, and other adverse sequelae from chylomicronemia, as well as to reduce the long-term risks of atherosclerosis. In this chapter, the author will focus on the therapy of patients identified to have increased plasma concentrations of LDL, VLDL remnants, and Lp(a); the treatment of combined hyperlipidemia and hypertriglyceridemic disorders will be discussed in Chapter 15.

Criteria for the diagnosis of hypercholesterolemia

Epidemiologic studies have demonstrated that lipid and lipoprotein concentrations vary among different populations, but are generally highest in those countries which consume a "Western diet" and lowest in those countries where the habitual consumption of fat and cholesterol is low [1]. There is general agreement [2] that plasma concentrations of total and LDL cholesterol in North America and western Europe are too high, and that a downward shift in the population mean would have a substantial impact on the development of coronary atherosclerosis. Indeed, the majority of cases of coronary heart disease occur in patients with plasma cholesterol concentrations between 200 and 270 mg/dl (5.2–7 mmol/l) and up to one-third of cases occur [3] in patients with total plasma cholesterol concentrations less than 200 mg/dl (5.2 mmol/l).

The National Cholesterol Education Program (NCEP) Expert Panel on Detection, Evaluation, and Treatment of high blood cholesterol in adults [4] has advocated the determination of total blood cholesterol

Table 14.1 Initial classification and recommended follow-up based on total blood cholesterol

Classification	Recommended follow-up
Desirable blood cholesterol <200 mg/dl	*Repeat within 5 years* Total cholesterol <200 mg/dl
Borderline-high blood cholesterol 200–239 mg/dl *High blood cholesterol* ≥240 mg/dl	*Dietary information; and recheck annually* Total cholesterol 200–239 mg/dl Without definite CHD or two other CHD risk factors (one of which can be male sex) *Lipoprotein analysis; further action based on LDL cholesterol level* Total cholesterol ≥240 mg/dl With definite CHD or two other CHD risk factors (one of which can be male sex)

CHD, coronary heart disease.

concentrations in every adult with a goal of identifying those at high risk. Recommended follow-up based upon initial determinations of a total serum cholesterol concentration is outlined in Table 14.1. The NCEP report [4] follows up on the recommendations of the 1985 Consensus Conference on lowering blood cholesterol to prevent heart disease [2] which recommended that severe hypercholesterolemia requiring diet and potentially drug therapy be considered to be present if cholesterol concentrations exceeded the 90th percentile for age. Moderate hypercholesterolemia was defined as serum cholesterol concentrations between the 75th and 90th percentiles. In contrast to the Consensus Conference report [2] the NCEP Panel as well as other expert panels in Europe [5], UK [6], and Canada [7] have defined more specific cutpoints for the diagnosis of hypercholesterolemia in adults, and have suggested that the primary target of therapy be directed at elevated levels of LDL cholesterol. Table 14.2 illustrates the recommended levels for consideration of diet and potentially drug therapy for individuals identified to have elevated levels of LDL cholesterol [4]. The NCEP Panel [4] has advocated a more aggressive approach to lipid-lowering therapy in patients with evidence of atherosclerosis, or those who have two or more known cardiovascular risk factors; in such patients, drug therapy may be considered when the LDL cholesterol concentration exceeds 160 mg/dl (4.2 mmol/l) on maximum dietary therapy. In patients who do not have evidence for coronary or peripheral vascular disease, the NCEP Panel advocated a therapeutic goal of under 160 mg/dl for LDL cholesterol, whereas in individuals with atherosclerosis or those with

Table 14.2 Classification and treatment decisions based on LDL cholesterol

Classification	Dietary treatment	Drug treatment
Desirable LDL cholesterol <130 mg/dl	*Initiation level* ≥160 mg/dl Without CHD or two other risk factors* ≥130 mg/dl With CHD or two other risk factors*	*Initiation level* ≥190 mg/dl Without CHD or two other risk factors* ≥160 mg/dl With CHD or two other risk factors*
Borderline-high-risk LDL cholesterol 130–159 mg/dl		
High-risk LDL cholesterol >160 mg/dl		
	Minimal goal <160 mg/dl† Without CHD or two other risk factors <130 mg/dl‡ With CHD or two other risk factors	*Minimal goal* <160 mg/dl Without CHD or two other risk factors* <130 mg/dl With CHD or two other risk factors*

* Patients have a lower initiation level and goal if they are at high risk because they already have definite coronary heart disease (CHD), or because they have any two of the following risk factors: male sex, family history of premature CHD, cigarette smoking, hypertension, low HDL cholesterol, diabetes mellitus, definite cerebrovascular or peripheral vascular disease, or severe obesity.
† Roughly equivalent to total cholesterol <240 mg/dl as goal for monitoring dietary treatment.
‡ Roughly equivalent to total cholesterol <200 mg/dl as goal for monitoring dietary treatment.

two other cardiovascular risk factors a lower level of LDL cholesterol (<130 mg/dl, 3.4 mmol/l) is considered desirable. Concentrations of LDL cholesterol below 100 mg/dl (2.5 mmol/l) may be necessary for the regression of atherosclerosis to occur in humans [8,9].

Evaluation of the patient with hypercholesterolemia

Increased levels of plasma cholesterol in the setting of normal triglyceride concentrations are usually attributable to an increased number of LDL particles in plasma. Less frequently, however, hypercholesterolemia may reflect cholestasis, in which an abnormal lipoprotein termed Lp(X) accumulates in plasma, or may be seen in patients with atypically high concentrations of Lp(a). The importance of establishing the causal factor(s) responsible for hypercholesterolemia in a given patient cannot be overemphasized; the characterization of and distinction between primary and secondary causes of hypercholesterolemia is paramount if a treatable secondary disorder is not to be overlooked. Evaluation of the patient with hypercholesterolemia should therefore include satisfactory exclusion of potentially treatable secondary factors (e.g., hypothyroidism), a detailed family history, and a careful clinical examination looking for characteristic physical findings. Increased concentrations of LDL cholesterol and normal triglyceride levels result from either an increase in the synthesis of LDL, as occurs in patients with familial combined hyperlipidemia, or from decreases in the rate of LDL catabolism, as occur in patients with either familial hyper-cholesterolemia (FH) or familial defective apoprotein (apo) B [10]. In addition to these disorders, many patients with modest primary hypercholesterolemia will not be genotypically definable, and are best characterized as having "polygenic hypercholesterolemia." Patients with heterozygous FH, which is inherited as an autosomal dominant trait with complete phenotypic expression in childhood, typically have two-to fourfold elevations in the plasma concentrations of LDL cholesterol, and total cholesterol concentrations range between 280 and 500 mg/dl (7.3–13 mmol/l). The high incidence of premature coronary artery disease in patients with FH is well documented [11] and appears to be further increased in families who concurrently have increased plasma concentrations of Lp(a) [12]. Biochemically, FH results from genetic mutations at the LDL receptor locus [11] and heterozygous patients have a 50% reduction in the number of high-affinity LDL receptors expressed on hepatic and peripheral cells which is responsible for the reduced fractional catabolic rate of LDL seen in this disorder. A reduction in LDL catabolism is also characteristically seen in patients with familial defective apo B, in which a single amino acid substitution of glutamine for arginine at position 3500 in apo B results in an apo B_{100} molecule with an impaired ability to bind to the LDL receptor [13]. In contrast to patients with FH, patients who are heterozygous for familial defective apo B have two populations of LDL particles in their plasma, one with normal and the other with defective binding properties to the LDL receptor. Some patients with this disorder have moderate hypercholesterolemia [13] but others may present with a phenotype similar to that seen in patients with FH including the presence of tendon xanthomas.

Familial combined hyperlipidemia, an autosomal dominant inherited trait, is characterized by an inherent overproduction of VLDL and LDL by the liver and different family members may present with increased levels of LDL, combined elevations of VLDL and LDL, or single elevations in the concentrations of VLDL. In contrast to FH, patients with familial combined hyperlipidemia do not typically have tendon xanthomas and there are no characteristic physical findings which alert the physician to this disorder. In many patients it is not possible to establish a precise

Table 14.3 The influence of drugs on plasma lipids and lipoproteins

Drug	Total chol	TG	LDL-Chol	HDL-Chol	Reference
	Lipid/lipoprotein				
Corticosteroids	↑	↑↑	±↑	±↑	[14]
Estrogens	↑	↑	↓	↑	[15]
Progestins	±↑	±↑	±↑	↓	[16]
Androgens	↓	±	±↑	↓	[17]
β-Blockers (without ISI)	↑	↑	±↑	↓	[18,19]
Thiazide diuretics	↑	↑	±↑	↓	[18,19]
Vitamin A derivatives	±↑	↑↑	↓	↓	[20,21]
Cimetidine	±↑	↑	↓	↓	[22]
Cyclosporine	↑	—	↑	—	[23]
Phenytoin	↑	—	—	↑	[24]
Barbiturates	↑	—	—	↑	[24]

TG, triglycerides; chol, cholesterol; ISI, intrinsic sympathomimetic activity.

genotypic diagnosis, and in discussing the treatment of primary hypercholesterolemia, no distinction will be made between the treatment of patients with familial combined hyperlipidemia who have a single elevation in LDL cholesterol concentrations and patients with polygenic causes of hypercholesterolemia. Treatment of patients with combined hyperlipidemia attributable to familial combined hyperlipidemia is discussed further in Chapter 15

In addition to endocrine, renal, and hepatic disorders which may result in secondary causes of hyperlipidemia, plasma concentrations of lipids and lipoproteins may also be influenced by a number of prescription drugs (Table 14.3) and it is important to consider these as potentially exacerbating causes of hyperlipidemia in a given patient.

Dietary treatment of hypercholesterolemia

Dietary restriction of saturated fats, cholesterol and, in patients who are overweight, total calories, represents the initial therapy for all patients with hypercholesterolemia including those who concurrently require drug therapy. Dietary therapy may be particularly effective in patients with Type III hyperlipidemia if they are overweight. In patients with primary hypercholesterolemia, dietary changes are aimed at reducing plasma concentrations of LDL cholesterol; dietary manipulations exert their lipid-lowering effects, alone or in combination, by either reducing the hepatic synthesis of VLDL and LDL or increasing the expression of hepatic LDL receptors with a concurrent stimulation in the rate of LDL

Table 14.4 Dietary therapy of hypercholesterolemia. (From [4])

Nutrient	Step-One Diet	Step-Two Diet
Total fat*	Less than 30%	Less than 30%
Fatty acids*		
Saturated	Less than 10%	Less than 7%
Polyunsaturated	Up to 10%	Up to 10%
Monounsaturated	10–15%	10–15%
Carbohydrates*	50–60%	50–60%
Protein*	10–20%	10–20%
Cholesterol	Less than 300 mg/day	Less than 200 mg/day
Total calories	To achieve and maintain desirable weight	To achieve and maintain desirable weight

* Percent of total calories.

removal from plasma. Hepatic LDL receptors are decreased by dietary saturated fatty acids and cholesterol [25,26]. The principal dietary modifications needed to reduce plasma LDL cholesterol concentrations involve decreased intakes of total fat (with a particular emphasis on the saturated fat content) and cholesterol and, in patients with Type III hyperlipidemia who are overweight, the avoidance of excess calories, particularly those derived from alcohol. Recommended changes advocated by the NCEP Panel are summarized in Table 14.4; in the Step-Two Diet the intake of saturated fatty acids is reduced to less than 7% of total calories and the daily cholesterol intake to below 200 mg. Replacement of saturated fats in the diet may be best achieved by increasing the intake of complex carbohydrates but moderate increases in the content of monounsaturated fatty acids and ω-6 polyunsaturated fatty acids may also be beneficial [27–29]. Although fish oils enriched in ω-3 fatty acids have a triglyceride-lowering effect when taken in doses of 3–5 g/day, such supplements increase LDL cholesterol concentrations in patients with primary hypercholesterolemia and cannot be recommended [30,31]. Consumption of greater than 15 g/day of ω-3 fatty acids has been shown to reduce concentrations of LDL cholesterol by 31% when substituted for saturated fats in the diet of patients with FH but, in the opinion of the author, such an intake is impractical and may pose risks from increased oxidation of lipoproteins [32].

The dietary changes outlined in Table 14.4 are practical and primarily involve substitution rather than complete changes in the eating style of the individual patient. The magnitude of lipid reduction achieved by these dietary changes depends on the individual dietary habits of the patient, the initial levels of total and LDL cholesterol, and individual diet responsiveness. Subjects with the apo E-IV allele also appear to be more diet responsive to reductions in the habitual intake of saturated fats and cholesterol [33]. Despite individual variability in the response to diet, a patient who has been consuming a typical Western diet containing 40–45% of their calories from fat, with a cholesterol intake of 400–500 mg/day, should see a reduction of 20–40 mg/dl in plasma cholesterol concentrations upon change to the Step-One Diet with a further 5–10 mg/dl decrease occurring in response to the Step-Two Diet [4]. Substantially larger changes have been obtained in response to a very low-fat vegetarian diet used in conjunction with moderate exercise [34].

In addition to the lipid-modifying effects which occur in response to changes in the amount and saturation of dietary fats, the cholesterol intake, and the total caloric intake, a number of other dietary components exert smaller effects on plasma lipid and lipoprotein concentrations. Thus, a mild hypercholesterolemic effect has been associated with the drinking of boiled, but not filtered, coffee [35], whereas a modest hypocholesterolemic effect has been observed in some [36] but not all [37] studies in which soluble fibers have been incorporated into a cholesterol-lowering diet. The frequency of meals also influences plasma lipid concentrations and a hypocholesterolemic effect has been observed in response to nibbling as compared to regular meal patterns [38].

For dietary treatment to be successful, it is important to allow an adequate trial (3–6 months) to enable the patient and his or her family to make the suggested changes in lifestyle. Consultation with a registered dietitian is particularly helpful and other family members should be actively involved in the nutritional education sessions. Their support is invariably helpful to the patient and they themselves are likely to benefit from increased knowledge concerning dietary treatment of hyperlipidemia.

Drug therapy for patients with primary hypercholesterolemia

Significant advances in our understanding of the pathophysiology and treatment of primary hypercholesterolemia have occurred in the last decade. Guidelines for the use of hypolipidemic drugs in the treatment of primary hypercholesterolemia have been established [4] but the importance of selecting a therapy appropriate for each individual patient cannot be overemphasized. Factors to be considered in the decision to use drugs as an adjunct to diet in reducing LDL cholesterol concentrations include the magnitude, duration and etiology of hypercholesterolemia, the family history of premature coronary artery disease and, if available, the concentrations of Lp(a), the age and sex of the patient, the presence or absence of atherosclerosis, the presence of other known cardiovascular risk factors, and last but not least, the attitude of the patient toward drug therapy and potential benefit to be derived from such treatment. Several factors need to be considered in selecting a drug for use as an initial therapeutic agent in adult patients with primary hypercholesterolemia. These include the magnitude of hypercholesterolemia, the age and lifestyle of the patient, relative contraindications to first-choice drugs, and the overall costs associated with purchase of the drugs and therapeutic monitoring.

The bile acid sequestrants, cholestyramine and colestipol, and nicotinic acid were advocated as drugs of first choice by the NCEP Panel [4] and both of these drugs have been shown to reduce cardiovascular morbidity and mortality and have a long-established record of clinical use. In my opinion, however, lovastatin, simvastatin, and pravastatin the currently available HMG-CoA reductase inhibitors available in the USA, also warrant inclusion as drugs of first choice for the treatment of adult patients with primary hypercholesterolemia (excluding women of child-bearing potential) because of their potent ability to lower LDL cholesterol concentrations and relatively low incidence of side-effects in short-term and moderately long-term use [39,40].

The bile acid sequestrants, cholestyramine and colestipol have been evaluated in a number of clinical trials and, in compliant patients, these drugs reduce plasma concentrations of LDL cholesterol in a dose-dependent manner by 15–30% [39]. Dose–response curves for these drugs are however nonlinear and in adult patients a 10–20% decrease in LDL cholesterol can often be achieved with doses of 10 g/day of colestipol or 8 g/day of cholestyramine. At these doses the drugs may be given once daily in the evening which tends to promote increased compliance. Cholestyramine and colestipol both act to bind bile acids in the intestinal lumen with a concurrent interruption in the enterohepatic circulation of bile acids and markedly increased excretion of fecal steroids. This depletion in the bile acid pool leads to an increased hepatic synthesis of bile acids, a decreased hepatic pool of cholesterol, and compensatory increases in hepatic cholesterol biosynthesis and in the number of high-affinity LDL receptors expressed on liver cell membranes. The ability of these drugs to reduce LDL cholesterol concentrations is due to an increased rate of LDL catabolism which results from the increased expression of high-affinity LDL receptors in the liver [41]. Bile acid sequestrants have the potential to reduce LDL cholesterol concentrations to under 130 mg/dl (3.4 mmol/l) in patients whose initial values are in the 175–200 mg/dl (4.5–5.2 mmol/l) range and such changes are often accompanied by small increases in HDL cholesterol and by a mild increase in plasma triglycerides.

The most common side-effects observed during treatment with bile acid sequestrants are changes in bowel function and a potential to exacerbate hemorrhoids. These drugs also have the potential to bind certain other coadministered charged drugs such as digitalis, thyroxine, and warfarin and may decrease the absorption of folic acid and fat-soluble vitamins. Cholestyramine and colestipol are however not absorbed from the gastrointestinal tract and their use does not require detailed monitoring for potential biochemical side-effects. The non-systemic nature of these drugs makes them the safest of the available hypocholesterolemic drugs and they are the drugs of choice for young women with primary hypercholesterolemia (e.g., FH) in whom drug therapy is deemed appropriate.

Nicotinic acid (niacin) was recommended as a drug of first choice by the NCEP Panel for the treatment of patients with primary hyper-cholesterolemia and theoretically is the drug of initial choice for patients with familial combined hyperlipidemia in whom increased concentrations of LDL cholesterol are attributable to an increased rate of VLDL and LDL synthesis [42]. The precise mechanism(s) by which nicotinic acid reduces lipoprotein concentrations is unclear but studies of LDL metabolism have indicated that the drug reduces the hepatic synthesis of VLDL and LDL [43]. Two preparations of nicotinic acid are available, regular and sustained release preparations; the latter are associated with a lower incidence of flushing but are inferior in their ability to lower LDL cholesterol concentrations and are more hepatotoxic [44,45]. Particular caution should be taken in advising patients not to change from regular to sustained-release formulations of nicotinic acid due to the increased risk of hepatotoxicity at the same total dose. The usual starting dose of nicotinic acid is 100−250 mg/day and the drug should be taken with meals in a progressively increasing dosage schedule until a dose of 1.5−2 g/day in divided doses has been achieved. The hypolipidemic effects of nicotinic acid vary from subject to subject and it is advisable to assess the therapeutic response and concurrently measure serum chemistries when patients have achieved a dose of 1.5−2 g daily. Further dose increase up to a maximum of 4.5−6 g/day may be made in incremental amounts but chemistry parameters and lipid measurements should be determined after each dose increase. When used as a single agent at doses of 3−6 g/day, nicotinic acid reduces plasma concentrations of LDL cholesterol by 20−35%, raises the concentrations of HDL by 10−20%, and reduces plasma triglycerides by 20−40% [42,44]. Increases in the plasma concentrations of HDL cholesterol are seen in response to low doses of nicotinic acid (1–1.5 g/day) but higher doses (2–6 g/day) are generally necessary to reduce LDL cholesterol concentrations [42,46].

Side-effects occur commonly in patients treated with nicotinic acid but can be minimized if patients are counseled concerning predictable side-effects and advised to take the medication with meals. In addition to the predictable cutaneous flushing, side-effects of concern include nausea, abdominal discomfort, dryness of the skin, and rarely blurred vision [44–46]. Nicotinic acid is contraindicated in patients with active liver disease, hyperuricemia, a prior history of peptic ulcer disease, or in patients who have previously had adverse reactions to this medication. The drug should be regarded as relatively contraindicated in patients with Type II diabetes. Laboratory abnormalities are more common in patients receiving doses of nicotinic acid which exceed 3 g/day and include increases in the serum concentrations of uric acid, glucose, aminotransferases, and alkaline phosphatase. It is essential that these biochemical parameters be monitored periodically during therapy with nicotinic acid. Nicotinic acid is the most cost effective of the hypolipidemic medications and favorably influences the plasma concentrations of all lipoproteins [47].

The development of specific competitive inhibitors of HMG-CoA reductase, the rate-limiting enzyme in cholesterol biosynthesis, has provided a new therapeutic modality for the treatment of patients with primary hypercholesterolemia and combined hyperlipidemia. Lovastatin was approved by the FDA in 1987 and simvastatin and pravastatin have recently been released. Figure 14.1 illustrates the structure of these drugs and highlights the similarity between the open acid portions and the structure of HMG-CoA. Lovastatin and simvastatin are administered as lactones and hydrolysis to the open acid form occurs in the liver; in contrast, pravastatin and fluvastatin are administered as the open acids. Despite differences in water solubility, all of these drugs are primarily taken up by the liver and exert their hypolipidemic effects by inhibiting hepatic HMG-CoA reductase. The ability of lovastatin and simvastatin to reduce plasma concentrations of total and LDL cholesterol have been well documented and, in patients with FH, both drugs reduce the rate of formation of mevalonic acid by 30–35% at doses of 40 mg/day [48,49]. This reduced formation of mevalonic acid is indicative of a decreased flux of HMG-CoA into the cholesterol biosynthetic pathway and is associated with a reduction in the cellular pool of cholesterol. This results in an increased expression of high-affinity LDL receptors on hepatocyte membranes which in turn stimulates an increase in the receptor-mediated catabolism of LDL and VLDL remnants [50]. Con-

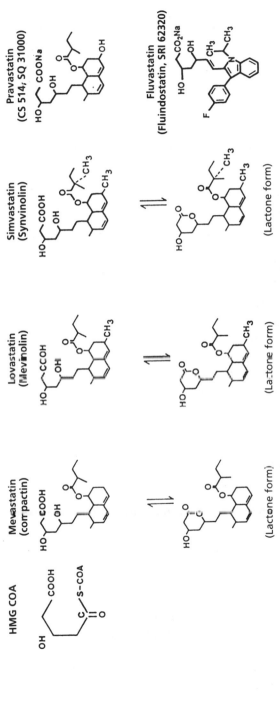

Fig. 14.1 Structure of some of the recently developed HMG-CoA reductase inhibitors highlighting the similarity between these agents and the structure of HMG-CoA.

Table 14.5 Comparative hypolipidemic effects of HMG-CoA reductase inhibitors in patients with heterozygous FH

Daily dose (mg)	Percent decrease in LDL cholesterol				
	Lovastatin		Simvastatin		Pravastatin
	a	b	c	d	e
10	20(13)	17(20)	28(8)	ND	19
20	28(13)	25(20)	30(4)	38(10)	26
40	35(13)	31(20)	37(7)	44(10)	32
80	38(13)	40(20)	42(4)	48(10)	39

FH, familial hypercholesterolemia; a, Illingworth and Sexton [52]; b, Havel *et al.* [53]; c, Mol *et al.* [54]; d, Illingworth and Bacon [39]; e, pravastatin monograph (to be published), number of patients not specified. Numbers in parentheses indicate the number of patients studied with each dose. ND, not determined.

current decreases in the hepatic synthesis of VLDL and LDL have also been reported during treatment with HMG-CoA reductase inhibitors [51]. The HMG-CoA reductase inhibitors are the most potent of the available drugs for maximally reducing LDL cholesterol concentrations in patients with primary hypercholesterolemia. The comparative efficacy of different doses of lovastatin, simvastatin, and pravastatin in reducing LDL cholesterol concentrations in patients with heterozygous FH is illustrated in Table 14.5. Simvastatin is twice as potent than either lovastatin or pravastatin on a weight-for-weight basis but with all three drugs, reductions in LDL cholesterol concentrations of 35–45% have been observed at maximal doses. The dose–response curves for all three drugs are however nonlinear and the greatest percentage of reduction in LDL occurs in response to the first 20 mg/day doses of lovastatin or pravastatin or the first 10 mg of simvastatin. Therapy with lovastatin, simvastatin, or pravastatin has been associated with a 20–30% decrease in the plasma concentrations of triglycerides and an overall tendency for HDL cholesterol to increase by 5–15% [52–55]. Adult patients with FH comprise less than 5% of the patient pool in whom LDL cholesterol concentrations are of sufficient magnitude to warrant drug therapy. The remaining group of patients with primary hypercholesterolemia have other less well characterized disorders including familial combined hyperlipidemia and polygenic causes of hypercholesterolemia. Despite considerable individual variability in the response to HMG-CoA reductase inhibitors, these drugs appear to be equally effective in reducing LDL cholesterol concentrations, when expressed as a percentage reduction from baseline, in patients with heterozygous FH as compared to patients with either familial combined hyperlipidemia or other less well characterized primary disorders [56, 57]. Although a preliminary report [58], suggested that patients with hypercholesterolemia due to familial defective apo B may not respond well to HMG-CoA reductase inhibitor therapy this response may be atypical. In the two patients reported by Corsini et al. [58], LDL cholesterol concentrations decreased by only 12 and 16%, respectively during treatment with simvastatin at doses of 20 and 40 mg/day; larger decreases have been observed in more recent studies with more patients [59].

The safety profile and tolerability of HMG-CoA reductase inhibitors in short-term and moderately long-term use have been good and reported side-effects have been uncommon [39,40,53,57]. Reported side-effects to date have included changes in bowel function, nausea, fatigue, insomnia, skin rashes, and, rarely, cholestasis and the development of myopathy [51]. Myopathy is uncommon but is more likely to occur when patients are receiving high doses of lovastatin (80 mg/day) [57]; the incidence of myopathy is increased in patients concurrently receiving cyclosporine, nicotinic acid, gemfibrozil, and erythromycin and HMG-CoA reductase inhibitors should be used very cautiously if at all in combination with these other drugs [60]. Lovastatin and other HMG-CoA reductase inhibitors are excreted primarily in bile and toxic levels could be obtained if these drugs were given at standard doses to patients with cholestasis or other disorders in which hepatic excretion and/or metabolism could be impaired. Initial concerns that HMG CoA reductase inhibitors would cause cataracts in humans have not been substantiated.

Biochemical tests to monitor the safety and efficacy of reductase inhibitors should be assessed at 6−8 week intervals for the first 9−12 months of therapy and at 3−4 monthly intervals thereafter. They should include assessments of liver function and possibly electrolytes. Determination of creatine kinase is appropriate in any patient who has symptoms suggestive of myopathy but the author does not advocate its use as a routine test to monitor safety during therapy with reductase inhibitors.

On the basis of their moderate hypocholesterolemic effects in patients with primary hypercholesterolemia, gemfibrozil and probucol are best regarded as second-choice agents, whereas the indications for clofibrate, neomycin, and D-thyroxine in the treatment of primary hypercholesterolemia are limited.

The hypolipidemic effects of the fibric acid class of drugs result from a number of different mechanism(s) including reductions in the synthesis of VLDL triglycerides, an increased activity of lipoprotein lipase, and an enhanced rate of receptor-mediated clearance of LDL from plasma [61]. Some of the second generation fibrates (e.g., bezafibrate, fenofibrate, and ciprofibrate) are more potent in their ability to lower LDL cholesterol concentrations than are gemfibrozil or clofibrate and if the former drugs become available these may have a role as potential first-choice drugs for the treatment of primary hypercholesterolemia. In contrast, however, clofibrate and gemfibrozil have been shown to reduce LDL cholesterol concentrations by 5 and 10%, respectively in patients with heterozygous FH and cannot be recommended as first-choice agents [61].

Probucol is a moderately effective drug for the treatment of primary hypercholesterolemia and at the recommended dose of 500 mg twice daily reduces LDL cholesterol concentrations by 8–15% [62–64]. Probucol is of equal efficacy in reducing LDL concentrations in patients with heterozygous FH as compared to other less well characterized causes of primary hypercholesterolemia. Probucol does not affect plasma triglyceride concentrations but reduces the levels of HDL cholesterol by up to 30% [62]. Probucol is a lipid-soluble drug whose mechanism of action in reducing LDL cholesterol concentrations has not been fully elucidated; however, in clinical use, probucol has been shown to induce regression of tendon xanthomas in patients with FH [65] and may exert other potentially beneficial effects on lipoproteins including the inhibition of LDL oxidation [66] and an increase in reverse cholesterol transport [67]. If antioxidant therapy in humans with hypercholesterolemia can be shown to be beneficial, then the therapeutic use of probucol in the prevention of atherosclerosis may increase. However, at the present time the drug has not been utilized in any primary or secondary prevention trials and it is unclear whether or not the antioxidant effects of this drug may have additional benefits over and above that due to the modest reduction in LDL which probucol facilitates.

Probucol is generally well tolerated and side-effects, which occur in less than 5% of patients, include changes in bowel function, abdominal discomfort, and nausea. Biochemical side-effects are uncommon. The lipid-soluble nature of probucol contributes to its storage in adipose tissue and the drug also has been shown to cause prolongation of the QT interval on the electrocardiogram.

Neomycin and D-thyroxine have both been used in the treatment of primary hypercholesterolemia but in the author's opinion neither can be recommended.

Combined drug therapy for severe hypercholesterolemia

Despite the ability of the first-choice drugs (bile acid sequestrants, nicotinic acid, and HMG-CoA reductase inhibitors) to reduce plasma concentrations of LDL cholesterol by 25–45% when used as monotherapy, many patients with severe hypercholesterolemia, particularly those with heterozygous FH, remain inadequately treated; in these patients the use of combination drug therapy utilizing two or more drugs with different mechanisms of action may be particularly effective [39,40,42,68]. The efficacy of some of the more established drug combinations for the treatment of severe hypercholesterolemia is summarized in Table 14.6. The most effective drug combinations have employed a bile acid sequestrant in combination with either nicotinic acid, lovastatin, or simvastatin. Combinations in which fibrates or probucol have been used with a bile acid sequestrant have also been evaluated although the LDL-lowering effects of probucol are quite variable. The dose–response curves for both bile acid sequestrants and HMG-CoA reductase inhibitors are nonlinear and the use of low doses of cholestyramine or colestipol in combination with lovastatin or simvastatin provides a therapeutic regimen that is usually well tolerated, shows additive lipid lowering, and is more cost effective than high-dose monotherapy [68]. Triple drug therapy has been utilized in selected patients with severe heterozygous FH and reductions of 60–70% in the plasma concentrations of LDL cholesterol have been observed in response to treatment with the ternary combination of lovastatin, colestipol, and nicotinic acid [39,69]. Not all drug combinations can be recommended due either to lack of efficacy or the potential for increased toxicity. No significant additional hypocholesterolemic effect has been observed with the combination of either lovastatin plus probucol [64] or lovastatin plus gemfibrozil [70] and use of the latter combination has been associated with an increased risk of myopathy [60]. Referral to a lipid specialist is appropriate for the management of most patients with severe hyper-

Table 14.6 Efficacy of combined drug regimens in severe primary hypercholesterolemia

Drug combination	Percent decrease in LDL cholesterol	Number of patients studied	Reference
Cholestyramine + nicotinic acid	48	6	[71]
Colestipol + nicotinic acid	47	11	[72]
Cholestyramine + bezafibrate	31	18	[73]
Colestipol + lovastatin	54	10	[74]
Cholestyramine + simvastatin	54	13	[75]
Cholestyramine + simvastatin	64	5	[76]
Lovastatin + nicotinic acid	49	8	[39]
Lovastatin + colestipol + nicotinic acid	67	21	[69]

cholesterolemia in whom combination drug therapy is warranted to obtain optimal control of the underlying lipid disorder [4].

Radical approaches to the treatment of severe hypercholesterolemia

In addition to diet and drug therapy, several other techniques have been employed in the treatment of patients with severe hypercholesterolemia. These include distal ileal bypass surgery, portocaval shunt or liver transplantation, and physical removal of lipoproteins by plasmapheresis or more selective forms of apheresis in which extracorporeal absorbants have been utilized to selectively remove apo B-containing lipoproteins from plasma. The use of any of these techniques is limited to patients seen in specialized lipid clinics and the number of patients likely to be treated by these techniques is small. Distal ileal bypass surgery reduces LDL cholesterol concentrations by 30–40% in patients with heterozygous FH [77] and, in patients with less severe degrees of hypercholesterolemia, has been associated with a reduction in cardiovascular morbidity and mortality [78]. Nonetheless, with the advent of potent LDL-lowering drugs such as lovastatin and simvastatin, this operation, which is ineffective in patients with homozygous FH, cannot be recommended. Liver transplantation and portocaval shunt surgery have both been utilized in the treatment of homozygous FH but in the opinion of the author selective LDL apheresis is the treatment of choice for this disorder [79,80]. Concentrations of LDL cholesterol can be reduced to under 40 mg/dl (1 mmol/l) by apheresis but increase in the ensuing days thereby necessitates repeat apheresis in 7–10 days in patients with homozygous FH and in 10–14 days in severe heterozygous patients. In addition to removing LDL from plasma, LDL apheresis also removes Lp(a) and may afford one mode of therapy for patients with FH in whom Lp(a) concentrations are substantially increased.

Therapy of Type III hyperlipoproteinemia

Type III hyperlipoproteinemia (dysbetalipoproteinemia) is an uncommon disorder of lipid metabolism in which VLDL and chylomicron remnants accumulate in plasma [81]. Untreated, patients with Type III hyperlipoproteinemia are at increased risk for the premature development of both coronary and peripheral vascular disease and the disorder is associated with characteristic xanthomas which regress in response to effective lipid-lowering therapy [81]. The pathophysiology of Type

III hyperlipoproteinemia has been elucidated and most patients who develop clinical expression of this disorder are homozygous for one allelic form of apo E (E-II) which has a reduced affinity for binding to LDL receptors. Clinical expression of Type III hyperlipoproteinemia normally requires the concurrent presence of an apo E variant, usually apo E-II, which has a reduced receptor-binding affinity together with an increase in the hepatic production of VLDL. Apo E is necessary for optimal hepatic metabolism of VLDL remnants, and when VLDL production is increased, this defective binding leads to the accumulation of chylomicron and VLDL remnants in plasma. These particles appear to be highly atherogenic.

Therapy of adult patients with Type III hyperlipoproteinemia involves, initially, the correction of secondary exacerbating factors, weight loss if the patient is overweight, and maximal dietary therapy with a concurrent restriction of alcohol intake. In patients in whom clinical expression of Type III hyperlipoproteinemia is due to secondary factors (e.g., obesity) which have promoted an increased synthesis of VLDL, diet, and weight loss may lead to complete correction of the hyperlipidemia. In other patients, particularly those in whom expression of Type III hyperlipoproteinemia is due to the presence of a separate monogenic lipid disorder, such as familial combined hyperlipidemia, dietary therapy alone is inadequate and the use of lipid-lowering drugs is necessary. Fibrate drugs are usually extremely effective in the therapy of patients with Type III hyperlipoproteinemia, and reductions of 30– 40% in the concentrations of plasma cholesterol together with 50–70% decreases in plasma triglycerides have been observed in response to treatment with gemfibrozil [82], clofibrate [83], or fenofibrate [84]. Nicotinic acid [85] and, in postmenopausal women, estrogens [86] may also be useful in the management of this disorder. In a recent study [83], the hypolipidemic effects of lovastatin and clofibrate were compared in 12 patients with Type III hyperlipoproteinemia. Both drugs were of equal efficacy in reducing plasma concentrations of VLDL and VLDL remnant particles, whereas lovastatin was superior in its ability to concurrently reduce concentrations of LDL cholesterol. An additional hypolipidemic effect was seen in six patients with severe Type III hyperlipoproteinemia when lovastatin was used in combination with clofibrate and, in these patients, total cholesterol concentrations decreased from 635 mg/dl (16.5 mmol/l) to 205 mg/dl (5.3 mmol/l). This combination may be particularly useful in those patients in whom expression of Type III hyperlipoproteinemia is due to the concurrent presence of familial combined hyperlipidemia plus homozygosity for apo E-II.

Treatment of the hypercholesterolemic patient with concurrently increased concentrations of Lp(a)

Increased plasma concentrations of Lp(a) represent an independent risk factor for accelerated atherosclerosis and accentuate the risk for premature coronary artery disease in patients with FH [12,87]. Published studies indicate that neither the bile acid sequestrants [88] nor the HMG-CoA reductase inhibitors (lovastatin, simvastatin, or pravastatin) [89,90] reduce plasma concentrations of Lp(a), even though these drugs are effective in reducing LDL cholesterol concentrations. Fibrates also appear to be ineffective in reducing plasma concentrations of Lp(a) [61], whereas nicotinic acid, at a dose of 4 g/day, has been reported to reduce Lp(a) concentrations by 38% [91]. Thus, of the currently available hypolipidemic drugs, nicotinic acid appears to be the only agent which effectively reduces plasma concentrations of Lp(a). Whether or not measures which reduce concentrations of both LDL cholesterol and Lp(a) will prove to be more effective than those which only reduce LDL remains to be established. The potential utility of N-acetylcysteine as a means of reducing plasma concentrations of Lp(a) [92,93], independent from any changes in LDL, as a therapeutic modality in patients with hypercholesterolemia and concurrently increased levels of Lp(a) warrants further investigation.

Treatment of secondary causes of hypercholesterolemia

Hypercholesterolemia with increased plasma concentrations of LDL cholesterol is seen as a secondary consequence of endocrine, renal, or hepatic diseases, and in some of these disorders the primary disorder may not be amenable to correction but the magnitude of hyper-cholesterolemia may warrant therapy aimed at reducing the risk of atherosclerosis. In the case of patients with primary hypothyroidism, treatment with L-thyroxine usually results in correction of the hypothyroid state and also normalization of the plasma lipid profile. However, in patients with secondary hypercholesterolemia due to the nephrotic syndrome or cholestasis associated with primary biliary cirrhosis the secondary disorder is not amenable to correction and the magnitude of hypercholesterolemia is often severe. The decision to use hypolipidemic drugs in patients with the nephrotic syndrome must be individualized, but the high incidence of premature atherosclerosis in patients with this disorder justifies selective use of hypolipidemic drugs in patients whose LDL cholesterol concentrations remain above 190–

230 mg/dl (5–6 mmol/l). Lovastatin and simvastatin have been shown to be effective in the treatment of patients with secondary hypercholesterolemia associated with the nephrotic syndrome [94,95] and these may be the optimal drugs for use in this patient population. Bile acid sequestrants often exacerbate mild hypertriglyceridemia whereas nicotinic acid may exacerbate preexistent hyperuricemia. Treatment of patients with cholestasis is difficult and none of the available hypolipidemic drugs is effective; bile acid sequestrants are often prescribed to relieve the pruritis associated with increased plasma concentrations in bile acids but these agents are relatively ineffective in reducing their hypercholesterolemia. HMG-CoA reductase inhibitors are excreted in bile and use of these drugs in patients with cholestasis is likely to result in significantly impaired hepatic excretion with a resultant increased risk for myopathy. Plasmapheresis appears to be the most effective treatment available for patients with severe hypercholesterolemia associated with cholestasis and should be considered in patients with xanthomatous neuropathy or evidence of coronary or peripheral vascular disease.

Treatment of hypercholesterolemia in children

Despite recommendations to the contrary [96] an increasing number of children in North America are being screened for hypercholesterolemia and consequently a small proportion are found to have hypercholesterolemia. As with adults, in any child identified to have hypercholesterolemia, it is important first to delineate the etiology of the lipid abnormality with the primary aims being directed at correction of secondary factors and, in most children, dietary therapy. Treatment of children identified to have heterozygous FH involves primarily a low-fat, low-cholesterol diet. At the present time, guidelines for the use of lipid-lowering drugs in children are incomplete [97] but, in the author's opinion, should be limited to the use of the nonsystemically acting bile acid sequestrants, cholestyramine, or colestipol. Clinical trials are currently evaluating the efficacy and safety of lovastatin in adolescent boys with FH; use of this class of drugs in the pediatric population must be regarded as investigational. In children with heterozygous FH the decision to begin drug therapy should depend on several factors including the magnitude of hypercholesterolemia, the family history of premature atherosclerosis, the sex of the child (boys warrant more aggressive treatment than girls), plasma concentrations of Lp(a), and the attitude of the child and his or her parents. Drug therapy should be individualized but is most appropriate for those children with LDL cholesterol concentrations which exceed 200–250 mg/dl on maximal dietary therapy. Monotherapy with bile acid sequestrants is unlikely to achieve normal lipid values, and, particularly in teenagers, compliance is poor. However, the risk of development of coronary artery disease before 30 years of age is very low and, in view of the lack of safety data available for systemically acting drugs, justifies waiting until the late teens before considering the use of more effective hypocholesterolemic drugs. Supplements of folic acid and fat-soluble vitamins may be advisable for children treated with cholestyramine and colestipol on a long-term basis. Drug therapy is ineffective for the rare child with homozygous FH and referral to a center specializing in the treatment of lipid disorders is mandatory for the effective management of these patients.

Acknowledgments

This work was supported in part by National Institutes of Health Research Grants HL 28399 and HL 37940, by the General Clinical Research Centers Program (RR334), and by the Clinical Nutrition Research Unit (P-30DK40566). I am grateful to Linda Seward and Marcia Hindman for the preparation of this manuscript and to patients and colleagues who have contributed to the work discussed in this review.

References

1 Stamler J. Population studies. In *Nutrition, Lipids and Coronary Heart Disease: a Global View* (eds RI Levy, BM Rifkind, BH Dennis, N Ernst). New York: Raven Press, 1979:25–88.
2 Consensus Conference. Lowering blood cholesterol to prevent heart disease. *JAMA* 1985;253:2080–6.
3 Miller M, Mead LA, Kwiterovich PO, Pierson TA. Dyslipidaemias with desirable plasma total cholesterol levels and angiographically demonstrated coronary artery disease. *Am J Cardiol* 1990;64:1–5.
4 The Expert Panel. Report of the National Cholesterol Education Program Expert Panel on detection, evaluation and treatment of high blood cholesterol in adults. *Arch Intern Med* 1988;148:36–69.
5 Study Group of the European Atherosclerosis Society. The recognition and management of hyperlipidaemia in adults. A policy statement of the European Atherosclerosis Society. *Eur Heart J* 1988;9:571–600.
6 Shepherd J, Betteridge DJ, Durrington P *et al*. Strategies for reducing coronary heart disease and desirable limits for blood lipid concentrations: guidelines from the British Hyperlipidaemia Association. *Br Med J* 1987;295:1245–6.
7 Canadian Lipoprotein Conference ad hoc Committee on Guidelines for Dyslipoproteinemias. Guidelines for the detection of high risk lipoprotein profiles and the treatment of dyslipoproteinemias. *Can Med Assoc J* 1990;142:1371–82.
8 Blankenhorn DH, Nessum SA, Johnson RL *et al*. Beneficial effects of combined

colestipol and niacin therapy on coronary atherosclerosis and coronary venous bypass grafts. *JAMA* 1987;257:3233−40.

9 Cashin-Hemphill L, Mack WJ, Pogoda JM *et al.* Beneficial effects of colestipol niacin on coronary atherosclerosis: four-year follow-up. *JAMA* 1990;264:3013−17.

10 Thompson GR. Primary hyperlipidemia. *Br Med Bull* 1990;46:986−1004.

11 Goldstein JL, Brown MS. Familial hypercholesterolemia. In *The Metabolic Basis of Inherited Disease,* 6th edn (eds CR Scriver, AL Beaudet, WS Sly, D Valle). New York: McGraw Hill, 1989:1215−50.

12 Seed M, Hoppichler F, Reaveley D *et al.* Relation of serum lipoprotein (a) concentration and apo (a) phenotype to coronary heart disease in patients with familial hypercholesterolemia. *N Engl J Med* 1990;322:1494−9.

13 Innerarity TL, Mahley RW, Weisgraber KH *et al.* Familial defective apolipoprotein B 100: A mutation of apo B that causes hypercholesterolemia. *J Lipid Res* 1990;31: 1337−49.

14 Ettinger WH, Hazzard WR. Prednisone increases very low density lipoprotein and high density lipoprotein in healthy men. *Metabolism* 1988;36:1055−8.

15 Molitch ME, Oill P, Odell WD. Massive hyperlipemia during estrogen therapy. *JAMA* 1974;227:522−5.

16 Crook D, Godsland I, Winn V. Oral contraceptives and coronary heart disease. Modulation of glucose tolerance and plasma lipids by progestins. *Am J Obstet Gynecol* 1988;158:1612−20.

17 Burry KA, Patton PE, Illingworth DR. Metabolic changes during medical treatment of endometriosis. Nafarelin acetate vs. danazol. *Am J Obstet Gynecol* 1989;160:1454−61.

18 Lardinois CK, Newman SL. The effects of antihypertensive agents on serum lipids and lipoproteins. *Arch Intern Med* 1988;148:1280−8.

19 Krone W, Nagele H. Effects of antihypertensives on plasma lipids and lipoprotein metabolism. *Am Heart J* 1988;116:1729−34.

20 Bershad S, Rubenstein A, Paterniti JR Jr *et al.* Changes in plasma lipids and lipoproteins during isotretinoin therapy for acne. *N Engl J Med* 1985;313:981−5.

21 Kata RA, Jorgensen II, Nigra TP. Elevation of serum triglyceride levels from oral isotretinoin in disorders of keratinization. *Arch Dermatol* 1980;116:1369−72.

22 Iverius PH, Brunzell JD. Chylomicronemia induced by cimetidine. *Gastroenterology* 1985;89:664−6.

23 Ballantyne CM, Podet EJ, Patsch WP *et al.* Effects of cyclosporine therapy on plasma lipoprotein levels. *JAMA* 1989;262:53−6.

24 Wallace RB, Hunninghake DB, Reiland S *et al.* Alterations of plasma high density lipoprotein cholesterol levels associated with consumption of selected medications. *Circulation* 1980;62(Suppl 4):77−85.

25 Spady DK, Dietschy JM. Dietary saturated triacylglycerols suppress hepatic low density lipoprotein receptor activity in the hamster. *Proc Natl Acad Sci USA* 1985;82:4526−30.

26 Spady DK, Dietschy JM. Interaction of dietary cholesterol and triglycerides in the regulation of hepatic low density lipoprotein transport in the hamster. *J Clin Invest* 1988;81:300−9.

27 Becker N, Illingworth DR, Alaupovic P, Sundberg EE, Connor WE. Effects of saturated, monounsaturated, and omega-6 polyunsaturated fatty acids on plasma lipids, lipoproteins and apoproteins in humans. *Am J Clin Nutr* 1983;37:355−60.

28 Grundy SM. Comparison of monounsaturated fatty acids and carbohydrates for lowering plasma cholesterol. *N Engl J Med* 1986;314:745−8.

29 Mattson FH, Grundy SM. Comparison of effects of dietary saturated, monounsaturated and polyunsaturated fatty acids on plasma lipids and lipoproteins in men. *J Lipid Res* 1985;26:194−202.

30 Harris WS. Fish oils and plasma lipids and lipoprotein metabolism in humans. A critical review. *J Lipid Res* 1989;30:785−807.

31 Wilt TJ, Lofgren RP, Nichol KL *et al.* Fish oil supplementation does not lower plasma

cholesterol in men with hypercholesterolemia. Results of a randomized placebo controlled crossover study. *Ann Intern Med* 1989;111:900−5.

32 Friday KE, Failor A, Childs MT, Bierman EL. Effects of n-3 and n-6 fatty acid enriched diets on plasma lipoproteins and apolipoproteins in heterozygous familial hypercholesterolemia. *Arterioscler Thromb* 1991;11:47−54.

33 Manttari M, Koskinen P, Ehnholm C, Huttunen JK, Manninen B. Apo E polymorphism influences the serum cholesterol response to dietary intervention. *Metabolism* 1991;40:217−21.

34 Ornish D, Brown SE, Scherwitz LW *et al.* Can life style changes reverse coronary heart disease? The Life Style Heart Trial. *Lancet* 1990;336:129−33.

35 Bak AAA, Grobbee D. The effect on serum cholesterol levels of coffee brewed by filtering or boiling. *N Engl J Med* 1989;321:1432−7.

36 Kay RM, Truswell AS. Effect of citrus pectin on blood lipids and fecal steroid excretion in men. *Am J Clin Nutr* 1977;30:171−5.

37 Swain JF, Rouse IL, Curley CB, Sacks FM. Comparison of the effects of oat bran and low fiber wheat on serum lipoprotein levels and blood pressure. *N Engl J Med* 1990;322:147−52.

38 Jenkins DJA, Wolever TMS, Vuksan V *et al.* Nibbling vs. gorging: Metabolic advantages of increased meal frequency. *N Engl J Med* 1989;321:929−34.

39 Illingworth DR, Bacon S. Treatment of heterozygous familial hypercholesterolemia with lipid lowering drugs. *Arteriosclerosis* 1989;9(Suppl 1):129−34.

40 Illingworth DR, Bacon SP, Larson KK. Long term experience with HMG CoA reductase inhibitors in the therapy of hypercholesterolemia. *Atherosclerosis Rev* 1988;18:161−87.

41 Shepherd J, Packard CJ, Bicker S *et al.* Cholestyramine promotes receptor mediated low density lipoprotein catabolism. *N Engl J Med* 1980;302:1219−22.

42 Illingworth DR. Drug therapy of hypercholesterolaemia. *Clin Chem* 1988;33:B123−B132.

43 Levy RI, Langer T. Hypolipidemic drugs and lipoprotein metabolism. *Adv Exp Med Biol* 1972;27:155−63.

44 Knopp RH, Ginsberg J, Albers JJ *et al.* Contrasting effects of unmodified and time release forms of niacin on lipoproteins in hyperlipidemic subjects: Clues to mechanism of action of niacin. *Metabolism* 1985;34:642−50.

45 Mullin GE, Greenson JK, Mitchell MC. Fulminant hepatic failure after ingestion of sustained release nicotinic acid. *Ann Intern Med* 1989;111:253−5.

46 Alderman JD, Pasternak RC, Sacks FM *et al.* Effect of a modified, well tolerated niacin regimen on serum total cholesterol, high density lipoprotein cholesterol, and the cholesterol:high density ratio. *Am J Cardiol* 1989;64:725−9.

47 Schulman KA, Kinosian B, Jacobson TA *et al.* Reducing high blood cholesterol level with drugs: Cost effectiveness of pharmacologic management. *JAMA* 1990;264:3025−33.

48 Pappu AS, Illingworth DR, Bacon S. Reduction in plasma low density lipoprotein cholesterol and urinary mevalonic acid by lovastatin in patients with heterozygous familial hypercholesterolemia. *Metabolism* 1989;38:542−9.

49 Hagamenas FC, Pappu AS, Illingworth DR. The effects of simvastatin on plasma lipoproteins and cholesterol homeostasis in patients with heterozygous familial hypercholesterolemia. *Eur J Clin Invest* 1990;20:150−7.

50 Brown MS, Goldstein JL. A receptor mediated pathway for cholesterol homeostasis. *Science* 1986;232:34−47.

51 Illingworth DR. HMG CoA reductase inhibitors. *Curr Opin Lipidol* 1991;2:24−30.

52 Illingworth DR, Sexton GJ. Hypocholesterolemic effects of mevinolin in patients with heterozygous familial hypercholesterolemia. *J Clin Invest* 1984;74:1972−8.

53 Havel RJ, Hunninghake DB, Illingworth DR *et al.* A multicenter study of lovastatin (mevinolin) in the treatment of heterozygous familial hypercholesterolemia. *Ann Intern Med* 1987;107:609−15.

54 Mol MJTM, Erkelens DW, Leuven JAG *et al.* Effects of synvinolin (MK733) on plasma lipids in familial hypercholesterolemia. *Lancet* 1986;ii:936−9.

55 Hoogerbrugge AnD, Mol MJTM, Van Dormaal JJ *et al.* The efficacy and safety of pravastatin compared to and in combination with bile acid-binding resins in familial hypercholesterolemia. *J Intern Med* 1990;228:261−6.

56 Hunninghake DB, Miller VT, Palmer RH *et al.* Therapeutic response to lovastatin (mevinolin) in nonfamilial hypercholesterolemia. *JAMA* 1986;256:2829−34.

57 Bradford RH, Shear CS, Chremos AN *et al.* Expanded clinical evaluation of lovastatin (EXCEL) study results 1) efficacy in modifying plasma lipoproteins and adverse event profile in 8245 patients with moderate hypercholesterolemia. *Arch Intern Med* 1991;151:43−9.

58 Corsini A, Mazzotti M, Fumagalli R *et al.* Poor response to simvastatin in familial defective apo B 100. *Lancet* 1991;337:305.

59 Illingworth DR, Vakar F, Mahley RW, Weisgraber KH. Hypocholesterolaemic effects of lovastatin in familial defective apolipoprotein B-100. *Lancet* 1992;1:598−600.

60 Pierce LR, Wysowski DK, Gross TP. Myopathy and rhabdomyolysis associated with lovastatin/gemfibrozil combination therapy. *JAMA* 1990;264:71−5.

61 Illingworth DR. Fibric acid derivatives. In *Drug Treatment of Hyperlipidemia* (ed. BM Rifkind). New York: Marcel Dekker, 1991:103−38.

62 Buckley MMT, Goa KL, Price AH, Brogden RN. Probucol: A reappraisal of its pharmacological properties and therapeutic use in hypercholesterolaemia. *Drugs* 1989;37:761−800.

63 Helve E, Tikkanen MJ. Comparison of lovastatin and probucol in treatment of familial and nonfamilial hypercholesterolemia: Different effects on lipoprotein profiles. *Atherosclerosis* 1988;72:189−97.

64 Witztum JL, Simmons D, Steinberg D *et al.* Intensive combination drug therapy of familial hypercholesterolemia with lovastatin, probucol, and colestipol hydrochloride. *Circulation* 1989;79:16−28.

65 Yamamoto A, Matsuzawa Y, Yokoyama S *et al.* Effects of probucol on xanthoma regression in familial hypercholesterolemia. *Am J Cardiol* 1986;57:29H−35H.

66 Steinberg D, Parthasarathy S, Carew TE, Khoo JC, Witztum JL. Beyond cholesterol: Modifications of low density lipoprotein that increase its atherogenicity. *N Engl J Med* 1989;320:915−24.

67 Franceschini T, Sirtori M, Vaccarino V *et al.* Mechanisms of HDL reduction after probucol: Changes in HDL subfractions and increased reverse cholesterol ester transfer. *Arteriosclerosis* 1989;9:462−9.

68 Illingworth DR. New horizons in combination drug therapy for hypercholesterolemia. *Cardiology* 1989;76(Suppl 1):83−100.

69 Malloy MJ, Kane JP, Kunitake ST *et al.* Complimentarity of colestipol, niacin, and lovastatin in treatment of severe familial hypercholesterolemia. *Ann Intern Med* 1987;107:616−23.

70 Illingworth DR, Bacon S. Influence of lovastatin plus gemfibrozil on plasma lipids and lipoproteins in patients with heterozygous familial hypercholesterolemia. *Circulation* 1989;79:590−6.

71 Packard CJ, Steward JM, Morgan HG, Lorimer AR, Shephard J. Combined drug therapy for familial hypercholesterolemia. *Artery* 1980;7:281−9.

72 Illingworth DR, Phillipson BE, Rapp JH, Connor WE. Colestipol plus nicotinic acid in treatment of heterozygous familial hypercholesterolaemia. *Lancet* 1981;i:296−8.

73 Curtis LD, Dickson AC, Ling KLE, Betteridge J. Combination treatment with cholestyramine and bezafibrate for heterozygous familial hypercholesterolaemia. *Br Med J* 1988;297:173−5.

74 Illingworth DR. Mevinolin plus colestipol in therapy for severe heterozygous familial hypercholesterolemia. *Ann Intern Med* 1984;101:598−604.

75 Lintott CJ, Scott RS, Nye ER, Robertson NC, Sutherland WHF. Simvastatin: An effective treatment for hypercholesterolaemia. *Aust N Z J Med* 1989;19:317−20.

76 Mölgaard J, VonSchenck H, Olsson, AG. Comparative effects of simvastatin and cholestyramine in treatment of patients with hypercholesterolaemia. *Eur J Clin Pharmacol* 1989;36:445−60.

77 Spengle FA, Jadhav A, Duffield RGM *et al.* Superiority of partial ileal bypass over cholestyramine in reducing cholesterol in familial hypercholesterolaemia. *Lancet* 1981;ii:768−71.

78 Buchwald H, Varco RL, Matts JP *et al.* The effect of partial ileal bypass surgery on mortality and morbidity from coronary heart disease in patients with hypercholesterolemia: Report of the program on the surgical control of the hyperlipidemias (POSCH). *N Engl J Med* 1990;323:946−55.

79 Bilheimer DW, Goldstein JL, Grundy SM, Starzl TE, Brown MS. Liver transplantation to provide low density lipoprotein receptors and lower plasma cholesterol in a child with homozygous familial hypercholesterolaemia. *N Engl J Med* 1984;311:1658−64.

80 Mabuchi H, Michishita I, Takeda M *et al.* A new low density lipoprotein apheresis system using two dextran sulphate cellulose columns in an automated column regenerating unit (LDL continuous apheresis). *Atherosclerosis* 1987;68:19−25.

81 Mahley RW, Rall SC Jr. Type III hyperlipoproteinemia (dysbetalipoproteinemia): The role of apolipoprotein E in normal and abnormal lipoprotein metabolism. In *The Metabolic Basis of Inherited Disease*, 6th edn (eds CR Scriber, AL Beaudet, WS Sly, D Valle). New York: McGraw-Hill, 1989:1195−213.

82 Houlston R, Quiney J, Watts GF *et al.* Gemfibrozil in the treatment of resistant familial hypercholesterolemia and Type III hyperlipoproteinemia. *J R Soc Med* 1988;81:274−6.

83 Illingworth DR, O'Malley JP. The hypolipidemic effects of lovastatin and clofibrate alone and in combination in patients with Type III hyperlipoproteinemia. *Metabolism* 1990;39:403−9.

84 Fruchart JC, Davignon J, Bard JM *et al.* Effect of fenofibrate treatment on Type III hyperlipoproteinemia. *Am J Med* 1987;83:71−4.

85 Hoogwerf BJ, Bantle JP, Kuba K *et al.* Treatment of type III hyperlipoproteinaemia with four different treatment regimens. *Atherosclerosis* 1984;51:251−9.

86 Kushwaha RS, Hazzard WR, Gagne C, Chait A, Albers AA. Type III hyperlipoproteinemia: Paradoxical hypolipidemic effects of estrogen. *Ann Intern Med* 1977;87:517−25.

87 Editorial. Lipoprotein Lp(a). *Lancet* 1991;337:397−8.

88 Vessby B, Costner G, Lithell H, Thomis J. Diverging effects of cholestyramine on apoprotein B and lipoprotein Lp(a). *Atherosclerosis* 1982;44:61−71.

89 Kostner GM, Gavish D, Leopold D *et al.* HMG CoA reductase inhibitors lower LDL cholesterol without reducing Lp(a) levels. *Circulation* 1989;80:1313−19.

90 Wiklund O, Angelin B, Olofsson SO *et al.* Apolipoprotein Lp(a) and ischemic heart disease in familial hypercholesterolemia. *Lancet* 1990;335:1360−3.

91 Carlson LA, Hamsten A, Asplund A. Pronounced lowering of serum levels of lipoprotein Lp(a) in hyperlipidaemic subjects treated with nicotinic acid. *J Intern Med* 1989;226:271−6.

92 Gavish D, Breslow JL. Lipoprotein Lp(a) reduction by *N*-acetylcysteine. *Lancet* 1991;337:203−4.

93 Stalenhoef AFH, Kroon AA, Demacker PNM. *N*-Acetylcysteine and lipoprotein. *Lancet* 1991;337:491.

94 Golper TA, Illingworth DR, Morris CD, Bennett WM. Lovastatin in the treatment of multifactorial hyperlipidemia associated with proteinuria. *Am J Kidney Dis* 1989;13:312−20.

95 Rabelink AJ, Hene RJ, Erkelens DW, Joles JA, Koomans HA. Effects of simvastatin and cholestyramine on lipoprotein profile in hyperlipidaemia of nephrotic syndrome. *Lancet* 1988;ii:1335−8.

96 Newman TB, Browner WS, Hulley SB. The case against childhood cholesterol screening. *JAMA* 1990;264:3039−43.

97 American Heart Association position statement. Diagnosis and treatment of primary hyperlipidemia in childhood. *Circulation* 1986;74:1181A−1188A.

Chapter 15
Treatment of Hypertriglyceridemia

HENRY N. GINSBERG

Introduction

Hypertriglyceridemia may be defined as the presence of a plasma triglyceride level above the 95th percentile for any age and sex, or by arbitrary cutpoints, such as 150 or 200 mg/dl, based on clinical experience. Because of the still uncertain role of plasma triglycerides as an independent risk factor for coronary artery disease [1], physicians do not have a clear picture of risk vs. triglyceride concentrations as they do for plasma cholesterol levels. Emerging data from ongoing research, however, suggest that plasma triglyceride levels above 120–130 mg/dl are associated with lower high-density lipoprotein (HDL) cholesterol levels and abnormalities of low-density lipoprotein (LDL) composition. Whether these findings will lead to much more aggressive therapeutic approaches to reduce plasma triglyceride concentrations remains to be determined.

In this chapter, normal triglyceride metabolism will be reviewed as a base for a discussion of very low-density lipoprotein (VLDL) metabolism in individuals with elevated plasma triglyceride levels. This will be followed by a description of dietary and pharmacologic approaches to therapy for hypertriglyceridemia.

Normal triglyceride metabolism

Intestinal triglyceride-rich lipoproteins

After consumption of a mixed meal consisting of typical foods, triglyceride and cholesterol are absorbed in the small intestine as fatty acids and cholesterol. Inside mucosal cells, reesterification to triglyceride and cholesteryl ester occurs and these hydrophobic lipids are incorporated into the core of nascent chylomicrons [2]. The chylomicron surface is composed of phospholipid and the apoproteins (apo) B_{48}, A-I, A-II, and A-IV. Apo B_{48} is necessary for the secretion of chylomicrons from the mucosal cell. Triglycerides comprise about 90%, by weight, of the chylomicron, which has a density less than that of plasma. This is the basis for the "chylomicron test," where plasma left standing at 4°C overnight will develop a cream layer on top if chylomicrons are present. In normal individuals this test is usually negative as chylomicrons are present for only a few hours after ingestion of fat.

After secretion into mesenteric lymphatics, chylomicrons make their way to the superior vena cava via the thoracic duct. In both lymph and plasma, chylomicrons acquire apo C-II, apo C-III, and apo E. These additional surface components are transferred from HDL. Apo E may be added to the chylomicron surface somewhat later than apo C-II and apo C-III. Cholesterol, both free and esterified, and phospholipids also transfer from HDL to chylomicrons. The apoprotein transfers or exchanges are linked to the initial plasma metabolism of chylomicron triglyceride by the enzyme lipoprotein lipase (LPL) [3]. Thus, after gaining apo C-II, the chylomicron can activate LPL and chylomicron core triglyceride can be hydrolyzed. Absence of either LPL or apo C-II results in lack of chylomicron triglyceride lipolysis and severe hyper-triglyceridemia (and hyperchylomicronemia). Apo C-III may modulate this step by its ability to inhibit LPL activity [4], although the kinetics of the interaction between LPL and both apo C-II and apo C-III are unclear. The hydrolysis of chylomicron triglycerides occurs in the capillary beds of adipose tissue, lung, and muscles. LPL is synthesized in those tissues and, after secretion from cells, binds to the luminal surface of capillary endothelial cells where triglyceride hydrolysis occurs.

Significant chylomicron triglyceride hydrolysis results in the formation of a chylomicron remnant which has a reduced core volume, and must, to maintain a spherical conformation, rid itself of excess surface [5]. This is actually a continuous process whereby phospholipid, free cholesterol, and apoproteins are transferred back to HDL, their initial source. Chylomicron remnants are relatively cholesteryl ester rich (both from dietary sources and from HDL-derived cholesteryl ester) in their core, and apo E rich on their surface. Remnants can interact with receptor(s) on hepatocytes and be rapidly removed from the circulation. The pathway(s) for uptake of chylomicron remnants by the liver is (are) poorly defined but may include LDL receptors that can recognize apo E, specific apo E receptors, and/or glycosaminoglycans that can bind apo E. It is clear that apo E is crucial in this process as individuals lacking apo E, or having the defective apo E-II isoform accumulate chylomicron remnants in plasma [6]. Apo B_{48} does not appear to play a role in remnant removal from plasma.

Hepatic triglyceride-rich lipoproteins

VLDL assembly takes place in the endoplasmic reticulum and Golgi body of hepatocytes [7,8]. Triglycerides, synthesized from fatty acids either taken up from plasma or newly synthesized in the liver, and cholesterol, synthesized from acetate or delivered to the liver by chylomicron remnants, are packaged together with apo B_{100} and phospholipids into nascent VLDL. Plasma VLDL also contain apo C-I, apo C-II, apo C-III, and apo E, and although some or all of these apoproteins may be added to the nascent VLDL particles as they are assembled in hepatocytes, the majority of these molecules are probably added to VLDL after their entry into plasma. The size of the VLDL seems to be determined mainly by the quantity of triglyceride available for packaging into these lipoproteins [7–9]. Hence, large triglyceride-rich VLDL will be secreted in situations where excess triglycerides are synthesized, such as obesity, diabetes mellitus, or alcohol consumption. Small VLDL, and possibly intermediate-density lipoprotein (IDL) and/or LDL-like particles may be secreted when triglyceride, but not cholesterol, availability is reduced.

The number of VLDL particles assembled and secreted by the liver appears to be regulated, but the mechanism for this regulation has not been defined. Because there appears to be only one apo B_{100} per VLDL particle, the rate of apo B_{100} synthesis might be rate limiting. Studies of hepatic apo B_{100} mRNA levels· under a variety of physiologic stimuli have not, however, demonstrated clear regulation at this point. On the other hand, posttranslational regulation of apo B_{100} secretion may be important [10]. Triglyceride flux, at least as determined in human studies, is not necessarily linked to increased apo B (and therefore VLDL) secretion by the liver [11]. Some recent studies, however, have suggested that cholesterol availability may regulate the number of VLDL particles secreted by the liver. The role of phospholipids in this pathway is also not known. The disorders called familial combined hyperlipidemia and hyperapobetalipoproteinemia appear to be characterized by increased rates of secretion of VLDL particles from the liver, while isolated familial hypertriglyceridemia seems to be caused by hepatic secretion of a normal number of VLDL particles which are triglyceride enriched [12,13].

In the plasma, VLDL lose triglycerides after interacting with LPL (activated by apo C-II). In doing so they become smaller and more dense, and are converted to IDL. The term VLDL remnant has also been used to describe this product of VLDL triglyceride catabolism in order to suggest a parallel with the chylomicron/chylomicron remnant system. Chylomicron remnants are quantitatively removed from plasma, while VLDL catabolism, in contrast, results in direct removal from plasma of some, but not all, particles [9,11,14]. We do not, as yet, have any method to clearly identify and isolate VLDL that are destined for removal from plasma from those that are converted to LDL. It appears, however, that larger VLDL are more likely to be removed directly from plasma while smaller, more dense VLDL are more efficiently converted to LDL.

VLDL catabolism has two significant consequences. First, as noted for chylomicron metabolism, loss of VLDL triglyceride results in the transfer of surface cholesterol, phospholipids, and apoproteins to HDL [5]. Efficient VLDL catabolism is associated with low plasma triglyceride concentrations and maximal availability of surface components for transfer to HDL. Hypertriglyceridemia, in contrast, is associated with reduced levels of HDL. Second, loss of triglyceride from VLDL generates IDL, which after interaction with the liver become LDL. Some LPL activity appears necessary for normal functioning of the metabolic cascade from VLDL to IDL to LDL [15]. It appears that both apo E and a second lipolytic enzyme, hepatic triglyceride lipase (HTGL), also play important roles in this process.

Apo E, acting as a ligand for one or more receptors, appears to be critical for both the direct removal of some VLDL particles from the circulation and for the conversion of other VLDL particles to IDL and LDL [16,17]. In patients who either lack apo E or who are homozygous for the E-II mutant isoform of apo E, apo B_{100} metabolism seems to stall at the remnant/IDL stage. In the majority of individuals who are E-II homozygous in the population but have normal lipids, there are increased numbers of cholesteryl ester-enriched VLDL remnants and reduced numbers of mature LDL in the plasma. A major unanswered question at this time relates to the mechanism whereby apo E can regulate both direct removal of VLDL from plasma and conversion of VLDL to LDL.

HTGL is an enzyme with homology to LPL. It is synthesized in the liver and can interact with several lipoprotein classes after binding to the luminal surface of endothelial cells in hepatic sinusoids. Studies suggests that HTGL plays a role in removing triglycerides from partially catabolized VLDL or IDL, and therefore in their conversion to LDL [18]. These data are supported by studies in a few subjects lacking HTGL who have increased VLDL remnant and IDL levels in plasma.

One other component of VLDL catabolism must be noted. During the period when VLDL triglycerides are being hydrolyzed, the VLDL particles become enriched in cholesteryl esters. This process, mediated by cholesterol ester transfer protein, generates a VLDL particle that has more cholesteryl ester molecules than are present in LDL. Two possible metabolic pathways can be invoked to explain how these VLDL can then give rise to LDL. First, the cholesteryl ester-enriched VLDL particles might deliver some of this core lipid to the liver (and/or other cells) without being internalized themselves. Second, a subset of VLDL particles might contain more cholesteryl ester than do LDL, and this subset (VLDL remnants) would not be converted to LDL. The potential atherogenicity of cholesteryl ester-enriched VLDL is discussed elsewhere in this book.

Pathophysiology of hypertriglyceridemic states

In the following section hypertriglyceridemia will be divided into two categories: isolated elevations of VLDL triglycerides, and elevations of VLDL triglycerides in combination with elevated levels of LDL cholesterol (Table 15.1). This division is somewhat arbitrary in that many subjects with isolated elevations of VLDL triglyceride can develop elevated LDL cholesterol concentrations when triglyceride levels are reduced by weight loss, diet modification, and/or drug therapy. Similarly, some subjects with consistently isolated elevations of plasma triglyceride may have first degree relatives with either isolated LDL cholesterol levels or combined hyperlipidemia. Hence, it is not easy to determine which of the two categories is appropriate for any individual patient. With this caveat in mind, the division is used to highlight differences in

Table 15.1 Characteristics of common hypertriglyceridemias

Type	Plasma lipid levels	Clinical signs
Isolated hypertriglyceridemia		
Mild	TG = 250–750 mg/dl (plasma may be cloudy). Elevations are in VLDL	Asymptomatic; may be associated with increased risk of vascular disease
Severe	TG >750 mg/dl (plasma may be milky). Elevations are in VLDL and chylomicrons	May be asymptomatic; may be associated with pancreatitis, abdominal pain, hepatosplenomegaly
Hypertriglyceridemia and hypercholesterolemia		
Combined hyperlipidemia	TG = 250–750 mg/dl; total cholesterol = 250–500 mg/dl; VLDL is elevated; LDL is >95th percentile	Usually asymptomatic until vascular disease develops. Familial form (FCHL) may present as isolated high TG or as isolated high LDL cholesterol
Dysbetalipoproteinemia	TG = 250–500 mg/dl; total cholesterol = 250–500 mg/dl; VLDL and IDL are elevated, LDL is normal or reduced	Usually asymptomatic until vascular disease develops; may have palmar or tuboeruptive xanthoma

lipoprotein physiology, and possibly in atherogenicity, between the two categories, and to set the stage for discussion of different approaches to pharmacotherapy for each.

It should also be noted that this presentation does not rely on the classical phenotype system, although those phenotypes are noted when appropriate. It is not that phenotypes are not helpful, but the genetic heterogeneity underlying each phenotype, together with similar (if not common) pathophysiology of the several phenotypes possible in combined hyperlipidemia, make a simpler classification system more manageable.

Hypertriglyceridemia with normal LDL cholesterol

In this group of disorders, elevated levels of fasting plasma triglycerides in the range of 250–750 mg/dl are generally associated with increased concentrations of only VLDL triglycerides (Type IV phenotype). When VLDL triglyceride levels are markedly elevated (regardless of etiology), or when LPL is either significantly reduced or totally deficient, chylomicron triglycerides may also be present, even after a 14-hour fast (Type V phenotype). Increased plasma levels of VLDL triglycerides are usually associated with excessive synthesis and secretion of VLDL triglyceride by the liver [19]. Hepatic triglyceride synthesis is regulated by substrate flow, particularly the availability of free fatty acids; by energy status, particularly the level of glycogen stores in the liver; and by hormonal status, particularly the balance between insulin and glucagon levels. It is therefore not surprising that obesity, excessive consumption of simple sugars and saturated fats, inactivity, alcohol consumption, and glucose intolerance or diabetes mellitus have been commonly associated with hypertriglyceridemia. Recent studies have also suggested a link between abnormal bile acid metabolism and overproduction of triglycerides in some subjects with hypertriglyceridemia [20]. Whatever the etiology, it is believed that in this disorder, sometimes referred to as primary hypertriglyceridemia, only hepatic triglyceride synthesis is increased and, therefore, a normal number of large, triglyceride-enriched VLDL particles are assembled and secreted by the liver. The secretion of a normal number of VLDL particles limits the rate of production of LDL particles, and these subjects do not develop coincident elevations of LDL cholesterol. However, because subjects with familial combined hyperlipidemia (see below) can present with isolated hypertriglyceridemia, the Type IV phenotype may result from either of these disorders. The importance of this statement derives from the apparently low risk for coronary heart disease (CHD) associated with primary hypertriglyceridemia compared to the significantly increased risk for CHD associated with combined hyperlipidemia.

The activity of the two key triglyceride hydrolyses, LPL and HTGL, will determine, to a significant degree, the severity of hypertriglyceridemia present in any individual. Most data suggest that LPL is normal in the majority of subjects with moderate hypertriglyceridemia (250–500 mg/dl), but that this enzyme activity may be reduced in more severely affected individuals (>750 mg/dl) [3]. When VLDL triglyceride concentrations are markedly elevated (>1000 mg/dl), LPL may be either saturated or actually "consumed." As a result, subjects with such levels of plasma triglycerides are relatively deficient in the enzyme during the postprandial period [21]. Accumulation of chylomicron triglycerides may then add to the hypertriglyceridemia in such patients. When LPL (or apo C-II) is totally deficient (Type I phenotype), plasma triglyceride concentrations >2000 mg/dl are commonly seen. In this case, both chylomicrons and VLDL make significant contributions to the hypertriglyceridemic state [22]. VLDL levels can be normal in the Type I phenotype, however, with only hyperchylomicronemia present. HTGL activity is frequently elevated in hypertriglyceridemic subjects and the meaning of this association is unclear, although it may be relevant to the reduced HDL cholesterol levels found in this condition [23]. Deficiency of HTGL is a rare disorder in humans which results in defective final catabolism and/or abnormal remodeling of small VLDL and IDL [24]. These individuals may resemble those with apo E-II homozygosity and the Type III phenotype.

Hypertriglyceridemia with elevated LDL cholesterol

Hypertriglyceridemia can also occur in two phenotypes in association with hypercholesterolemia. In the first, called combined hyperlipidemia (Type IIB phenotype), both total plasma triglycerides and LDL cholesterol concentrations must, by definition, be greater than the 90th percentiles for age- and sex-matched controls [25]. Combinations of regulatory defects in lipid and/or apoprotein metabolism are likely to account for a significant number of individuals with this phenotype. A familial form of combined hyperlipidemia (FCHL) has been identified, however, in which probands may present with combined hyperlipidemia, with only hypertriglyceridemia, or with only elevated levels of LDL cholesterol [26]. This disorder appears to be transmitted as an autosomal dominant gene, and the diagnosis rests on the presentation, at some point in time, of combined hyperlipidemia in the proband. The presence of various lipid phenotypes (Types IIa, IIb, or IV) in first degree family members, along with either isolated hypertriglyceridemia or an isolated elevation of LDL cholesterol in the proband, can also form the basis for diagnosis. It should be noted that more than one single-gene disorder may result in the same FCHL phenotype. Additionally, individuals who have inherited two separate genes associated with lipid disorders can present with combined hyperlipidemic phenotypes.

FCHL (as well as the undefined combined hyperlipidemic phenotype) is associated with increased secretion of VLDL particles (as determined by the flux of VLDL apo B_{100}) [12,13,27]. Since apo B_{100} is required for the secretion of hepatic lipids in VLDL, individuals with FCHL will have higher levels of plasma VLDL triglycerides if, for any other reason (see above), they synthesize triglycerides at an increased rate. Once they have assembled and secreted increased numbers of triglyceride-rich VLDL, these individuals will have plasma triglyceride concentrations determined by their ability to hydrolyze VLDL triglyceride with LPL and/or HTGL. The ability to hydrolyze VLDL triglycerides will also regulate the generation of LDL in plasma. Thus, subjects with FCHL who have very high VLDL triglyceride concentrations (and are not able to efficiently catabolize VLDL) may have normal or actually reduced numbers of LDL particles in the circulation and a normal LDL cholesterol concentration. If these same individuals are able to efficiently catabolize the increased numbers of VLDL particles that are entering the plasma, they will generate increased numbers of LDL particles and present, therefore, with both hypertriglyceridemia and increased plasma levels of LDL cholesterol. Finally, subjects with FCHL who are synthesizing only normal quantities of triglycerides will still tend to generate increased numbers of LDL particles. These individuals can present with only elevated plasma LDL cholesterol concentrations. FCHL may occur in as many as 1/50 to 1/100 Americans, and is the most common familial lipid disorder found in survivors of myocardial infarction [26].

Dysbetalipoproteinemia (Type III phenotype) is the second type of hyperlipidemia in which elevations of both plasma triglycerides and cholesterol can occur. This is a rare disorder affecting 1/10 000 people which results from mutations in the gene for apo E. These mutations (there are several) result in the synthesis of defective forms of this apoprotein, called apo E-II. Since apo E appears to play crucial roles in the catabolism of chylomicron and VLDL remnants [6], subjects with defective apo E accumulate these cholesteryl ester-enriched remnant lipoproteins in their plasma. VLDL triglyceride and VLDL cholesterol are both elevated in this disorder. Chylomicron remnants are also present in fasting plasma from dysbetalipoproteinemic subjects [28]. In contrast, LDL cholesterol levels are not elevated in this disorder. Of interest are the data indicating that 1/100 people are homozygous for the mutant apo E-II isoform; 99% of these apo E-II/E-II subjects have normal plasma triglyceride and cholesterol levels. They do, however, have increased VLDL remnants and reduced LDL cholesterol levels (possibly a consequence of their inability to normally process VLDL). Thus, in the 1/10 000 individuals with the clinically relevant entity, dysbetalipo-proteinemia, a second defect in lipid metabolism must be present.

Low HDL cholesterol in hypertriglyceridemia

The pathophysioloy and treatment of low HDL cholesterol levels will be addressed in the next chapter. It is only necessary at this point to note that plasma levels of HDL cholesterol are inversely related to plasma triglyceride levels and that reduced HDL levels are common in both isolated hypertriglyceridemia and in hypertriglyceridemia combined with elevated LDL cholesterol levels. Hence, even though plasma triglycerides have not been shown clearly to be independently associated with risk for CHD, patients with hypertriglyceridemia can also be viewed as patients with low HDL cholesterol concentrations. The reduced HDL cholesterol concentrations are associated with increased exchange of HDL cholesteryl esters for VLDL triglycerides, and this process results in cholesteryl ester enrichment of VLDL. These potentially atherogenic VLDL may, in fact, be the link between reduced HDL cholesterol levels and increased risk for CHD.

Dietary therapy

The National Cholesterol Education Program has recommended a two-step approach to lower plasma total cholesterol concentrations by progressively reducing intakes of saturated fatty acids and cholesterol. The Step-One Diet, which is similar to the guidelines recommended by the American Heart Association, is a population-based approach for lowering blood cholesterol. The recommendations (Table 15.2) include a total fat intake of less than 30% of total calories; an intake of saturated fat less than 10% of calories; an intake of polyunsaturated fat up to 10% of calories; and an intake of the rest of fat calories as monounsaturates. Cholesterol intake should be less than 300 mg/day. Dietary treatment should be aimed to achieve and maintain ideal body weight and healthy eating patterns, with a permanent change in eating behavior.

There is some controversy over the use of low total fat, high carbohydrate diets to treat hypertriglyceridemia. Although diets high in simple sugars can elevate plasma triglyceride concentrations [11], several

Table 15.2 Diet therapy of hypertriglyceridemia

Nutrient	Recommended dietary intake	
	Step-One Diet	Step-Two Diet
Total fat	Less than 30% of total calories	
Saturated fatty acids	<10% total calories	<7% total calories
Polyunsaturated fatty acids	Up to 10% of total calories	
Monounsaturated fatty acids	10−15% of total calories	
Carbohydrates	50−60% of total calories	
Protein	10−20% of total calories	
Cholesterol	<300 mg/day	<200 mg/day
Total calories	To achieve and maintain desirable weight	

studies have demonstrated that this rise does not occur when complex carbohydrates, with adequate soluble fiber content, are used. In addition, since elevations of LDL (such as in combined hyperlipidemia) certainly add significantly to any risk associated with hypertriglyceridemia, reductions in dietary saturated fat and cholesterol must be the focus of any dietary therapy. Finally, there is concern that alternatives to increased dietary carbohydrate, which would necessarily be higher in monounsaturated or polyunsaturated fat, would be associated with weight gain.

The Step-One Diet should be followed for a minimum of 3 months to maximize the time for the desired response expected with good adherence. If the response is not achieved, the NCEP recommendation is to progress to the Step-Two Diet (Table 15.2). The Step-One Diet should reduce plasma total and LDL cholesterol levels about 10% from baseline, depending on previous diet pattern and inherent characteristics of responsiveness [29]. Advancement to the Step-Two Diet may achieve a further 5% drop in plasma total cholesterol. The Step-Two Diet is recommended if the response to the Step-One Diet is not optimum. It calls for reducing further the saturated fatty acid intake to less than 7% of calories and cholesterol intake to less than 200 mg/day. Both the Step-One and Step-Two Diets recommend that patients achieve and maintain ideal body weight.

The Step-Two Diet may require intensive nutrition counseling in order to lower the saturated fat and cholesterol content of the diet even further without jeopardizing food palatability and acceptability. The total fat intake, however, can be maintained at 30% of total calories (Table 15.2). This would allow the individual to use monounsaturated sources of fat (olive and canola oils) as a replacement for the additional removal of saturated fats, thereby providing satiety attributable to the fat content of the meal.

Special considerations for hypertriglyceridemic individuals

Patients with hypertriglyceridemia will benefit by the addition of various strategies to the Step-One Diet plan. These include weight reduction, exercise, and abstention from alcohol. These adjuncts to diet will be particularly beneficial to patients who may be particularly sensitive to the increases in dietary carbohydrate associated with the Step-One and Step-Two Diets. Treatment of associated medical problems which can cause clinically significant hypertriglyceridemia in individuals with underlying predispositions can be very useful. These disorders include diabetes mellitus, hypothyroidism, chronic renal disease, and liver disease. As noted above, there is controversy concerning the use of high-carbohydrate diets in the treatment of hypertriglyceridemia. This is particularly true for individuals who are also diabetic. More studies of dietary therapy are needed in this patient group.

Severe hypertriglyceridemia and chylomicronemia (plasma levels of triglyceride >1000 mg/dl) should be treated with a very low-fat diet (10–20% of total calorie intake as fat) to prevent the patient from getting pancreatitis. These patients should also be told that if they are very sensitive to fatty foods, one meal comprising prime ribs, baked potato topped with sour cream, and cheesecake can precipitate an attack of pancreatitis. Fish oils as a supplement to a low-fat diet may help further reduce serum triglyceride levels in some patients. The widespread use of ω-3 fatty acid supplements in the treatment of hypertriglyceridemia cannot, however, be recommended because of the lack of large, long-term clinical trial results.

Drug therapy

General approach

If maximal efforts at dietary therapy have failed to achieve goals set by the physician and patient, intervention with pharmacologic agents may be initiated. The goals set for any individual patient will, of course, depend on several criteria. These include the presence or absence of CHD, the presence or absence of other risk factors (including family history of CHD), the age, and the sex of the patient. Because, as stated earlier, it has not been determined fully whether or not the plasma triglyceride concentration is an independent risk factor for CHD, an individual's LDL cholesterol and/or HDL cholesterol level can also be used to guide drug therapy. This can be true both in terms of goals and in terms of the initial choice of pharmacologic agent.

Nicotinic acid

Niacin (or nicotinic acid) is a water-soluble vitamin that has been used to treat hyperlipidemias for over three decades. Niacin therapy results in lower plasma levels of total and LDL cholesterol, and reductions in total plasma triglyceride concentrations. Dramatic increases in HDL cholesterol levels can occur during niacin therapy as well. Long-term effects of this treatment have been well described and documented. Niacin was used in a study of middle-aged men who had survived a myocardial infarction, and this therapy was associated with a reduction in coronary events [30]. A subsequent follow-up study of the men involved in this study showed, furthermore, that the niacin-treated group of men had increased survival [31]. Niacin was also used successfully in the CLAS [32] and FATS [33] protocols.

Pharmacology and metabolism

Niacin is readily absorbed from the gastrointestinal tract and peak blood levels are reached by 15–40 minutes after ingestion. Much of the dose is removed via the liver, before it reaches the circulation [34]. This high first-pass extraction of niacin by the liver may be responsible for much of the drug's mechanism of action, although niacin also has important effects on peripheral tissues. Nicotinic acid does not appear to interact with other drugs.

Mechanism of action

Niacin therapy affects the circulating levels of all major classes of lipoproteins. Plasma VLDL concentrations can fall dramatically, as reflected by decreases in plasma triglyceride levels. LDL cholesterol levels also fall during niacin treatment, while the levels of HDL cholesterol, the putative antiatherogenic lipoprotein, increase. Although the mechanisms underlying these changes are not completely defined, several possible mechanisms are described below.

Niacin decreases circulating levels of free fatty acids due to a decrease in intracellular lipolysis and release of fatty acids from adipose tissue [35]. This in turn reduces fatty acid uptake by the liver and may, in part, be responsible for decreased hepatic VLDL production. Of interest is the theoretical possibility that reduced fatty acid release from adipose tissue would be associated with increased insulin sensitivity in muscle and liver. The finding that nicotinic acid treatment can exacerbate glucose intolerance or diabetes mellitus suggests decreased, not increased, insulin sensitivity during niacin therapy, however.

LDL levels appear to fall as a result of decreased production of this particle [36]. This may be due to either a decrease in hepatic production and secretion of VLDL or to reduced conversion of precursor VLDL to LDL. Decreased production of LDL directly by the liver is another possible basis for niacin's effect on plasma LDL concentrations. Niacin has been shown to decrease the fractional catabolism of HDL apo A-I without affecting its production [37]. Because hypertriglyceridemia is associated with increased fractional catabolism of HDL apo A-I, reductions in plasma triglyceride concentrations during niacin therapy may result in decreased fractional clearance of HDL from plasma, and increased plasma HDL levels [38].

Additional actions of niacin have been described which may relate to its beneficial effects in preventing coronary events. Niacin therapy is associated with release of large amounts of prostaglandins, some of which may be associated with the decreased platelet aggregability seen with this drug.

Clinical efficacy

Because it is a vitamin, niacin is available as a nonprescription tablet which can be purchased in most pharmacies or health food stores in 50–500 mg tablets. Niacinamide, an alternative vitamin form of this compound, is not effective as a lipid-lowering agent. Slow-release forms of niacin, which some patients prefer because they tend to be associated with less flushing, are available at increased cost. They may cause more gastrointestinal and hepatic problems, however. There are also limited data related to the clinical efficacy of the slow-release forms, and the data that are available suggest that they are less effective than the short-acting agents [39].

Response to therapy may be somewhat variable. However, in general, reductions of approximately 15–25% in total plasma and LDL cholesterol can be expected in most patients. HDL cholesterol increases of 15–25% have been reported. In patients with hypertriglyceridemia, niacin therapy may be associated with 30–40% decreases in plasma triglyceride concentrations, with reductions in circulating triglycerides to normal levels in some cases. The response to niacin is variable with good cholesterol lowering occurring in some cases at less than 1 g/day, but occasional patients require up to 9 g/day. It is not clear if different doses are necessary for effective lowering of triglycerides, HDL, or LDL.

The most troubling side-effect of this medication is a benign vasodilatation of peripheral capillaries that occurs about 30 minutes after niacin administration. This "flush" may be avoided by starting with small amounts of niacin (e.g., 100–250 mg) and gradually increasing the dose by 250 mg every 3–5 days until the level of 1 g, two or three times a day, is attained. The medication should be taken with meals to decrease flushing and to avoid gastrointestinal irritation.

Toxicity

Niacin therapy is associated with a number of either inconvenient or potentially harmful side-effects. As noted above, the most common inconvenient side-effect is the "flush." This sensation, like a mild sunburn, occurs 15–30 minutes after a dose and lasts 30–60 minutes. Occasional patients may actually develop postural hypotension and will complain of light-headedness. This can be clinically significant if niacin therapy is initiated at a full dose. Fortunately, patients usually develop tachyphylaxis to the vasodilation and should be told that the worst flushing will occur upon initiating the therapy or when increasing the dose. The flushing is thought to be prostaglandin mediated and can be reduced or sometimes totally eliminated by prior ingestion of aspirin or ibuprofen. As described above, initial use of small doses, followed by a gradual build-up to the full dose of 1–4 g/day will also minimize flushing.

Niacin is also a gastric irritant and can worsen or precipitate peptic ulcer disease. Peptic ulcer disease should be an absolute contraindication to use of niacin. Increases in liver transaminase levels are common with niacin, occurring in 3–5% of patients. Increases up to threefold above normal levels of these enzymes, in the absence of symptoms, is not considered an absolute indication to stop therapy. Occasionally, a patient will develop a clinical picture compatible with acute hepatitis with fever, fatigue, right upper quadrant pain, and marked elevations of liver function tests. This is dose related and resolves after discontinuation of therapy. Liver function tests should, therefore, be obtained several weeks after the patient has been placed on niacin, and after increasing the dose. Dry skin and mucous membranes and pruritis can occur, and may be quite troubling in patients with dermatologic disorders. Blood uric acid levels invariably increase during niacin treatment, due to decreased renal clearance, and in predisposed individuals acute attacks of gout may be precipitated. Additional side-effects include decreased glucose tolerance, atrial tachycardia, and toxic amblyopia.

Effect on atherosclerosis

Niacin alone or in combination with resins has been used in several important secondary prevention studies. In the Coronary Drug Project Follow-Up study, the group treated with niacin during the original 7-year study was found to have increased survival 8 years later [31]. Combined with colestipol, niacin treatment of patients in the CLAS [32] and FATS [33] protocols was associated with angiographically proven reductions in progression of CHD. In some subjects in each of these studies actual regression of coronary lesions occurred as well.

Fibrates

The fibric acid derivatives can significantly reduce plasma total and VLDL triglyceride levels. They are a widely prescribed group of agents that also can reduce total plasma and LDL cholesterol levels, although these effects are more variable. Thus, modest to significant reductions in total and LDL cholesterol levels may be observed in normotriglyceridemic individuals, while unchanged or actually increased LDL cholesterol levels may be seen in hypertriglyceridemic subjects during therapy. Fibrates do, however, appear to consistently increase HDL cholesterol levels in hypertriglyceridemic subjects. Effects on HDL cholesterol concentrations in individuals with low HDL levels and normal plasma triglyceride concentrations may be inconsistent, however.

Pharmacology and metabolism

The fibrates are a group of hypolipidemic compounds characterized structurally by their phenoxyisobutyrate group. Clofibrate, the first of the fibric acid derivatives to be used clinically, gained additional potency with the addition of a Cl at the *para* position of the aromatic ring. Bezafibrate and fenofibrate both have the *para*Cl functions, while gemfibrozil does not. Bezafibrate and gemfibrozil are both in the acid form, while clofibrate and fenofibrate are not. Modification of the benzoyl group in bezafibrate and in fenofibrate appears to have significantly increased their hypolipidemic activity. The increased chain spacing in gemfibrozil appears to have done likewise to this drug's potency [40].

In general, the fibrates are well absorbed and are bound to plasma albumin and, interestingly, to apo B-containing lipoproteins. Because of the relatively high affinity of fibrates for circulating proteins, significant drug interactions between fibrates and other agents are common. The most important of these interactions has been with coumarin derivatives and some antiinflammatory agents. The concomitant use of a fibrate and coumarin anticoagulants raises the possibility of hemorrhage due to prolongation of the prothrombin time. This must be considered when fibrates are used in patients receiving this class of anticoagulants. Once in the bloodstream, all the fibrates are effectively removed and accumulated by the liver.

The modest modifications of structure of the different fibrates have significant effects on drug metabolism [40]. Clofibrate undergoes conversion to free clofibric acid which is excreted mainly through the kidneys in either unchanged or conjugated forms; 60–80% of plasma clofibrate is conjugated to glucuronic acid. The half-life of clofibrate is between 13 and 19 hours, and may be significantly prolonged in subjects with renal failure. Gemfibrozil is mainly free in plasma, circulating either in the unchanged form or after oxidation to a benzoic form. Plasma half-life is between 1 and 2 hours. Fenofibrate has several metabolic fates, including conversion to both free fenofibric acid and to a hydroxylated form of fenofibrate. Fenofibric acid is the major form of the drug in plasma and has a half-life of 20–24 hours. Bezafibrate does not undergo significant metabolic modification in plasma and has a half-life of only 1.5 hours.

Mechanism of action

Several effects of the fibrates on both hepatic triglyceride and cholesterol metabolism have been suggested by *in vitro* and *in situ* studies in rats and, to a lesser degree, in rabbits. There are conflicting data regarding differences among the various fibrates, but since the reported data for any one drug are from different laboratories using different protocols and methods, no firm conclusions can be drawn concerning any single agent.

Fibrates appear to inhibit triglyceride synthesis in the liver. Both reductions in fatty acid synthesis and reduced incorporation of glycerol and oleate into triglycerides have been demonstrated in livers from rats treated with fibrates [41]. Fatty acid oxidation also appears to be increased in both mitochondria and in peroxisomes. Decreased incorporation of acetate into cholesterol has also been observed and the activity of hydoxymethylglutaryl-CoA reductase (HMG-CoAR) is reduced in livers from rats treated with fibrates. Direct addition of fibrates to liver cells in culture does not, however, affect HMG-CoAR activity [41]. Hence, any effect of fibrates on cholesterol synthesis via the rate-limiting enzyme, HMG-CoAR, must be secondary to other direct effects.

Studies of triglyceride and cholesterol metabolism conducted *in vivo* support some of the *in vitro* data cited above. Glycerol incorporation into VLDL triglyceride, measured in kinetic studies of subjects treated with fibrates, demonstrates modest reductions in the rates of secretion of VLDL triglycerides into plasma compared to the untreated state [42, 43]. These turnover studies have also indicated increased fractional catabolism (FCR) of VLDL triglycerides during fibrate treatment [43]. Postheparin plasma LPL activity has been increased at the same time, consistent with the kinetic data [44]. In contrast, HTGL activity is not affected by fibrate therapy. Hence, the marked reductions in plasma triglycerides associated with fibric acid therapy results mainly from increased hydrolysis of VLDL triglycerides, with modest, additive reductions in VLDL secretion into plasma.

Cholesterol metabolism during fibrate therapy can be quite complex. Total body sterol balance studies indicate reduced cholesterol synthesis and increased biliary cholesterol excretion [43]. In hypercholesterolemic subjects who have normal triglycerides in the untreated state, fibrate therapy appears to reduce plasma LDL cholesterol levels by increasing receptor-mediated removal of LDL [42]. This finding is consistent with reduced hepatic cholesterol synthesis during treatment and concomitant increased hepatic LDL receptor activity. On the other hand, when hypertriglyceridemic subjects (in whom LDL cholesterol levels are normal or even reduced) are treated with fibrates, the cholesteryl ester content of their LDL increases and the FCR of LDL apo B is reduced to normal [42]. As a result, plasma LDL cholesterol levels can remain unchanged, or actually rise, during fibrate treatment of hypertriglyceridemia.

Increases in HDL cholesterol and apo A-1 concentrations are commonly seen during fibrate treatment, particularly in subjects presenting initially with hypertriglyceridemia. *In vivo* studies of HDL metabolism have been inconsistent. Gemfibrozil and fenofibrate treatment appear to be associated with increased production of apo A-I [42], while bezafibrate therapy had no effect on this parameter [42]. The FCR of HDL apo A-I is frequently increased in hypertriglyceridemic subjects, but there are no data indicating that this abnormality is affected by fibric acid therapy. As in the case of LDL, fibrate therapy does result in reduced HDL triglyceride and increased HDL cholesteryl ester content. It is fair to state at this time that we do not know why HDL cholesterol rises during fibrate treatment.

Clinical efficacy

There does not seem to be any significant difference between the triglyceride lowering of any of the available fibric acid derivatives. All of them can reduce plasma and VLDL triglycerides by 30–40%. The effects of individual fibrates on LDL cholesterol levels do appear to differ, at least in individuals with normal plasma triglyceride levels. Fenofibrate and bezafibrate appear to be significantly more effective in reducing LDL cholesterol in normotriglyceridemic subjects than are clofibrate or gemfibrozil. In hypertriglyceridemic subjects. LDL cholesterol levels, as noted above, either remain unchanged or actually increase during fibric acid therapy, and there do not seem to be any differences among the agents in this regard. HDL cholesterol levels are increased 5–15% by all the fibric acid derivatives, although clofibrate appears to be less effective in this regard than the other agents.

Toxicities

Proliferation of peroxisomes and development of neoplastic nodules in the liver during fibrate therapy have been the focus of most animal toxicity studies [40]. True carcinomas of the liver have been identified in some of these studies. While the basis of peroxisomal proliferation is unknown, it is thought to be secondary to increased β-oxidation of fatty acids in hepatic mitochondria. Concerns about potential carcinogenicity of fibrates in humans have been prominent, but no evidence for hepatic cancer or significant hepatomegaly or liver dysfunction has surfaced in clinical trials.

In the World Health Organization (WHO) study of clofibrate, increased total mortality was observed in the treated group [45], and this was associated, in part, with an increased incidence of gastrointestinal cancers. In the Helsinki Heart Study, therapy with gemfibrozil was not associated with increases in cancers of any type [46].

All of the fibric acid derivatives appear to increase the lithogenicity of bile. This arises from increased delivery of cholesterol to bile and reduced conversion of cholesterol to bile acids [47,48]. Although there was an increased incidence of gallstones noted in the WHO study treatment group [45], there was no such occurrence in the Helsinki Heart Study [46]. Long-term clinical experience with fenofibrate and bezafibrate in Europe has failed to uncover significant gallstone disease concomitant with use of these fibrates.

Effect on atherosclerosis

Two of the fibrates, clofibrate and gemfibrozil, have been used to treat hyperlipidemia in primary and secondary intervention trials. Clofibrate was used in several trials with varying results. Overall, reduced numbers of nonfatal myocardial infarctions and/or cardiovascular mortality were associated with clofibrate treatment in those studies, without reduction in total mortality. The largest clofibrate trial was carried out by WHO (see above). Various categories of nonfatal coronary artery ischemic events were found to be reduced by clofibrate treatment. Fatal myocardial infarctions were not reduced, however, and total mortality was increased, secondary to increased deaths related to malignant and nonmalignant gastrointestinal disease [45].

In the Helsinki Heart Study, in which gemfibrozil was used, treatment was associated with significant reductions in total coronary artery disease endpoints, including total cardiovascular mortality [46]. In this study, 2000 males received gemfibrozil and 2000 males received placebo over a 5-year period. Increasing differences in cardiovascular endpoints, including total cardiovascular mortality, became evident after 3 years in the Helsinki Study. At the end of the study, the gemfibrozil-treated group had a 35% reduction in endpoints compared to the placebo group. Drug therapy was associated with 11% lower LDL cholesterol and 12% higher HDL cholesterol levels in the treated group versus the placebo group. Multivariate analysis suggested that these changes could account for the differences in endpoint rates. Plasma triglycerides were also reduced by 35% in the gemfibrozil group as well. Subgroup analysis indicated that subjects with isolated elevations of LDL cholesterol, with combined elevations of LDL cholesterol and triglycerides, or with isolated elevations of triglycerides did equally well. These results indicate that different patients, with varying pathophysiologies, may respond differently to fibrates in terms of lipid lowering, but may benefit similarly from such treatment.

HMG-CoAR inhibitors

HMG-CoAR inhibitors, which are competitive inhibitors of this rate-limiting enzyme in the biosynthetic pathway for cholesterol synthesis, can lower plasma total and LDL cholesterol levels by 25–50%. Clinical trials of this class of agents have demonstrated that they also reduce plasma triglyceride levels 15–25%. HDL cholesterol concentrations increase 5–10% during therapy with these agents.

Pharmacology

Mevastatin, initially called compactin, was the first of these fungal lactones and was found to be a potent inhibitor of cholesterol bio-synthesis [49]. This was followed by fermentation or synthesis of a series of similar lactone compounds, many of which have been used in humans. Lovastatin and simvastatin differ from mevastatin by the addition of, respectively, one or two methyl groups. Pravastatin differs from the parent compound in that the lactone ring is open, forming the dihydroxycarboxylate form of the compound. This is the active form of the drug. A fully synthesized compound, fluvastatin, is similar to the acid form of the drug except that it has an additional benzene ring with an attached fluorine.

The reductase inhibitors are administered as either the lactone or the acid salt. It appears that at higher doses, the hydroxyacid form of the drug is better absorbed; only about 30% of the lactone form is absorbed. In the case of the absorbed lactone forms, conversion to the active hydroxyacid derivative occurs primarily within the liver. The liver takes up the lactone form very efficiently during the first pass of the blood from the portal system [49]. More of the acid salt forms pass through the liver into the peripheral circulation after oral administration and can be measured in peripheral blood. However, the acid forms are not taken up well by tissues other than the liver, and so the relevance of their presence in the peripheral circulation is unclear. In the bloodstream, reductase inhibitors are bound to albumin. Final metabolism of these compounds is in the liver, and there is no evidence for enterohepatic recirculation of drug. After oral or intravenous administration, less than 10% of the drug lovastatin was found to be excreted in the urine. Whether or not clinically relevant tissue selectivity is a characteristic of any of the available HMG-CoAR inhibitors remains to be determined.

Although it was originally thought that reductase inhibitors would not interact with other drugs, it now appears that lovastatin may increase the efficacy of coumarin anticoagulants. Further studies of drug interaction will be required.

Mechanism of action

These compounds are competitive inhibitors of the enzyme HMG-CoAR, the rate-limiting enzyme in cholesterol biosynthesis. Studies in animals have suggested that as a response to decreased cholesterol biosynthesis, cells and organs respond by increasing their synthesis of both HMG-CoAR [50] and LDL receptors [51]. Thus, although a decrease in total body cholesterol biosynthesis may not be apparent [52,53], plasma LDL cholesterol levels may decrease as a result of increased receptor-mediated fractional removal of LDL by the liver [54]. This appears to account for the response to these drugs in subjects with heterozygous familial hypercholesterolemia who have only one-half of the normal number of receptors. Subjects with moderate hypercholesterolemia (polygenic) or with combined hyperlipoproteinemia have normal LDL receptors, however, and the benefits of HMG-CoAR inhibitor treatment in these patients appear to derive from decreased hepatic production of apo B-containing lipoproteins. These patients do not consistently demonstrate increased fractional catabolism of circulating LDL during treatment with reductase inhibitors [55,56]. The results of several studies suggest, therefore, that there is coordinate regulation of cholesterol synthesis with the assembly and packaging of preformed apo B into VLDL and LDL. Interestingly, reduced rates of secretion of VLDL triglycerides are also observed in subjects with hypertriglyceridemia treated with HMG-CoAR inhibitors [57]. Whether this is a concomitant of reduced VLDL apo B secretion or a direct effect of reductase inhibitors on hepatic triglyceride synthesis remains to be determined.

Clinical efficacy

Lovastatin, pravastatin, and simvastatin are presently the HMG-CoAR inhibitors approved for general use in the USA. All of these drugs appear, at this time, to have similar clinical efficacy, although long-term studies (more than 1 year) of any reductase inhibitors are lacking. Using 5–40 mg/day of lovastatin twice daily the dose–response decrease in total and LDL cholesterol ranged from 21 to 32% and 25 to 39%, respectively [58], and the presently recommended dose range is 20–80 mg daily, given either four times daily for the 20–40 mg doses or twice daily for larger doses. Similar doses of the other reductase inhibitors appear to be equally efficacious. Although there was no evidence of tachyphylaxis to the effects of these agents in clinical trials, some physicians have been reporting loss of efficacy after several months of treatment. While it is likely that reduced patient compliance with drug and diet regimens is the basis for these observations, increased synthesis of HMG-CoAR by the liver may be involved.

Of particular relevance to the treatment of hypertriglyceridemia is the observation that lovastatin therapy is associated with modest reductions of plasma triglyceride (15–25%), and small, but not insignificant, increases in HDL (5–10%). The use of this drug in the treatment of elevated plasma triglycerides, or reduced levels of HDL cholesterol, will probably be driven by the coexisting level of LDL cholesterol in any individual patient. Hence, if LDL is high in a patient with a combined hyperlipidemic phenotype, lovastatin may be a rational first choice. Niacin or a fibric acid derivative may be added later if needed (see below for possible toxicity). If LDL is normal or low-normal in a hyper-triglyceridemic subject, niacin or a fibric acid derivative would be the appropriate first choice for therapy.

Toxicity

The clinical trials conducted thus far for all of the reductase inhibitors have been very comforting. Most of the longer trials that have been reported have involved lovastatin, including a recent 48-week trial with over 8000 subjects [59]. In that study, lovastatin was associated with increases in liver transaminases more than three times the upper limit of normal in approximately 1% of patients. Symptoms compatible with hepatitis are very unusual. The biochemical disorder usually is alleviated after discontinuing the medication. Severe myositis, with fever, myalgias, and creatinine phosphokinase levels of >1000 IU occurred in 0.1–0.2% of patients taking lovastatin alone [59]. This adverse reaction is more frequent in patients also taking cyclosporine (25–30%), gemfibrozil (3–5%), and niacin (3–5%). Low rates of complaints such as gastrointestinal upset, insomnia, and headache have been reported in clinical trials of lovastatin. There is no evidence of long-term toxicity or oncogenic potential in humans, although long-term data are very limited at this time. Clinical trials with pravastatin, simvastatin (which has been widely used in Europe for several years), and fluvastatin have, in general, revealed similar low profiles of adverse reactions.

Effect on atherosclerosis

The limited time since introduction of these agents has not allowed their use in primary or secondary prevention trials. Such studies are, however, currently in progress.

Combination therapy

If pharmacologic therapy for isolated hypertriglyceridemia is required, an adequate response is usually achieved with either niacin or a fibrate.

If significant elevations in plasma triglycerides persist after an adequate trial of either of these agents, combined treatment using both together might be worthwhile. There is little documented experience with this combination, however, and so their use together must be undertaken with caution. In addition, since a dose relationship between plasma triglyceride concentrations and risk for CHD has not been clearly established, therapeutic goals in the treatment of hypertriglyceridemia remain vague. On the other hand, if elevated plasma triglycerides are associated (as they commonly are) with reduced plasma levels of HDL cholesterol, the combination of niacin and gemfibrozil might be tried if both agents alone reduced triglycerides without significantly affecting HDL levels. Again, there is little, if any, reported experience with this approach.

In the treatment of hypertriglyceridemia combined with elevated levels of LDL cholesterol, niacin alone may be adequate. If not, niacin plus a fibrate may achieve lowering of LDL that is not attainable with either alone. If significant elevations of LDL cholesterol are present in a patient who also has markedly elevated plasma triglyceride levels, a reductase inhibitor may have to be used in combination with either niacin or a fibrate. As noted above, both of these combinations carries a risk of severe myositis (3–5% incidence). The use of either combination should be limited to individuals with severe combined hyperlipidemia and either multiple other risks for CHD or the presence of CHD itself. Careful patient education as to the risks involved in such treatment is required.

As noted earlier in this chapter, use of ω-3 fatty acid supplements to lower plasma triglycerides cannot be recommended at present. Their use as adjuncts in patients with plasma triglyceride levels >1000 mg/dl that persist despite fibrate treatment may be useful. There are no reports of the long-term efficacy of such a combination, however.

References

1 Austin MA. Plasma triglyceride and coronary heart disease. *Arterioscler Thomb* 1991; 11:2–14.
2 Green PHR, Glickman RM. Intestinal lipoprotein metabolism. *J Lipid Res* 1980;21: 942–52.
3 Olivecrona T, Olivecrona-Bengtsson G. Lipoprotein lipase from milk—The model enzyme in lipoprotein lipase research. In *Lipoprotein Lipase* (ed. J Borensztajan). Chicago: Evener Publishers, 1987:15–58.
4 Ginsberg HN, Le NA, Goldberg IJ *et al.* Apolipoprotein B metabolism in subjects with deficiency of apolipoprotein CIII and AI: Evidence that apolipoprotein CIII inhibits catabolism of triglyceride-rich lipoproteins by lipoprotein lipase *in vivo. J Clin Invest* 1986;78:1287–95.
5 Tall AR, Small DM. Plasma high density lipoproteins. *N Engl J Med* 1978;299:1232–6.

6 Schneider WJ, Kovanen PT, Brown MS *et al.* Familial dysbetalipoproteinemia: Abnormal binding of mutant apoprotein E to low density lipoprotein receptors of human fibroblasts and membranes from liver and adrenal of rats, rabbits, and cows. *J Clin Invest* 1981;68:1075−85.

7 Janero DR, Siuta-Mangano P, Miller KW, Lane MD. Synthesis, processing and secretion of hepatic very low density lipoprotein. *J Cell Biochem* 1984;24:131−52.

8 Olofsson SO, Bjursell G, Bostrom K *et al.* Apolipoprotein B: structure, biosynthesis and role in the lipoprotein assembly process. *Atherosclerosis* 1987;68:1−17.

9 Ginsberg HN, Le NA, Gibson JC. Regulation of the production and catabolism of plasma low density lipoproteins in hypertriglyceridemic subjects: Effects of weight loss. *J Clin Invest* 1985;75:614−23.

10 Dixon J, Furakowa S, Ginsberg HN. Oleic acid stimulates secretion of apoB-containing lipoproteins from HepG2 cells by reducing intracellular degradation of apoB. *J Biol Chem* 1991;266:5080−6.

11 Ginsberg HN, Le NA, Melish J, Steinberg D, Brown WV. Effect of a high carbohydrate diet on apoprotein B catabolism in man. *Metabolism* 1981;30:347−53.

12 Chait A, Albers JJ, Brunzell JD. Very low density lipoprotein overproduction in genetic forms of hypertriglyceridemia. *Eur J Clin Invest* 1980;10:161−72.

13 Teng B, Sniderman AD, Soutar AK, Thompson GR. Metabolic basis of hyperapobetalipoproteinemia. Turnover of apolipoprotein B in low density lipoprotein and its precursors and subfractions compared with normal and familial hypercholesterolemia. *J Clin Invest* 1986;77:663−72.

14 Gotto AM, Pownall HJ, Havel RA. Introduction to the plasma lipoproteins. In *Methods of Enzymology*, Vol. 128 (eds JP Segrest, JJ Albers). New York: Academic Press, 1986: 3−40.

15 Goldberg IJ, Le NA, Ginsberg HN, Krauss RM, Lindgren FT. Lipoprotein metabolism during acute inhibition of lipoprotein lipase in the cynomolgus monkey. *J Clin Invest* 1988;81:561−8.

16 Mahley RW. Apolipoprotein E: cholesterol transport protein with expanding role in cell biology. *Science* 1988;240:622−30.

17 Mahley RW, Innerarity TL, Rall SC Jr, Weisgraber KH. Plasma lipoproteins: alolipo- protein structure and function. *J Lipid Res* 1984;25:1277−94.

18 Goldberg IJ, Le NA, Paterniti JR Jr *et al.* Lipoprotein metabolism during acute inhibition of hepatic triglyceride lipase in the cynomolgus monkey. *J Clin Invest* 1982;70:1184−92.

19 Reaven GM, Hill DB, Gross RC, Farquhar JW. Kinetics of triglyceride turnover of very low density lipoproteins of human plasma. *J Clin Invest* 1965;44:1826−33.

20 Angelin B, Hershon KS, Brunzell JD. Bile acid metabolism in hereditary forms of hypertriglyceridemia: evidence for an increased synthesis rate in monogenic familial hypertriglyceridemia. *Proc Natl Acad Sci USA* 1987;84:5434−8.

21 Goldberg IJ, Kandel JJ, Blum CB, Ginsberg HN. Association of plasma lipoproteins with postheparin lipase activities. *J Clin Invest* 1986;78:1523−8.

22 Fredrickson DS, Goldstein JL, Brown MS. The familial hyperlipoproteinemias. In *The Metabolic Basis of Inherited Disease* (eds JB Stanburg, JB Wyngaarden, DS Fredrickson). New York: McGraw-Hill, 1978:604−55.

23 Kinnunen PKJ. Hepatic endothelial lipase: Isolation, some characteristics, and physiological role. In *Lipases* (eds B Borgstrom, HL Brockman). New York: Elsevier, 1984:307−28.

24 Breckenridge WC, Little JA, Alaupovic P *et al.* Lipoprotein abnormalities associated with a familial deficiency of hepatic lipase. *Atherosclerosis* 1982;45:161−79.

25 The Lipid Research Clinics. Population Studies Data Book. Vol. I The prevalence Study. US Department of Health and Human Services, Public Health Service, National Institutes of Health.

26 Goldstein JL, Schrott HG, Hazzard WR, Bierman EL, Motulsky R. Hyperlipidemia in coronary heart disease: Genetic analysis of lipid levels in 176 families and delineation

of a new inherited disorder combined hyperlipidemia. *J Clin Invest* 1973;52:1544—68.

27 Kissebah AH, Alfarsi A, Adams PW. Integrated regulation for very low density lipoprotein triglyceride and apolipoprotein B kinetics in man: Normolipidemic subjects, familial hypertriglyceridemia and familial combined hyperlipidemia. *Metabolism* 1981;20:856—68.

28 Morganroth J, Levy RI, Fredrickson DS. The biochemical, clinical and genetic features of type III hyperlipoproteinemia. *Ann Intern Med* 1975;82:158—74.

29 Ginsberg HN, Barr SL, Karmally W *et al.* Reduction of plasma cholesterol levels in normal men on an American Heart Association Step 1 diet or a Step 1 diet with added monounsaturated fat. *N Engl J Med* 1990;322:574—9.

30 Coronary Drug Project. Clofibrate and niacin in coronary heart disease. *JAMA* 1975;231:360—81.

31 Canner PL, Berge KG, Wenger NK *et al.* Fifteen year mortality in coronary drug project patients: Long-term benefit with niacin. *J Am Coll Cardiol* 1968;8:1245—55.

32 Blankenhorn DH, Nessim SA, Johnson RL *et al.* Beneficial effects of combined colestipol—niacin therapy on coronary atherosclerosis and coronary venous bypass grafts. *JAMA* 1987;257:3233—40.

33 Brown G, Albers JJ, Fisher LD *et al.* Regression of coronary artery disease as a result of intensive lipid-lowering therapy in men with high levels of apolipoprotein B. *N Engl J Med* 1990;323:1289—98.

34 Greengard P. Water-soluble vitamins: The vitamin B complex. In *Pharmacological Basis of Therapuetics*, 5th edn (eds LS Goodman, A Gilman). New York: MacMillan Publishing Co., 1975:1549—63.

35 Carlson LA, Oro L. Effects of treatment with nicotinic acid for one month on serum lipids in patients with different types of hyperlipidemia. *Atherosclerosis* 1973;18:1—9.

36 Langer T, Levy RI. The effect of nicotinic acid on the turnover of low density lipoproteins in type II hyperlipoproteinemia. In *Metabolic Effects of Nicotinic Acid and its Derivatives* (eds KK Gey, LA Carlson). Bern: Hans Huber, 1971.

37 Shepherd J, Packard CJ, Patsch JR, Gotto AM Jr, Taunton OD. Effects of nicotinic acid therapy on plasma high density lipoprotein subfraction distribution and composition and on apolipoprotein A metabolism. *J Clin Invest* 1979;63:858—67.

38 Le AN, Gibson JC, Ginsberg HN. Independent regulation of plasma apolipoprotein CII and CIII concentrations in very low density and high density lipoproteins: Implications for the regulation of the catabolism of these lipoproteins. *J Lipid Res* 1988;29:669—77.

39 Knopp RH, Ginsberg J, Albers JJ *et al.* Contrasting effects of unmodified and time-released forms of niacin on lipoproteins in hyperlipidemic subjects: Clues to mechanism of action of niacin. *Metabolism* 1985;34:642—50.

40 Sirtori CR, Franceschini G. Effects of fibrates on serum lipids and atherosclerosis. *Pharmacol Ther* 1988;37:167—91.

41 Kloer HU. Structure and biochemical effects of fenofibrate. *Am J Med* 1987;83:3—8.

42 Ginsberg HN. Changes in lipoprotein kinetics during therapy with fenofibrate and other fibric acid derivatives. *Am J Med* 1987;83:66—70.

43 Grundy SM, Vega GL. Fibric acids: Effects on lipids and lipoprotein metabolism. *Am J Med* 1987;83:9—20.

44 Boberg J, Boberg M, Gross R *et al.* The effects of treatment with clofibrate on hepatic triglyceride and lipoprotein lipase activities of postheparin plasma in male patients with hyperlipoproteinemia. *Arteriosclerosis* 1977;267:499—503.

45 Oliver MF, Heady JA, Morris JN *et al.* Report from the committee of principal investigators: A cooperative trial in the primary prevention of ischaemic heart disease using clofibrate. *Br Heart J* 1978;40:1069—118.

46 Frick MH, Elo O, Haapa K *et al.* Helsinki heart study: Primary-prevention trial with gemfibrozil in middle-aged men with dyslipidemia. *N Engl J Med* 1987;317:1237—45.

47 Palmer RH. Effects of fibric acid derivatives on biliary lipid composition. *Am J Med* 1987;83:37—43.

48 Pertsemlids D, Penveliwalla D, Aherns EJ Jr. Effects of clofibrate and of an estrogen—

progestin combination on fasting biliary lipids and cholic acid kinetics in man. *Gastroenterology* 1974;66:565−73.

49 Alberts AW. HMG-CoA reductase inhibitors—the development. In *Atherosclerosis Reviews* Vol. 18 (eds J Stokes III, M Mancini). New York: Raven Press, 1988:123−32.

50 Mehrabian M, Callaway KA, Clarke CF *et al.* Regulation of rat liver 3-hydroxy-3-methylglutaryl coenzyme A synthase and the chromosomal localization of the human gene. *J Biol Chem* 1986;261:16249−55.

51 Kovanen PT, Bilheimer DW, Goldstein JL, Jaramillo JJ, Brown MS. Regulatory role for hepatic low density lipoprotein receptors *in vivo* in the dog. *Proc Natl Acad Sci USA* 1981;78:1194−8.

52 Grundy SM, Bilheimer DW. Inhibition of 3-hydroxy-3-methylglutaryl-CoA reductase by mevinolin in familial hypercholesterolemia heterozygotes: Effects on cholesterol balance. *Proc Natl Acad Sci USA* 1984;81:2538−42.

53 Goldberg IJ, Holleran S, Ramakrishnan R *et al.* Lack of effect of lovastatin therapy on the parameters of whole body cholesterol turnover. *J Clin Invest* 1990;86:801−18.

54 Bilheimer DW, Grundy SM, Brown MS, Goldstein JL. Mevinolin and colestipol stimulate receptor-mediated clearance of low density lipoprotein from plasma in familial hypercholesterolemia heterozygotes. *Trans Assoc Am Physicians* 1983;96:1−9.

55 Grundy SM, Vega GL. Influence of mevinolin on metabolism of low density lipoproteins in primary moderate hypercholesterolemia. *J Lipid Res* 1985;26:1464−75.

56 Arad Y, Ramakrishnan R, Ginsberg HN. Lovastatin therapy reduces low density lipoprotein apoB levels in subjects with combined hyperlipidemia by reducing the production of apoB-containing lipoproteins: implications for the pathophysiology of apoB production. *J Lipid Res* 1990;31:567−82.

57 Arad Y, Ramakrishnan R, Ginsberg HN. Effects of lovastatin therapy on very low-density lipoprotein triglyceride metabolism in subjects with combined hyperlipidemia: Evidence for reduced assembly and secretion of triglyceride-rich lipoproteins. *Metabolism* 1992;41:487−93.

58 Therapeutic response to lovastatin (mevinolin) in nonfamilial hypercholesterolemia. A multicenter study. The Lovastatin Study Group II. *JAMA* 1986;256:2829−34.

59 Bradford RH, Shear CL, Chremos AN *et al.* Expanded clinical evaluation of lovastatin study results. *Arch Intern Med* 1991;151:43−9.

Chapter 16
The Management of Low HDL States

PHILIP J. BARTER & KERRY-ANNE RYE

Introduction

Although it is well established that a low concentration of high-density lipoprotein (HDL) cholesterol is a powerful predictor of premature coronary heart disease (CHD) [1,2], the mechanism underlying the association is obscure. Furthermore, there is no definitive information to suggest that interventions which increase or decrease the concentration of HDL cholesterol translate into changes in coronary risk. Thus, to address the issue of the management of low HDL states, it is necessary to reach some conclusions regarding possible mechanisms by which HDL may influence the development of CHD. To this end, it is worth briefly reviewing the role played by HDL in plasma cholesterol transport and how this is related to the development of CHD. In the first instance, the processes which influence the concentration of HDL will be considered before turning to other potentially atherogenic factors for which a low concentration of HDL may be a marker. Finally, the issue of the practical management of subjects with low concentrations of HDL cholesterol will be addressed.

Role of HDL in plasma cholesterol transport

HDL play a fundamental role in the pathway known as reverse cholesterol transport. This is the process by which cholesterol is transported from peripheral tissues to the liver, where it may either be recycled or excreted as a component of bile. It is frequently stated that the capacity of HDL to protect against CHD relates to their involvement in reverse cholesterol transport; specifically, it has been concluded that elevated concentrations of HDL increase the removal of cholesterol from the arterial wall. It should be noted, however, that there is no evidence that the rate of reverse cholesterol transport is actually increased in subjects with high concentrations of HDL.

The initial step in the pathway of reverse cholesterol transport involves the transfer of cellular cholesterol to specific subpopulations of HDL where it is esterified by the enzyme lecithin cholesterol acyltransferase (LCAT) [3]. The cholesteryl esters which are formed in this reaction are incorporated into the core of HDL, thus leaving their surfaces depleted of unesterified cholesterol. This creates a concentration gradient down which unesterified cholesterol moves from cell membranes to be the surface of HDL.

Most of the cholesteryl esters incorporated into HDL are transferred to other lipoprotein fractions in a process which is facilitated by the cholesteryl ester transfer protein (CETP) [4]. Thus, the ultimate fate of the cholesteryl esters which are generated as components of HDL is linked to the metabolism of all plasma lipoprotein fractions. A large proportion of the cholesteryl esters in HDL are transferred by CETP to very low-density lipoproteins (VLDL) in exchange for triglyceride [5]. However, since VLDL are catabolized to low-density lipoproteins (LDL), it is the latter fraction which transports the major proportion of the cholesteryl esters in plasma. In other words, in the presence of CETP, most of the unesterified cholesterol acquired by HDL from peripheral tissues is removed from the plasma as cholesteryl esters in the potentially atherogenic LDL fraction. In this sense, it is difficult to view the pathway of reverse cholesterol transport as being protective against CHD.

Explanation for the inverse relationship between HDL and CHD

The observation that a low concentration of HDL is predictive of coronary risk suggests that either:
1   a high level of HDL cholesterol protects against CHD;
2   a low level of HDL cholesterol is harmful; or
3   a low level of HDL cholesterol is a marker for some other factor which is a direct cause of CHD.
Each of these possibilities will be considered.

Does an increased concentration of HDL protect against CHD?

As outlined above, one common view holds that the HDL fraction protects against CHD by virtue of its role as the initial acceptor of tissue cholesterol in the pathway of reverse cholesterol transport. According to this view an increase in the concentration of HDL promotes an increase in the efflux of cholesterol from peripheral tissues. Since this efflux is dependent on the concentration gradient which is generated and maintained by the esterification of cholesterol in the LCAT reaction, it follows that the movement of cholesterol from peripheral tissues into the plasma is, in part, regulated by whatever regulates the LCAT reaction. Although HDL are the preferred lipoprotein substrates for LCAT, there is no evidence that the rate of plasma cholesterol esterification increases with increasing concentrations of HDL. Indeed, the rate of plasma cholesterol esterification has been shown to decrease in subjects with increased concentrations of HDL cholesterol [6]. This may relate to the fact that subjects with elevated HDL tend also to have high concentrations of the HDL_2 subfraction, which is a competitive inhibitor of LCAT [7]. Thus, in subjects with high concentrations of HDL cholesterol, the rate of plasma cholesterol esterification and, by inference, the pathway of reverse cholesterol transport, is decreased. This is in total conflict with the popular view that a high concentration of HDL protects against CHD by increasing the rate of efflux of cholesterol from the arterial wall. While it is conceivable that HDL may protect against CHD in ways which are unrelated to cholesterol transport, there is little evidence to support such a proposition. On the basis of currently available knowledge, therefore, it is reasonable to conclude that a high concentration of HDL *per se* is probably not directly protective against CHD.

Does a decreased concentration of HDL cause CHD?

The HDL in subjects with a low concentration of HDL cholesterol are generally smaller than those found in subjects with normal concentrations of HDL cholesterol [8]. Since the rate of cholesterol esterification catalyzed by LCAT correlates inversely with HDL particle size [9], it follows that the rate of plasma cholesterol esterification will also correlate inversely with the concentration of HDL cholesterol. Thus, subjects in whom the concentration of HDL cholesterol is low are likely to have an increased rate of plasma cholesterol esterification and the rate at which cholesterol is transferred into the plasma from peripheral tissues will be correspondingly enhanced. Since a large proportion of this cholesterol is incorporated into the LDL fraction, as cholesteryl esters, it is conceivable that low concentrations of HDL may increase the flow of cholesterol into the atherogenic LDL fraction and thus increase the risk of CHD.

Is a decreased concentration of HDL a marker for the presence of other factors which cause CHD?

It could be argued that HDL neither cause nor protect against CHD but that the concentration of HDL cholesterol reflects the presence of some other factor which is the true cause of CHD.

To address this issue it is necessary to understand something of the factors which influence the concentration of HDL.

Factors which influence the concentration of HDL

Five categories of factors will be considered: genetic factors, metabolic factors, lifestyle factors, drugs, and disease states. Although there is an obvious overlap between these categories, each will be considered separately.

Genetic factors

The apolipoprotein (apo) A-I gene exists in a cluster with the genes for apo C-III and apo A-IV on chromosome 11 [10]. Restriction fragment length polymorphisms (RFLP) have been used as markers to investigate the genetic determinants of HDL concentration. Overall, the data have been conflicting, although there is general agreement that variation in the apo A-I–C-III–A-IV gene region does contribute to a small proportion of the variation in the concentration of HDL [11]. An interesting recent observation is that variations in the apo B gene are associated with increased concentrations of HDL cholesterol and apo A-I [12]. The mechanism underlying such an association is not known, although it has been postulated that variations in the apo B molecule may influence the rate at which lipids are transferred between HDL and apo B-containing lipoproteins [11].

While the search continues for a genetic basis of the variation in HDL concentration in the general population, there has emerged a growing list of rare specific genetic disorders which have profound effects on HDL concentration and composition. These include the marked elevations of HDL associated with a familial deficiency of CETP [13], the decreased concentration of HDL accompanying familial deficiencies of LCAT [14], and the increased concentration of HDL triglyceride in familial hepatic lipase deficiency [15]. In Tangier disease, an as yet unidentified genetic defect is responsible for an extremely rapid rate of HDL catabolism, which results in a virtual absence of plasma HDL [16]. There is also a variety of other genetic abnormalities which compromise apolipoprotein synthesis or function. These are manifested as either a complete absence or a deficiency of apo A-I, apo A-I, and apo C-III, or apo A-I, apo C-III, and apo A-II [17]. Some, but not all, of these familial low HDL states are associated with premature CHD [17]. However, they are all very rare and only account for a small proportion of the subjects with low con-

Table 16.1 Metabolic factors involved in the regulation of HDL

Factor	Effect on HDL
Lecithin cholesterol acyltransferase	Increase HDL cholesteryl esters Increase particle size of HDL
Lipoprotein lipase + triglyceride-rich lipoproteins	Increase HDL phospholipid and unesterified cholesterol, increase particle size of HDL
Hepatic lipase	Decrease HDL phospholipid and triglyceride Decrease particle size of HDL
Cholesteryl ester transfer protein + triglyceride-rich lipoproteins	Decrease HDL cholesteryl esters Increase HDL triglyceride Increase particle size of HDL
Cholesterol ester transfer protein + triglyceride-rich lipoproteins + hepatic lipase	Decrease HDL cholesteryl esters Decrease HDL apo A-I Reduce particle size of HDL
Cholesterol ester transfer protein + nonesterified fatty acids + either triglyceride-rich lipoproteins or LDL	Decrease HDL cholesteryl esters Decrease HDL apo A-I Reduce particle size of HDL

centrations of HDL. As such these disorders do not represent a major management challenge.

Metabolic factors (Table 16.1)

The concentration, composition, and subpopulation distribution of HDL are regulated by interactions with a range of plasma proteins and other lipoprotein fractions. An understanding of the mechanisms underlying such interactions may provide insights into how the concentration of HDL is controlled and give clues regarding the identity of possible atherogenic factors which may also lead to low concentrations of HDL.

LECITHIN CHOLESTEROL ACYLTRANSFERASE

LCAT catalyzes the transfer of an acyl group from lecithin to unesterified cholesterol to form lysolecithin and cholesteryl esters. Since HDL are the major substrates of LCAT in plasma, the reaction increases the cholesteryl ester content and the size of the particles in this lipoprotein fraction.

Insights into the physiologic function of LCAT have been obtained from the investigation of subjects with an inherited deficiency of the enzyme. The plasma of such subjects is totally deficient in cholesterol esterifying activity and, as a consequence, most of the circulating cholesterol exists in the unesterified form [14]. The plasma of these subjects contains HDL which are either very small spheres or disks [14,18]. The disks consist of apolipoproteins, phospholipids, and unesterified cholesterol and are deficient in cholesteryl esters. The absence of cholesterol esterifying activity in the plasma of these subjects translates into an inability to transport cholesterol from cell membranes into HDL; as a consequence, their cell membranes are markedly enriched in cholesterol [14].

When the plasma of LCAT-deficient subjects is incubated *in vitro* with an exogenous source of LCAT, the discoidal and small spheroidal HDL are converted into spheres of a size similar to normal HDL_3 [14,18]. It has also been suggested that LCAT is of major importance in the conversion of HDL_3 to HDL_2 [19], although others have concluded that LCAT alone has little effect on HDL subpopulation distribution and that an additional source of unesterified cholesterol such as LDL is required before LCAT is able to promote significant increases in the particle size of HDL [20]. It should be noted that the HDL_2 formed *in vitro* by the action of LCAT on HDL_3 are markedly enriched with cholesteryl esters and depleted of phospholipids and unesterified cholesterol when compared with native HDL_2. Furthermore, they possess a ratio of apo A-I to apo A-II which resembles that of the parent HDL_3 and is much lower than in native HDL_2. Thus, while LCAT is clearly capable of increasing the size of HDL_3, additional factors must operate *in vivo* in the formation of HDL_2. Furthermore, with the exception of the relatively rare states of LCAT deficiency, it is unlikely that the concentration of LCAT is a rate-limiting factor in the regulation of either HDL concentration or subpopulation distribution.

LIPOPROTEIN LIPASE

Lipoprotein lipase (LPL) is a heparin-releasable endothelial lipase which hydrolyzes triglyceride and, to a lesser extent, phospholipids in triglyceride-rich lipoproteins (TGRLP). While HDL are not the preferred substrates for LPL, the concentration of HDL is influenced by variations in activity of the enzyme. The concentration of both total HDL and HDL_2 correlate positively and significantly with the activity of LPL in post-heparin plasma and adipose tissue [21,22]. It has been suggested that hydrolysis of the lipids in TGRLP by LPL results in the generation of surplus surface components which are incorporated into HDL_3. This process favors the conversion of HDL_3 to HDL_2 [23]. According to this view, an increased activity of LPL will result in an increased concentration of HDL_2. It is also known, however, that the concentration of HDL cholesterol varies inversely with that of TGRLP [24]. On this basis, the correlation between HDL concentration and LPL activity may reflect the fact that activity of LPL is a major determinant of the concentration of TGRLP and that it is the concentration of TGRLP which determines the concentration of HDL.

HEPATIC LIPASE

Hepatic lipase (HL) is an endothelial enzyme which, like LPL, is released into the circulation after intravenous injection of heparin. In contrast to LPL, activity of HL in postheparin plasma correlates inversely with the concentration of HDL [25]. It is possible that the lower HDL concentrations in males than females may relate to the capacity of androgens to increase [26] and estrogens to decrease [27] activity of HL. HL promotes hydrolysis of both triglyceride and phospholipids in all lipoprotein fractions, with a particular preference *in vitro* for HDL [28]. Insights into the function of HL *in vivo* have been obtained from investigation of a small number of human subjects with a familial deficiency of the enzyme. These subjects have triglyceride enrichment of LDL and HDL and increased concentrations of intermediate-density lipoproteins (IDL) and HDL_2 [15].

Further insights into the function of HL have been obtained by injecting animals with specific antibodies against HL [29,30]. Although the results of the animal studies have been variable, there have generally been increases in the concentration of HDL phospholipids which coincided with inhibition of the enzyme. These changes are short-lived, however, and may not necessarily be representative of those associated with a chronic deficiency of HL. Some of the effects of chronic deficiency *in vivo* have been deduced from studies of rabbits, an animal species naturally deficient in activity of HL [31]. Compared with human HDL, rabbit HDL are enlarged, enriched in triglyceride, and depleted of cholesteryl esters [31]. When rabbit plasma is incubated *in vitro* with HL, there is substantial hydrolysis of the HDL triglyceride which results in the composition of HDL becoming similar to that of human subjects [31]. The HL-mediated hydrolyses of rabbit HDL trigyceride is accompanied by a reduction in the HDL particle size and a decrease in the concentration of apo A-I [32]. The latter finding has been attributed to a reduction in the HDL core volume which leads to the loss of redundant surface components. A comparable finding in human plasma has been shown to represent an interaction between HL and CETP [33] (see below). Overall, the available data are consistent with the proposition that activity of HL is an important determinant of the concentration of HDL.

CETP promotes the transfer of cholesteryl esters from HDL, where they are synthesized in the LCAT reaction, to both VLDL and LDL [4]. This is accompanied by a reciprocal transfer of triglyceride from VLDL to HDL [4]. Since CETP has been shown to account for all of the cholesteryl ester and triglyceride transfer activity in human plasma [34], this protein may play an important role in regulating the concentrations of cholesterol and triglyceride in each of the lipoprotein fractions. Some insights into the physiologic significance of CETP have been obtained from deficiency states in both animals and humans.

Activity of CETP varies widely between different animal species [35]. For example, activity of CETP in rabbits is much higher than in humans but is not detectable in rat plasma [35]. In rat plasma, therefore, the cholesteryl esters incorporated into HDL remain with this fraction, which is the dominant transport vehicle for plasma cholesterol in this species [36]. Rat HDL tend to be larger and less dense than human HDL [36,37]. In fact, rat HDL contain a subfraction of very large, cholesteryl ester-rich particles, designated HDL_1, which are not normally detectable in human plasma. When rats are injected intravenously with human CETP [37,38] the HDL_1 subfraction disappears and the particle size of the rat HDL_2 subfraction decreases.

There have been reports of human subjects with increased concentrations of HDL in whom cholesterol ester transfers are reduced. Not all of these subjects have a deficiency of CETP. Kurasawa et al. [39] and Yokoyama et al. [40] have described a male subject with a high concentration of HDL cholesterol and a decreased rate of cholesteryl ester transfer. The HDL of this subject were much larger than normal and were relatively deficient in triglyceride. In addition, the VLDL were deficient in cholesteryl esters. In this case, however, the abnormality was caused by the inability of HDL to participate in the transfer process and not by a deficiency of CETP activity in the plasma [40].

On the other hand, there have been two reports of subjects with hyperalphalipoproteinemia in whom high concentrations of HDL were associated with a complete absence of activity of CETP in the plasma [13,41]. The plasma of both of the subjects reported by Koizumi et al. contained very large HDL which were cholesteryl ester rich and depleted of triglyceride [13]. In the three cases of CETP deficiency reported by

Yamashita *et al.* [41], the enlarged, cholesteryl ester-rich HDL were shown also to be enriched with apo E. In addition, the LDL of these subjects were heterogeneous and contained subpopulations of very small particles [41]. Overall, the lipoproteins in these CETP-deficient humans are very similar to those of rats. These examples show that a complete deficiency of CETP has profound effects on the concentration, composition, and subpopulation distribution of HDL. In human subjects, however, a complete deficiency of CETP is rare and there is little evidence to suggest in most human subjects that variations in HDL concentration are caused by variations in the concentration of plasma CETP. On the other hand, there is evidence that the activity of CETP is subject to modulation by a variety of plasma factors and that interactions between CETP and other plasma factors may be important determinants of the concentration of HDL.

INTERACTIONS OF CETP, HL, AND VLDL WITH HDL (Fig. 16.1)

As outlined above, CETP promotes the heteroexchange of cholesteryl ester and triglyceride between HDL and VLDL. This results *in vitro* in the formation of a cholesteryl ester-depleted, triglyceride-enriched HDL fraction. Since triglyceride molecules are larger than cholesteryl ester molecules, these triglyceride-enriched HDL are also enlarged [42]. HL, on the other hand, promotes the hydrolysis of HDL triglyceride and abolishes the CETP-mediated triglyceride enrichment of HDL [43]. The combination of HL, CETP, and VLDL therefore modifies HDL such that not only are they depleted of cholesteryl esters but they are no longer enriched in triglyceride; such HDL are reduced in particle size [43,44].

In addition to hydrolyzing triglyceride in HDL, HL has also been found to enhance the capacity of CETP to promote transfers of cholesteryl esters from HDL to VLDL [33]. The potential importance of this synergism is highlighted by the observation that HDL which are incubated in the presence of HL, CETP, and VLDL not only become depleted of core lipids and reduced in size but also sustain a significant loss of apo A-I [33]. Thus, interactions between HDL, VLDL, CETP, and HL may be of importance in regulating not only the concentration of lipid constituents but also the apolipoproteins of HDL and may explain why the concentration of HDL is frequently reduced in subjects with hypertriglyceridemia [24]. While the mechanism of the synergism is still uncertain, there is some evidence that it represents an interaction between CETP and the nonesterified fatty acids (NEFA) generated during the hydrolysis of HDL triglyceride by HL.

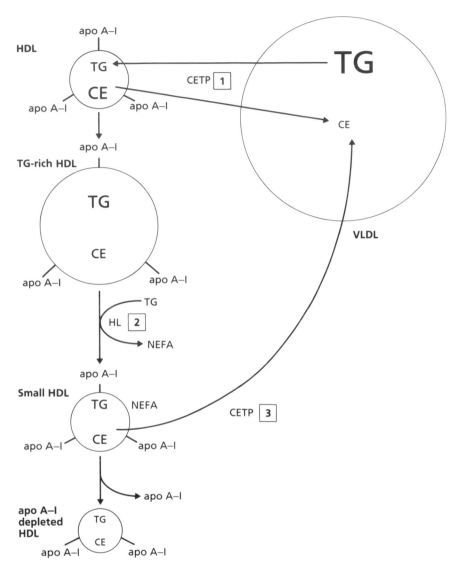

Fig. 16.1 Interactions of HDL with CETP, HL, and VLDL. **1** CETP promotes the heteroexchange of cholesteryl esters (CE) and triglyceride (TG) between HDL and VLDL. This results in enlarged TG-enriched HDL particles which are depleted of CE. **2** HL hydrolyzes a proportion of the HDL TG to form small, core lipid-depleted HDL particles which are enriched in NEFA. **3** The interaction between NEFA and CETP results in an enhancement of the transfer of CE from HDL to VLDL which leads to a further reduction in core volume and a consequent shedding of redundant apo A-I from the surface of the HDL particles.

MODULATION OF THE EFFECTS OF CETP BY NEFA

When incubated *in vitro* with HDL and LDL, CETP promotes an exchange of cholesteryl esters between the two lipoprotein fractions but minimal net mass transfer in either direction. However, when NEFA are added to the incubation mixture, a net mass transfer of cholesteryl esters from HDL to LDL is observed [45]. As a consequence, the HDL become depleted of core lipids and reduced to a size which is similar to the HDL formed during the incubation of HDL, VLDL, CETP, and HL [44,45]. NEFA also mimic the effects of HL on HDL when they are present in incubations of HDL, VLDL, and CETP. As outlined above, CETP promotes approximately equimolar heteroexchanges of cholesteryl esters for triglyceride between HDL and VLDL [5]. In the presence of NEFA, these CETP-mediated transfers are modified such that there is an increase in the net mass transfer of cholesteryl esters from HDL to VLDL but a decrease in the amount of triglyceride transferred from VLDL to HDL [46]. This leaves HDL particles which are depleted of core lipids and reduced in particle size. The effect of NEFA on the activity of CETP is abolished by fatty acid-free albumin but not by fatty acid-rich albumin [45]. Thus, it is reasonable to postulate that the presence of NEFA on the surface of lipoproteins converts a CETP-mediated process of neutral lipid exchange between HDL and other lipoproteins into one of net mass transfer of core lipids from HDL to both LDL and VLDL. The mechanism by which NEFA interact with CETP to deplete HDL of core lipids is not known, although it may relate to the capacity of NEFA to enhance the binding of CETP to lipoproteins [47]. Regardless of the mechanism, it may be speculated that any circumstance which increases the concentration of lipoprotein-associated NEFA may also favor a net efflux of core lipids out of HDL and thus a reduced concentration of HDL constituents. Such a mechanism may underlie the low concentration of HDL cholesterol in obesity [48] and diabetes mellitus [49], and explain the increase in HDL cholesterol which follows the cessation of smoking [50].

Lifestyle factors (Table 16.2)

Several lifestyle factors are known to influence the concentration of HDL cholesterol. In most cases, however, the underlying mechanism is poorly understood.

DIET

It is generally accepted that dietary modification is the first line of treatment of most hyperlipidemic states. Diets low in saturated fat

Table 16.2 Lifestyle factors which influence HDL

Factors which increase HDL cholesterol
Diet
    Saturated fat
    Cholesterol
    Alcohol
Exercise

Factors which decrease HDL cholesterol
Diet
    Polyunsaturated fat
    Carbohydrate
Obesity
Smoking

and cholesterol and relatively high in carbohydrate are commonly recommended as therapy for hypercholesterolemia, as is a partial replacement of saturated fat by monounsaturated or polyunsaturated fat. It should be noted, however, that such diets not only reduce the concentration of LDL but also that of HDL [51–54]. Indeed, diets enriched with cholesterol have been shown to be associated with an increase in HDL cholesterol [52]. The mechanisms underlying these dietary effects on HDL are not clear. Nor are the implications in terms of CHD risk.

If it were to be argued that dietary measures which increase the concentration of HDL cholesterol should be encouraged, it would follow that the diet should be rich in saturated fat and cholesterol and low in carbohydrate. However, such diets also raise the concentration of LDL and may actually increase the risk of CHD. Thus, given the current state of ignorance regarding the mechanism underlying the relationship between the concentration of HDL cholesterol and development of CHD, it is not possible to make specific dietary recommendations on the management of low HDL states. A possible exception to this is the management of the low concentration of HDL associated with obesity since it is known that the weight loss accompanying a reduction in energy intake by obese subjects leads to an increase in HDL cholesterol concentration [55].

OBESITY

The concentration of HDL cholesterol correlates negatively and significantly with body weight [48]. It is not known, however, whether obesity *per se* predisposes to low HDL or whether the low concentration of HDL in such subjects is a function of other factors such as elevated plasma concentrations of triglyceride [56] and increased activity of HL [57]. Long-term but not short-term weight reduction of obese subjects is accompanied by an increase in HDL concentration and a decrease in plasma triglyceride concentrations [55,58]. However, the time course of the increase in concentration of HDL during long-term weight reduction is not related to the decrease in plasma triglyceride [55,58]. This observation casts doubt on the suggestion that the low concentration of HDL in obesity is solely the consequence of an increased concentration of TGRLP. The concentration of NEFA is also increased in obesity [59], possibly as a consequence of insulin resistance. Given the capacity of NEFA to promote the CETP-mediated net mass transfer of cholesteryl esters from HDL to LDL (see above) [45], it is possible that the elevated concentrations of NEFA and TGRLP as well as the increased activity of HL in obesity are cooperatively responsible for the low concentration of HDL in such subjects.

ALCOHOL CONSUMPTION

Several studies have shown that a high to moderate intake of alcohol increases the concentration of HDL cholesterol [60]. While it has been suggested that an alcohol-induced increase in HDL may be protective against CHD, the mechanism of this association has not yet been established beyond reasonable doubt. For this reason it would be irresponsible to advocate the use of alcohol as a measure to protect against CHD.

SMOKING

Smoking is a well recognized major risk factor for CHD. Smoking is also known to reduce the concentration of HDL cholesterol [50], although whether the low HDL contributes to the coronary risk in smokers is uncertain. The mechanism underlying the low concentration of HDL in smokers is not understood but it may be related to the increased concentrations of plasma triglyceride in such subjects. This is unlikely to be the whole explanation, however, since hypertriglyceridemia in smokers tends to be mild. When smoking is stopped the concentration of HDL rises within a few weeks [50].

EXERCISE

An association between exercise and high concentrations of HDL is now well established. Long-term aerobic exercise programs in previously sedentary people increase the concentration of HDL cholesterol [61]. In addition, subjects who are habitually physically active tend to have higher HDL concentrations than do sedentary subjects [62]. The mechanism responsible for this relationship may be related to an increased activity of LPL induced by exercise [63] which, in turn, reduces the concentration of TGRLP. The increase in HDL may be secondary to these events.

Drugs (Table 16.3)

A variety of drugs are known to influence the concentration of HDL. In most cases neither the mechanism nor the implications for CHD are completely understood.

DRUGS USED TO TREAT DYSLIPIDEMIAS

These agents fall into two categories with respect to their effects on the concentration of HDL: those that increase and those that decrease the concentration of HDL.

Agents which increase the concentration of HDL

The drugs which most effectively raise the level of HDL also reduce the concentration of plasma triglyceride. Thus, agents such as nicotinic acid [64], its analog, acipimox [65], and fibrates such as clofibrate [66], gemfibrozil [67], fenofibrate [68], and bezafibrate [69] all increase the concentration of HDL while decreasing the concentration of TGRLP. The bile acid sequestering agents, cholestyramine and colestipol, and the hydoxymethylglutaryl-CoA reductase (HMG-CoAR) inhibitors, lovastatin, simvastatin, and pravastatin, primarily lower the concentration of LDL but may also promote small increases in the concentration of HDL cholesterol [70,71]. In this case the magnitude of the increase in HDL concentration tends to be less than that observed with the triglyceride-lowering agents.

Nicotinic acid and acipimox. These agents reduce the concentration of plasma triglyceride and increase that of HDL cholesterol [64,65]. Nicotinic acid also reduces the concentration of LDL cholesterol [64]. Although the mechanism of action of these agents is uncertain, it may be related to their antilipolytic activity [72]. These agents inhibit lipolysis in adipose tissue. This leads to a decrease in the concentration of plasma NEFA and, as a consequence, a decreased hepatic synthesis of triglyceride and a decreased plasma concentration of TGRLP. The increased

Table 16.3 Effects of hypolipidemic drugs on concentration of HDL cholesterol

Drugs which induce major increases in HDL
Antilipolytic agents
  Nicotinic acid
  Acipimox
Fibrates
  Bezafibrate
  Fenofibrate
  Gemfibrozil
  Ciprofibrate

Drugs which induce mild increases in HDL
Bile acid sequestering agents
  Cholestyramine
  Colestipol
HMG-CoAR inhibitors
  Lovastatin
  Simvastatin
  Pravastatin

Drugs which reduce concentrations of HDL Probucol

concentration of HDL may simply be secondary to the reduction in TGRLP, although nicotinic acid-induced changes in the two lipoprotein fractions may be dissociated [73]. It is tempting to speculate that the increased concentration of HDL in subjects being treated with nicotinic acid or acipimox may be a direct function of the reduced concentration of plasma NEFA. It should be noted, however, that the reduction in plasma NEFA concentration promoted by nicotinic acid is transient [72] whereas the associated increase in concentration of HDL is both substantial and long-lived.

Fibrates.   Clofibrate has been used as a hypolipidemic drug for many years. Its main effect is to lower plasma triglyceride and, in some subjects, the concentration of plasma cholesterol. Clofibrate also promotes a modest increase in the concentration of HDL cholesterol. The newer fibrates, especially gemfibrozil [74], are, by contrast, potent elevators of HDL cholesterol. There is general agreement that the fibrates act by stimulating the activity of LPL [75]. At present it is not known whether the increased concentration of HDL cholesterol is secondary to the LPL-mediated reduction in TGRLP or whether the fibrates modify HDL synthesis or catabolism.

Bile acid sequestering agents.   Cholestyramine and colestipol bind bile acids and increase their elimination in the feces. The consequent channeling of hepatic cholesterol into bile acid synthesis depletes the hepatocytes of cholesterol. This translates into an increase in hepatocyte LDL receptor activity and a consequent reduction in plasma LDL cholesterol concentration. While these agents may increase the concentration of plasma triglyceride in some subjects, they can also be associated with a modest increase in the concentration of HDL cholesterol [70]. Many studies, however, have failed to reveal an increase in HDL cholesterol during treatment with bile acid sequestering agents [76].

HMG-CoAR inhibitors.   Drugs such as lovastatin, simvastatin, and pravastatin inhibit the synthesis of cholesterol in hepatocytes. This stimulates the synthesis of LDL receptors and reduces the concentration of LDL in plasma. These agents may also promote a slight increase in the concentration of HDL cholesterol [71], although the effect is much less than that observed with the newer fibrates.

Agents which decrease the concentration of HDL

The most obvious example in this category is probucol, an antioxidant which lowers the concentration of cholesterol in both LDL and HDL [77]. The reduction in HDL cholesterol has been attributed to an increased activity of CETP in subjects taking probucol [78], although whether or not this is the only mechanism is uncertain. The capacity of probucol to reduce the concentration of HDL has been the source of concern, although there is no evidence to suggest that the effect is detrimental. In fact, probucol has been shown to reduce tendon xanthomas in human subjects [79] and to have powerful antiatherogenic properties in animals [80]. It has been suggested that the antiatherogenic properties of probucol may be unrelated to its lipid-lowering action but rather that they are due to its ability to prevent the formation of oxidized LDL [81]. In this case the low HDL may be coincidental and possibly of little consequence. Given the potential importance of probucol as an antiatherogenic agent, this is an issue which should be resolved by further research.

ANTIHYPERTENSIVE AGENTS

Several of the noncardioselective beta-blocking agents which are used to treat hypertension increase plasma triglyceride and reduce HDL cholesterol concentration [82]. Similar effects have been reported for a range of diuretics [83]. While this is not a problem of the newer antihypertensive agents, it is still an issue worth remembering if only to ensure that plasma lipids are measured at regular intervals in subjects who are being treated for hypertension.

ANTICONVULSANTS

The concentration of HDL cholesterol in epileptic patients treated with phenytoin has been found to be significantly higher than that in control subjects [84]. This effect has been attributed to the action of phenytoin as an inducer of microsomal enzymes [85]. An elevation of HDL cholesterol has also been observed in subjects treated with carbamezepine [86] and phenobarbital [87]. The implications of therapy with anti-convulsants in terms of coronary risk are not known.

Low HDL as a component of disease states

DIABETES MELLITUS

In insulin-dependent diabetes mellitus (IDDM) the main lipid abnormality is an elevation of plasma triglyceride which tends to return to normal when the diabetes is controlled by insulin. The concentration of HDL cholesterol in IDDM is variable. In noninsulin-dependent diabetes mellitus (NIDDM) the lipoprotein profile tends to resemble that found in obesity, with elevated TGRLP and reduced HDL cholesterol [49,88]. The mechanism underlying the decreased concentration of HDL cholesterol in NIDDM is uncertain, but, as in obese subjects, it may be secondary to the increased concentrations of TGRLP or NEFA. The concentration of HDL cholesterol in NIDDM has been reported to correlate inversely with the level of endogenous insulin [89] suggesting that the low HDL in such subjects may be a function of the hyperinsulinism or the insulin resistance.

RENAL DISEASE

Subjects with chronic renal failure have a high rate of CHD despite being controlled by maintenance dialysis [90]. Such subjects tend to have increased concentrations of plasma triglyceride and decreased concentrations of HDL cholesterol which are not normalized by dialysis [91]. The mechanism responsible for the reduced HDL cholesterol is uncertain and its role in the susceptibility of these subjects to atherosclerosis remains to be determined.

OTHER DISORDERS

The concentration of HDL cholesterol has been reported to be low during acute infections [92], in some malignancies [93], and in a variety of diseases of the liver [94].

Potential atherogenic factors associated with low HDL

Recognizing that there is no conclusive evidence either that a high concentration of HDL is directly protective against CHD or that a low concentration is a direct cause, it is worth considering what other atherogenic factors may be present in subjects with low HDL. Many subjects with low concentrations of HDL also have elevated concentrations of TGRLP [24]. This combination of hypertriglyceridemia and low HDL cholesterol concentration is highly predictive of CHD [95]. As outlined above (see Fig. 16.1), the low concentration of HDL in such subjects is probably a direct consequence of the elevated TGRLP concentration. Thus, low levels of HDL may be regarded as a reflection of the increased concentration of TGRLP and, to the extent that TGRLP are atherogenic, as a marker for a state of increased atherogenicity.

Whether or not TGRLP are atherogenic has been the subject of much debate. Overall, there is little or no evidence to suggest that either chylomicrons or VLDL are atherogenic. It should be noted, however, that the TGRLP fraction also includes the partially catabolized remnants of chylomicrons and VLDL. Circumstantial evidence suggests that these remnants may be highly atherogenic [96]. Thus, it is possible that an increased predisposition to CHD in subjects with hypertriglyceridemia may exist only if the TGRLP fraction contains a significant proportion of remnants. If these remnants were to lower the concentration of HDL to a greater extent than do comparable levels of chylomicrons or VLDL, it would then be possible to explain why the concentration of HDL in subjects with hypertriglyceridemia is such a powerful predictor of CHD risk.

According to the scheme outlined in Fig. 16.1, the low concentration of HDL in subjects with hypertriglyceridemia is the consequence of a synergism between TGRLP, CETP, and HL. The extent of the HDL modification is dependent on the concentration of TGRLP and the activities of CETP and HL [44]. We postulate that the remnants of TGRLP differ from both chylomicrons and VLDL in that they stimulate activity of HL. If this were so, it would be predicted that an accumulation of remnants would be more effective than either chylomicrons or VLDL in terms of reducing the concentration of HDL. In other words, a low concentration of HDL in subjects with mild to moderate hypertri-glyceridemia would indicate that the TGRLP fraction is significantly contaminated by atherogenic remnant particles. We suggest that it is the increased level of remnant particles rather than the decreased level of HDL which represents the true cause of CHD in such cases. If this is so, any therapy should logically be directed primarily at the remnant particles rather than the low HDL concentration.

Clinical states of low HDL: management in relation to CHD prevention

In any discussion of the management of low HDL states, it must be emphasized that there is no conclusive evidence to suggest that increasing the concentration of HDL *per se* protects against CHD. For this reason, a decision to embark on therapy designed primarily to raise HDL should be made only with caution. Rather, the major thrust of management should be directed against accompanying elevated concentrations of LDL and TGRLP.

General guidelines

There are several general principles of management of low HDL states which are not controversial. For example, smokers should be encouraged to stop smoking, obese subjects should be advised about diet and helped to lose weight, and attention should be paid to diabetic control In circumstances where it is not contraindicated, sedentary subjects should be encouraged to embark on a long-term program of aerobic exercise. However, in many cases, such approaches are either inapplicable, inappropriate, or unsuccessful. Under these circumstances, the concentration of HDL may remain low unless drug treatment is instituted.

Familial HDL deficiency

There are some rare conditions in which basic genetic defects are manifested as very low concentrations or complete absence of HDL. These conditions are not necessarily associated with premature athero-sclerosis and effective therapy designed to increase the concentration of HDL in these disorders has not been reported.

Low HDL associated with elevated plasma triglyceride

It has long been recognized that the concentration of HDL cholesterol correlates negatively with the concentration of plasma triglyceride [24]. Indeed, low HDL concentration associated with mild to moderate hypertriglyceridemia is a relatively common disorder. Evidence is now emerging that the combination of mild hypertriglyceridemia with a low concentration of HDL cholesterol may be associated with a very high CHD risk [95]. At present it is not known whether the increased risk of CHD in such subjects is caused by the low HDL, by the elevated triglyceride or, as suggested above, by increased concentrations of the atherogenic remnants of TGRLP. In the Helsinki Heart Study, therapy with gemfibrozil resulted in a reduction in the concentration of LDL cholesterol and plasma triglyceride and an increase in the concentration of HDL cholesterol [74]. The changes in both LDL and HDL, but not plasma triglyceride, were found to contribute to a reduction in CHD. In this study the greatest reduction in CHD risk was observed in the subjects with the lowest baseline levels of HDL cholesterol. In contrast, gemfibrozil had virtually no effect on the development of CHD in subjects with higher baseline levels of HDL cholesterol.

Given that the combination of a high concentration of plasma triglyceride and a low concentration of HDL is associated with a high risk of CHD [95] and given that intervention which lowers triglyceride and raises HDL cholesterol in such subjects has been found to translate into reduced risk [74], there is a powerful case for treating such subjects. General measures such as stopping smoking and, if indicated, weight reduction and a controlled exercise program should be applied. If these measures fail to correct the dyslipidemia, drug therapy is indicated, using either: (i) one of the fibrate group of drugs (newer agents include gemfibrozil, fenofibrate, and bezafibrate); or (ii) nicotinic acid or its analog, acipimox. Each of these categories of drug is effective in lowering plasma triglyceride and, to varying extents, raising HDL cholesterol.

Low HDL in obesity

The concentration of HDL cholesterol is frequently low in obese subjects. These individuals also tend to have high concentrations of both plasma triglycerides and NEFA. The pathologic significance of the elevated NEFA in obesity and their relationship with low concentrations of HDL has yet to be defined. Given that both obesity and a low concentration of HDL are associated with an increased CHD risk, the discovery of a low concentration of HDL in an obese subject is cause for concern and warrants strong encouragement for weight reduction. Drug therapy should be reserved for subjects who also have elevated LDL or TGRLP and who do not respond to nonpharmacologic measures. If LDL are elevated the drug of choice is either a bile acid sequestering agent, one of the HMG-CoAR inhibitors, or nicotinic acid; if TGRLP are increased the appropriate drugs include a fibrate or one of the nicotinic acid-type agents. It is probable that successful lowering of both TGRLP and LDL will be associated with increased concentration of HDL. Nevertheless, without accompanying loss of weight, the HDL may remain low despite drug therapy.

Low HDL in diabetes mellitus

The concentration of HDL cholesterol is frequently reduced in NIDDM [49]. In fact, the plasma lipid profiles of these subjects is often similar to that encountered in obesity and may relate in part to insulin resistance. As in obesity, patients with NIDDM tend to have increased concentrations of TGRLP, reduced concentrations of HDL cholesterol, and increased concentrations of NEFA. The fact that many patients with NIDDM are also overweight is a further reflection of the overlap between NIDDM and obesity.

Patients with NIDDM are at increased risk of CHD. Whether this is a consequence of the associated dyslipidemia or to a primary vasculopathy or to both is not known. However, given the increased predisposition to CHD of nondiabetic subjects with the combination of hypertriglyceridemia and low HDL, there is nothing to suggest that a comparable lipid disorder in diabetics is any less atherogenic. As such, therapy for the lipid disorder is indicated. If after taking measures to control the diabetes, including (if applicable) a program of weight loss, the plasma triglyceride remains elevated and the HDL cholesterol remains low, consideration should be given to drug therapy along the same principles as outlined above for obese subjects. Care should be exercised in the choice of drug, since some agents (e.g., nicotinic acid) have been reported to compromise diabetic control [97].

Low HDL in subjects taking probucol

Despite the concern about the reduction in concentration of HDL in subjects taking probucol, there is no evidence that this effect is detrimental. Given that probucol reduces tendon xanthomas in humans [79] and is directly antiatherogenic in animals [80], on balance it seems more than reasonable to ignore the reduction in concentration of HDL which occurs during therapy with this agent.

Low HDL unassociated with elevations of other lipoprotein fractions

It has been found in population studies that for any given plasma concentration of HDL cholesterol, the risk of CHD increases with increasing concentrations of total plasma or LDL cholesterol; conversely, for any given concentration of plasma or LDL cholesterol, the risk of CHD increases with decreasing HDL cholesterol levels [74,98–100]. Thus, it could be argued that even in the absence of other lipoprotein disturbances, a low concentration of HDL cholesterol should be cause for concern. However, as discussed above, it is also known that the consumption of low-fat, low-cholesterol, high-carbohydrate diets tends to be associated with lower concentrations of HDL cholesterol. Given that populations in which such diets are habitually consumed generally do not have an increased risk of CHD in association with the low concentrations of HDL cholesterol, any decision to initiate treatment on the basis of an isolated low HDL concentration should be made with great caution.

It is not yet known whether the risk of CHD is reduced by intervention in subjects with isolated low HDL. Indeed, it is uncertain what intervention, if any, should be employed under these circumstances. Until much more is known regarding the mechanism underlying the negative correlation between HDL concentration and CHD risk, it could be argued that intervention with drugs is not yet indicated for these individuals. However, if the family history of CHD is very strong or if the subject already has evidence of active CHD, consideration may be given to the use of either nicotinic acid or one of the newer fibrates. It should be emphasized, however, that there is no evidence to support the use of drugs in subjects with isolated low HDL and that it is imperative to conduct more research in order to understand the mechanism responsible for the increased risk of CHD in such subjects.

References

1 Miller GJ, Miller NE. Plasma high-density-lipoprotein concentration and the development of ischaemic heart disease. *Lancet* 1975;i:16–19.
2 Gordon T, Castelli WP, Hjortland MC, Kannel WB, Dawber TR. High density lipoprotein as a protective factor against coronary heart disease. The Framingham Study. *Am J Med* 1977;62:707–14.

3 Castro GR, Fielding CJ. Early incorporation of cell-derived cholesterol into prebeta-migrating high density lipoprotein. *Biochemistry* 1988;27:25—9.

4 Barter PJ, Hopkins GJ, Calvert GD. Transfers and exchanges of esterified cholesterol between plasma lipoproteins. *Biochem J* 1982;208:1—7.

5 Nichols AV, Smith L. Effects of very low density lipoproteins on lipid transfer in incubated serum. *J Lipid Res* 1965;6:206—10.

6 Wallentin L, Vikrot O. Lecithin:cholesterol acyl transfer in plasma of normal persons in relation to lipid and lipoprotein concentration. *Scand J Clin Lab Invest* 1975;35:669—76.

7 Barter PJ, Hopkins GJ, Gorjatschko L, Jones ME. Competitive inhibition of plasma cholesterol esterification by human high-density lipoprotein-subfraction 2. *Biochim Biophys Acta* 1984;793:260—8.

8 Chang LBF, Hopkins GJ, Barter PJ. Particle size distribution of high density lipoproteins as a function of plasma triglyceride concentration in human subjects. *Atherosclerosis* 1985;56:61—70.

9 Barter PJ, Hopkins GJ, Gorjatschko L. Lipoprotein substrates for plasma cholesterol esterification. Influence of particle size and composition of high density lipoprotein subfraction 3. *Atherosclerosis* 1985;58:97—107.

10 Karathanasis SK. Apolipoprotein multigene family: tandem organization of apolipoprotein A IV, A I and C III genes. *Proc Natl Acad Sci USA* 1986;82:6374—8.

11 Humphries S, Paul H, Jeenah M, Rosseneu M, Miller N. The contribution of variation at the apo A I—C III—A IV gene locus to the determinants of HDL cholesterol and apo A I levels. In *Disorders of HDL* (ed. LA Carlson). London: Smith-Gordon, 1990:63—70.

12 Myant NB, Gallagher J, Barbir M *et al.* Restriction fragment length polymorphisms in the apo B gene in relation to coronary heart disease. *Atherosclerosis* 1989;77:193—201.

13 Koizumi J, Mabuchi H, Yoshimura A *et al.* Deficiency of serum cholesteryl-ester transfer activity in patients with familial hyperalphalipoproteinaemia. *Atherosclerosis* 1985;58:175—86.

14 Glomset JA, Norum KR, Gjone E. Familial lecithin·cholesterol acyltransferase deficiency. In *The Metabolic Basis of Inherited Disease*, 5th edn (eds JB Stanbury, JB Wyngaarden, DS Fredrickson, JL Goldstein, MS Brown). New York: McGraw-Hill, 1983:643—54.

15 Breckenridge WC. Deficiencies of plasma lipolytic activities. *Am Heart J* 1987;113:567—72.

16 Schaefer EJ, Blum CB, Levy RI *et al.* Metabolism of high density apolipoproteins in Tangier disease. *N Engl J Med* 1978;299:905—10.

17 Breslow JL. Genetic basis of lipoprotein disorders. *J Clin Invest* 1989;84:373—80.

18 Chen C, Applegate K, King WC. Study of the small spherical high-density lipoproteins of patients afflicted with familial lecithin:cholesterol acyltransferase deficiency. *J Lipid Res* 1984;25:269—82.

19 Daerr WH, Greten H. *In vitro* modulation of the distribution of normal human plasma high density lipoprotein subfractions through the lecithin:cholesterol acyltransferase reaction. *Biochim Biophys Acta* 1982;710:128—33.

20 Rajaram OV, Barter PJ. Increases in the particle size of high-density lipoproteins induced by purified lecithin:cholesterol acyltransferase: effect of low density lipoproteins. *Biochim Biophys Acta* 1986;877:406—14.

21 Nikkila EA. Metabolic and endocrine control of plasma high density lipoprotein concentration. In *High Density Lipoproteins and Atherosclerosis* (eds AM Gotto Jr, NE Miller, MF Oliver). Amsterdam: Elsevier/North Holland Biomedical Press, 1984;177—92.

22 Taskinen MR, Nikkila EA. High density lipoprotein subfractions in relation to lipoprotein lipase activity in tissues in man—evidence for reciprocal regulation of HDL_2 and HDL_3 levels by lipoprotein lipase. *Clin Chim Acta* 1981;112:325—32.

23 Eisenberg S. High density lipoprotein metabolism. *J Lipid Res* 1984;25:1017—58.

24 Nichols AV. Human serum lipoproteins and their interrelationships. *Adv Biol Med Phys* 1967;11:109−58.
25 Kuusi T, Saarinen P, Nikkila EA. Evidence for the role of hepatic endothelial lipase in the metabolism of plasma high density lipoprotein₂ in man. *Atherosclerosis* 1980;36:589−93.
26 Taggart HM, Applebaum-Bowden D, Haffner S *et al*. Reduction in high density lipoproteins by anabolic steroid (Stanozolol) therapy for post-menopausal osteoporosis. *Metabolism* 1982;31:1147−52.
27 Tikkanen MJ, Nikkila EA, Kuusi T, Sipinen S. High density lipoprotein-2 and hepatic lipase: reciprocal changes produced by estrogen and norgestrel. *J Clin Endocrinol Metab* 1982;54:1113−17.
28 Groot PHE, Scheck LM, Jansen H. Liver lipase and high-density lipoprotein. Lipoprotein changes after incubation of human serum with rat liver lipase. *Biochim Biophys Acta* 1983;751:393−400.
29 Kuusi T, Kinnunen PJK, Nikkila EA. Hepatic endothelial lipase antiserum influences rat plasma low and high density lipoproteins *in vivo*. *FEBS Lett* 1979;104:384−8.
30 Murase T, Itakura H. Accumulation of intermediate density lipoprotein in plasma after intravenous administration of hepatic triglyceride lipase antibody in rats. *Atherosclerosis* 1981;39:293−300.
31 Clay MA, Hopkins GJ, Ehnholm CP, Barter PJ. The rabbit as an animal model of hepatic lipase deficiency. *Biochim Biophys Acta* 1989;1002:173−81.
32 Clay MA, Rye KA, Barter PJ. Evidence *in vitro* that hepatic lipase reduces the concentration of apolipoprotein A-I in rabbit high density lipoproteins. *Biochim Biophys Acta* 1990;1044:50−6.
33 Clay MA, Newnham HH, Barter PJ. Hepatic lipase promotes a loss of apolipoprotein A-I from triglyceride-enriched human high density lipoproteins during incubation *in vitro*. *Arteriosclerosis* 1991;11:415−22.
34 Yen FT, Deckelbaum RJ, Mann CJ *et al*. Inhibition of cholesteryl ester transfer protein activity by monoclonal antibody. Effects on cholesteryl ester formation and neutral lipid mass transfer in human plasma. *J Clin Invest* 1989;83:2018−24.
35 Ha YC, Barter PJ. Differences in plasma cholesteryl ester transfer activity in sixteen vertebrate species. *Comp Biochem Physiol* 1982;71B:265−9.
36 Oschry Y, Eisenberg S. Rat plasma lipoproteins: re-evaluation of a lipoprotein system in an animal devoid of cholesteryl ester transfer activity. *J Lipid Res* 1982;23:1099−106.
37 Ha YC, Chang LBF, Barter PJ. Effects of injecting exogenous lipid transfer protein into rats. *Biochim Biophys Acta* 1985;833:203−10.
38 Ha YC, Barter PJ. Effects of sucrose feeding and injection of lipid transfer protein on rat plasma lipoproteins. *Comp Biochem Physiol* 1986;83B:463−6.
39 Kurasawa T, Yokoyama S, Miyake Y, Yamamura T, Yamamoto A. Rate of cholesteryl ester transfer between high and low density lipoproteins in human serum and a case with decreased transfer rate in association with hyperalphalipoproteinemia. *J Biochem* 1985;98:1499−508.
40 Yokoyama S, Kurasawa T, Nishikawa O, Yamamoto A. High density lipoproteins with poor reactivity to cholesteryl ester transfer reaction observed in a homozygote of familial hyperalphalipoproteinemia. *Artery* 1986;14:43−51.
41 Yamashita S, Matzuzawa Y, Okazaki M *et al*. Small polydisperse low density lipoproteins in familial hyperalphalipoproteinemia with complete deficiency of cholesteryl ester transfer activity. *Atherosclerosis* 1988;70:7−12.
42 Hopkins GJ, Chang LBF, Barter PJ. Role of lipid transfers in the formation of a subpopulation of small high density lipoproteins. *J Lipid Res* 1985;26:218−29.
43 Hopkins GJ, Barter PJ. Role of triglyceride-rich lipoproteins and hepatic lipase in determining the particle size and composition of high density lipoproteins. *J Lipid Res* 1986;27:1265−77.

44 Newnham HH, Barter PJ. Synergistic effects of lipid transfers and hepatic lipase in the formation of very small high density lipoproteins during incubation of human plasma. *Biochim Biophys Acta* 1990;1044:57–64.

45 Barter PJ, Chang LBF, Rajaram OV. Sodium oleate promotes a redistribution of cholesteryl esters from high to low density lipoproteins. *Atherosclerosis* 1990;84:13–24.

46 Barter PJ, Chang LBF, Rajaram OV. Sodium oleate dissociates the heteroexchange of cholesteryl esters and triacylglycerol between HDL and triacylglycerol-rich lipoproteins. *Biochim Biophys Acta* 1990;1047:294–7.

47 Sammett D, Tall AR. Mechanisms of enhancement of cholesteryl ester transfer protein activity by lipolysis. *J Biol Chem* 1985;260:6687–97.

48 Glueck CJ, Taylor HL, Jakobs D *et al*. Plasma high-density lipoprotein cholesterol: association with measurement of body mass. *Circulation* 1980;62(Suppl IV):62–9.

49 Taylor KG, Wright AD, Carter TJ *et al*. High density lipoprotein cholesterol and apolipoprotein A-I levels at diagnosis in patients with non-insulin-dependent diabetes. *Diabetologia* 1981;20:535–9.

50 Stubbe I, Eskilsson J, Nilsson-Ehle P. High-density lipoprotein concentrations increase after stopping smoking. *Br Med J* 1982;284:1511–13.

51 Katan MB. Diet and HDL. In *Clinical and Metabolic Aspects of High-density Lipoproteins* (eds NE Miller, GJ Miller). Amsterdam, New York, Oxford: Elsevier, 1984:103–31.

52 Schonfeld G, Patsch W, Rudel LL *et al*. Effects of dietary cholesterol and fatty acids on plasma lipoproteins. *J Clin Invest* 1982;69:1072–80.

53 Brussaard JH, Katan MB, Groot PHE, Havekes LM, Hautvast JGAJ. Serum lipoproteins of healthy persons fed a low fat diet or a polyunsaturated fat diet for three months: a comparison of two cholesterol-lowering diets. *Atherosclerosis* 1982;42:205–19.

54 Shepherd J, Packard CJ, Patsch JR, Gotto AM, Taunton OD. Effects of dietary polyunsaturated and saturated fat on the properties of high density lipoproteins and the metabolism of apolipoprotein A-I. *J Clin Invest* 1978;61:1582–92.

55 Wolf RN, Grundy SM. Influence of weight reduction on plasma lipoproteins in obese patients. *Arteriosclerosis* 1983;3:160–9.

56 Albrink MJ, Meigs JW. The relation between serum triglycerides and skinfold thickness in obese subjects. *Ann N Y Acad Sci* 1965;131:673–5.

57 Harno K, Nikkila EA, Kuusi T. Plasma HDL-cholesterol and postheparin plasma hepatic endothelial lipase (HL) activity: relationship to obesity and non-insulin-dependent diabetes (NIDDM). *Diabetologia* 1980;19:281.

58 Zimmerman J, Kaufmann NA, Fainaru M *et al*. Effect of weight loss in moderate obesity on plasma lipoprotein and apolipoprotein levels and on high density lipoprotein composition. *Arteriosclerosis* 1984;4:115–23.

59 Dole VP. A relation between non-esterified fatty acids in plasma and the metabolism of glucose. *J Clin Invest* 1956;35:150–4.

60 Castelli WP, Doyle JT, Gordon T *et al*. Alcohol and blood lipids: the Cooperative Lipoprotein Phenotyping Study. *Lancet* 1977;ii:153–5.

61 Lopez SA, Vial R, Balart L, Arroyave G. Effect of exercise and physical fitness on serum lipids and lipoproteins. *Atherosclerosis* 1974;20:1–9.

62 Gordon DJ, Witztum JL, Hunninghake D, Gates S, Glueck CJ. Habitual physical activity and high-density lipoprotein cholesterol in men with primary hypercholesterolemia. *Circulation* 1983;67:512–20.

63 Peltonen P, Marniemi J, Hietanen E, Vuori I, Ehnholm C. Changes in serum lipids, lipoproteins and heparin releasable lipolytic enzymes during moderate physical training in man. A longitudinal study. *Metabolism* 1981;30:518–25.

64 Shepherd J, Packard CJ, Patsch JR, Gotto AM Jr, Taunton OD. Effects of nicotinic acid therapy on plasma high density lipoprotein subfraction distribution and composition and on apolipoprotein A metabolism. *J Clin Invest* 1979;63:858–67.

65 Sirtori CR, Gianfranceschi G, Sirtori M *et al*. Reduced triglyceridemia and increased high density lipoprotein cholesterol levels after treatment with acipimox, a new inhibitor of lipolysis. *Atherosclerosis* 1981;38:267–71.

66 Nichols AV, Strisower EH, Lindgren FT. Analysis of change in ultracentrifugal lipoprotein profiles following heparin and ethyl-*p*-chloro-phenoxyisobutyrate administration. *Clin Chim Acta* 1968;20:277–83.

67 Kaukola S, Manninen V, Malkonen M, Ehnholm C. Gemfibrozil in the treatment of dyslipidaemias in middle-aged survivors of myocardial infarction. *Acta Med Scand* 1981;209:69–73.

68 Rossner S, Oro L. Fenofibrate therapy of hyperlipoproteinaemia. *Atherosclerosis* 1981;38:273–82.

69 Olsson AG, Lang PD. One-year study of the effect of bezafibrate on serum lipoprotein concentration in hyperlipoproteinaemia. *Atherosclerosis* 1978;31:429–33.

70 Vessby B, Kostner G, Lithell J, Thomis H. Diverging effects of cholestyramine on apolipoprotein B and lipoprotein Lp (a). *Atherosclerosis* 1982;44:61–71.

71 Olsson AG, Molgaard J, von Scherk H. Synvinolin in hypercholesterolaemia. *Lancet* 1986;ii:390–1.

72 Carlson LA. Inhibition of the mobilization of free fatty acids from adipose tissue. *Ann N Y Acad Sci* 1965;131:119–42.

73 Fears R. Drug treatment of hyperlipidaemia. *Drugs of Today* 1984;20:257–94.

74 Manninen V, Huttunen JK, Heimonen OP, Tenkanen L, Frick MH. Relation between baseline lipid and lipoprotein values and the incidence of coronary heart disease in the Helsinki Heart Study. *Am J Cardiol* 1989;63:42H–47H.

75 Nikkila EA, Huttunen JK, Ehnholm C. Effect of clofibrate on post-heparin plasma triglyceride lipase activities in patients with hypertriglyceridemia. *Metabolism* 1977;26:179–86.

76 Sirtori CR, Franceschini G. Drug effects on HDL. In *Clinical and Metabolic Aspects of High-density Lipoproteins* (eds NE Miller, GJ Miller). Amsterdam, New York, Oxford: Elsevier, 1984:341–79.

77 LeLorier J, Du Breuil-Quidoz S, Lussier-Cacon S, Yung-Shen H, Davignon J. Diet and probucol in lowering cholesterol concentrations. *Arch Intern Med* 1977;137:1429–34.

78 Franceschini G, Sirtori M, Vaccarino V *et al*. Mechanisms of HDL reduction after probucol. Changes in HDL subfractions and increased reverse cholesteryl ester transfer. *Arteriosclerosis* 1989;9:462–9.

79 Yamamoto A, Matsuzawa Y, Yokoyama S *et al*. Effects of probucol on xanthomata regression in familial hypercholesterolemia. *Am J Cardiol* 1986;57:29H–35H.

80 Kita T, Nagamo Y, Yokode M *et al*. Probucol prevents the progression of atherosclerosis in Watanabe heritable hyperlipidemic rabbit, an animal model for familial hypercholesterolemia. *Proc Natl Acad Sci USA* 1987;84:5928–37.

81 Parthasarthy S, Young SG, Witztum JL, Pittman RC, Steinberg D. Probucol inhibits oxidative modification of low density lipoprotein. *J Clin Invest* 1986;77:641–4.

82 Leren P, Foss PO, Helgeland A *et al*. Effects of propranolol and prazosin on blood lipids. The Oslo Study. *Lancet* 1980;ii:4–6.

83 Ames RP. The effects of antihypertensive drugs on serum lipids and lipoproteins. I. *Diuretics Drugs* 1986;32:260–78.

84 Nikkila EA, Kaste M, Ehnholm C, Viikari J. Elevation of high-density lipoprotein in epileptic patients treated with phenytoin. *Acta Med Scand* 1978;204:517–20.

85 Conney AH. Pharmacological implications of microsomal enzyme induction. *Pharmacol Rev* 1967;19:317–66.

86 O'Neill B, Callaghan N, Stapleton M, Molloy W. Serum elevation of high density lipoprotein (HDL) cholesterol in epileptic patients taking carbamazepine or phenytoin. *Acta Neurol Scand* 1982;65:104–9.

87 Luoma PV, Myllyla VV, Hokkanen E. Relationship between plasma high-density lipoprotein cholesterol and anticonvulsant levels in epileptics. *J Cardiovasc Pharmacol* 1982;4:1024–7.

88 Howard BV. Lipoprotein metabolism in diabetes mellitus. *J Lipid Res* 1987;28:613–28.
89 Jiao S, Kameda K, Matsuzawa Y *et al.* Influence of endogenous hyperinsulinism on high density lipoprotein$_2$ in Type 2 (non-insulin-dependent) diabetes mellitus and impaired glucose tolerance. *Atherosclerosis* 1986;60:279–86.
90 Goldberg AP, Harter HR, Patsch W *et al.* Racial differences in plasma high-density lipoproteins in patients receiving hemodialysis. A possible mechanism for accelerated atherosclerosis in white men. *N Engl J Med* 1983;308:1245–52.
91 Bagdade JD, Albers JJ. Plasma high density lipoprotein concentrations in chronic hemodialysis and renal transplant patients. *N Engl J Med* 1977;296:1436–9.
92 Miller GJ, Koplan JP, Morgan P *et al.* High-density lipoprotein cholesterol concentration and other serum lipids in an isolated island community free of coronary heart disease. *Int J Epidemiol* 1979;8:219–25.
93 Barclay M, Escher GC, Kaufman RJ *et al.* Serum lipoproteins and human neoplastic disease. *Clin Chim Acta* 1964;10:39–47.
94 Kanel GC, Radvan G, Peters RL. High-density lipoprotein cholesterol and liver disease. *Hepatology* 1983;3:343–8.
95 Castelli WP. The triglyceride issue: A view from Framingham. *Am Heart J* 1986;112:432–7.
96 Mahley RW. Atherogenic lipoproteins and coronary artery disease: Concepts derived from recent advances in cellular and molecular biology. *Circulation* 1985;72:943–8.
97 Molnar GD, Berge KG, Rosevear JW, McGuckin WF, Achor RWP. The effect of nicotinic acid in diabetes mellitus. *Metabolism* 1964;13:181–90.
98 Pocock SJ, Shaper AG, Phillips AN. HDL-cholesterol, triglycerides and total cholesterol in ischaemic heart disease. *Br Med J* 1989;298:998–1002.
99 Abbott RD, Wilson PWF, Kannel WB, Castelli WP. High density lipoprotein, total cholesterol screening and myocardial infarction. The Framingham Study. *Arteriosclerosis* 1988;8:207–11.
100 Assmann G, Schulte H, Funke H, von Eckardstein A, Seedorf U. The prospective cardiovascular Munster (PROCAM) Study: identification of high risk individuals for myocardial infarction and the role of HDL. In *High Density Lipoproteins and Atherosclerosis* (ed. NE Miller). Amsterdam, New York, Oxford: Excerpta Medica, 1989:51–65.

Index

Page numbers in **bold** refer to tables; in *italics* refer to figures.